Vascular Access in Neonates and Children

Daniele G. Biasucci
Nicola Massimo Disma • Mauro Pittiruti
Editors

Vascular Access in Neonates and Children

Springer

Editors
Daniele G. Biasucci
Intensive Care Unit, Department
of Emergency, Anesthesiology
and Intensive Care
Fondazione Policlinico Universitario
"A. Gemelli" IRCCS
Rome, Italy

Nicola Massimo Disma
Head of Research and Innovation
Unit, Department of Anesthesia
Istituto Giannina Gaslini
Genova, Italy

Mauro Pittiruti
Department of Surgery
Catholic University Hospital
Rome, Italy

ISBN 978-3-030-94708-8 ISBN 978-3-030-94709-5 (eBook)
https://doi.org/10.1007/978-3-030-94709-5

This Springer imprint is published by the registered company Springer Nature Switzerland AG
The registered company address is: Gewerbestrasse 11, 6330 Cham, Switzerland

Contents

List of Contributors

Giovanni Barone Neonatal Intensive Care Unit, Ospedale 'Infermi', Rimini, Italy

James Bennett Anesthesia Department, Birmingham Children's Hospital, Birmingham, UK

Daniele G. Biasucci Intensive Care Unit, Department of Emergency, Anesthesiology and Intensive Care, Fondazione Policlinico Universitario "A. Gemelli" IRCCS, Rome, Italy

Christian Breschan Klinikum Klagenfurt, Klagenfurt, Austria

Claudio Carlini Alessandria Children Hospital, AON SS Antonio e Biagio e Cesare Arrigo, Alessandria, Italy

Davide Celentano Pediatric Intensive Care Unit, Fondazione Policlinico Universitario "A. Gemelli" IRCCS, Rome, Italy

Roberta Centorrino Division of Pediatrics and Neonatal Critical Care, Medical Centre "A.Béclère", South Paris University Hospital, APHP and South Paris-Saclay University, Paris, France

Elisa Cerchia Alessandria Children Hospital, AON SS Antonio e Biagio e Cesare Arrigo, Alessandria, Italy

Alessandro Crocoli Operative Unit of General and Thoracic Surgery, Bambino Gesù Children's Hospital IRCCS, Rome, Italy

Vito D'Andrea Neonatal Intensive Care Unit, University Hospital Fondazione Policlinico Gemelli IRCCS, Rome, Italy

Valentina Dell'Orto Division of Pediatrics and Neonatal Critical Care, Medical Centre "A.Béclère", South Paris University Hospital, APHP and South Paris-Saclay University, Paris, France

Nicola Massimo Disma Anesthesia and Intensive Care, Pediatric Hospital 'G.Gaslini', Genova, Italy

Thomas Engelhardt Department of Anesthesia, Royal Aberdeen Children's Hospital, Aberdeen, UK

Massimo Lamperti Anesthesiology Institute, Cleveland Clinic, Abu Dhabi, UAE

Daniele De Luca Division of Pediatrics and Neonatal Critical Care, Medical Centre "A.Béclère", South Paris University Hospital, APHP and South Paris-Saclay University, Paris, France

Gurinder Singh Malhi Anesthesia Department, Birmingham Children's Hospital, Birmingham, UK

Diego Neuhaus Department of Anesthesia, University Children's Hospital, Zurich, Switzerland

Thierry Pirotte Department of Anesthesia, Cliniques Universitaires Saint-Luc—Université Catholique de Louvain, Brussels, Belgium

Mauro Pittiruti Department of Surgery, Catholic University Hospital, Rome, Italy

Department of Surgery, Fondazione Policlinico Universitario "A. Gemelli" IRCCS, Rome, Italy

Alessio Pini Prato Alessandria Children Hospital, AON SS Antonio e Biagio e Cesare Arrigo, Alessandria, Italy

Elizabeth Prentice Department of Anesthesia, Royal Children's Hospital, Melbourne, VIC, Australia

Giorgia Prontera Neonatal Intensive Care Unit, University Hospital Fondazione Policlinico Gemelli IRCCS, Rome, Italy

Serena Rubortone Neonatal Intensive Care Unit, University Hospital Fondazione Policlinico Gemelli IRCCS, Rome, Italy

Giancarlo Scoppettuolo Department of Infective Diseases, Fondazione Policlinico Universitario "A. Gemelli" IRCCS, Rome, Italy

Pierre Tissières Pediatric Intensive Care and Neonatal Medicine, Le Kremlin-Bicêtre, France

Xavier Torterüe Pediatric Intensive Care and Neonatal Medicine, Le Kremlin-Bicêtre, France

Part I
General Considerations on Venous Access in Neonates and Children

Chapter 1
Vascular Access in Pediatric Patients: Classification and Indications

Mauro Pittiruti

1.1 Venous Access in Neonates: Classification

In neonates, as in adults, venous access devices (VADs) are mainly classified in two categories, central venous access devices and peripheral venous access devices, depending on the position of the tip. A VAD with its tip located in the superior vena cava, or in the right atrium or in the inferior vena cava is defined as 'central'. All VADs with tips located in other sites of the vasculature must be regarded as 'peripheral'.

Other criteria of classification include (a) the technique of insertion (i.e., percutaneous venous access, either 'blind' or ultrasound-guided or guided by Near-Infra-Red technology; direct insertion in a patent vein, as it occurs with umbilical venous catheters; surgical cutdown of the vein; etc.); (b) the vein utilized as entrance in the vasculature (i.e., a superficial vs. a deep vein; a vein located in the upper limb, in the lower limb or at the scalp; etc.); (c) the location of the exit site of the catheter (i.e., the chest area, or the groin, or mid-arm, or mid-thigh, etc.). Last but not least, venous access devices may be further classified according to specific structural features regarding their design or the material they are made of.

1.1.1 Peripheral Venous Access Devices

Peripheral VADs in neonates are mainly represented by short cannulas.

Short cannulas are inserted by direct venipuncture, with or without the aid of visualization by NIR technology (Near Infra-Red); small bore, 24G or 26G cannulas are used. Polyurethane cannulas with pre-assembled extension and wide soft

M. Pittiruti (✉)
Department of Surgery, Catholic University Hospital, Rome, Italy

D. G. Biasucci et al. (eds.), *Vascular Access in Neonates and Children*,
https://doi.org/10.1007/978-3-030-94709-5_1

wing (so-called 'integrated' cannulas) will have chances of longer duration. The choice of the superficial vein to be cannulated will be guided preferably by the RaSuVA protocol, which involves a systematic examination of the superficial veins of the newborn, from the foot to the head, first on the right side and then on the left side, evaluating the seven sites where it is more likely to identify a vein: (1) medial malleolus, (2) lateral malleolus, (3) retro popliteal area, (4) hand and wrist, (5) antecubital area, (6) preauricular zone, (7) post-auricular zone.

1.1.2 Central Venous Access Devices

Central VADs in neonates can be classified as follows: (a) Umbilical venous catheters (UVC) inserted in the umbilical vein soon after birth; (b) epicutaneo-cava catheters (ECC) inserted by percutaneous puncture/cannulation of superficial veins; (c) central VADs inserted by ultrasound guided venipuncture in deep veins of the infra/supraclavicular area (Centrally Inserted Central Catheters = CICCs) or in the groin (Femorally Inserted Central Catheters = FICC); (d) central VADs surgically inserted by venous cutdown of deep veins.

All central lines will allow the safe infusion of any solutions, including solutions potentially associated with endothelial damage. Though, other performances of central venous access will depend on the type of device: UVC, CICC and FICC are usually appropriate also for administration of blood and blood products, for blood sampling and—depending on the exact location of the tip—also for hemodynamic monitoring; in contrast, ECC will not be appropriate for these purposes.

The umbilical venous catheter (UVC) is the only central VAD that is positioned by direct placement of the catheter into the vein, without the need for percutaneous puncture. Positioning is only possible at the time of birth or within few hours after birth, when the umbilical cord vessels are still accessible; the position of the tip—which is traditionally verified with relatively inaccurate systems such as radiology—should be nowadays more appropriately verified by echocardiography. In fact, UVC malposition is potentially associated with very serious complications, so that the correct placement of the tip should be assessed as accurately as possible. The choice between single and double lumen is mainly related to the clinical conditions of the newborn: in the stable preterm newborn a single lumen UVC is sufficient, while the acutely ill newborn requires a double lumen UVC. All UVC are made of polyurethane, though they are not certified as 'pressure injectable'. Recent evidence (see SHEA guidelines) suggests that UVC made of polyurethane treated with silver ions may be preferable, in order to reduce the risk of infection, especially in newborns with a gestational age less than or equal to 30 weeks. The caliber of UVC is between 2.5Fr and 8Fr for the single lumens and between 4Fr and 8Fr for the double lumen. The UVC allows high flow, blood sampling, and hemodynamic monitoring. UVC < 4Fr, however, have a relevant risk of occlusion. UVC is a central catheter potentially burdened by severe complications, both infectious and thrombotic. Within few days after birth, it should be removed and replaced with an appropriate venous access, which may differ depending on the clinical conditions of the neonate.

Epicutaneo-cava catheters (ECC) are peripherally inserted central catheters inserted into superficial veins; they are different from ultrasound-guided PICCs, which are peripherally inserted central catheters inserted in the deep veins of the arm. The first-choice material of ECC is polyurethane. Most ECCs are single lumen, with caliber ranging between 1Fr and 2.7Fr; double lumen 2Fr ECC are also available, although less frequently used. Insertion is performed by direct percutaneous cannulation of visible/palpable superficial veins, with or without the aid of the visualization by NIR (Near Infra-Red) technology. The choice of vein should be guided by the RaSuVA protocol (Rapid Superficial Vein Assessment), which involves a systematic examination of the superficial veins of the newborn, from the foot to the head, first on the right side and then on the left side, evaluating the seven sites where it is most likely to identify a vein: (1) medial malleolus, (2) lateral malleolus, (3) retro popliteal area, (4) hand and wrist, (5) antecubital area, (6) preauricular zone, (7) post-auricular zone. Echocardiography plays an increasingly important role in the correct placement of such catheters, as a method of both tip navigation and tip location. According to the latest evidence, ECC are appropriate when the expected duration of i.v. treatment does not exceed 2 weeks; due to the small size, they are not appropriate for blood sampling or for high flows or for hemodynamic monitoring: therefore, they should be used in stable newborns who need only intravenous hydration/nutrition. In case of failure of the positioning of the ECC (lack of suitable peripheral veins, repeated malpositions, repeated ineffective attempts, etc.), a CICC or a FICC should be used.

Centrally Inserted Central Catheters (CICCs) are inserted by ultrasound-guided puncture and cannulation of different veins of the infra/supra-clavicular area (axillary, subclavian, internal jugular, external jugular, brachio-cephalic). In the newborn, the easiest and safest supra-clavicular vein available for ultrasound-guided puncture and cannulation is always the brachio-cephalic vein. Even in premature infants, the caliber of this vein is approximately 3 mm, which allows the placement of a 3Fr power injectable polyurethane catheter. Insertion must be carried out according to the SICA-Ped protocol developed by GAVeCeLT: ultrasound evaluation of all central veins according to the RaCeVA protocol (Rapid Central Vein Assessment); maximum barrier precautions; skin antisepsis with chlorhexidine 2% in alcohol; ultrasound-guided venipuncture (in case of brachio-cephalic vein: visualization in long axis and 'in plane' puncture); tip navigation by supra-clavicular ultrasound scan; tip location by intracavitary ECG technique and/or echocardiography; sutureless securement; coverage of the exit site with cyanoacrylate glue and transparent semipermeable dressing with high transpirability. Furthermore, in the newborn it is always advisable to tunnel the catheter so that the exit site is in the infra-clavicular area, even if the puncture site is in the supraclavicular area. For best tunneling, we recommend the off-label use of central catheters marketed as PICC (3Fr single lumen or 4Fr bi-lumen): these catheters are in power injectable polyurethane, high flow, and they are inserted by modified Seldinger technique (which makes the tunneling easier). Pressure injectable CICCs can be used not only for normal infusions, but also for high flow infusions, for blood transfusion, for blood sampling and for hemodynamic monitoring (as long as the tip is positioned in the right atrium).

Femorally Inserted Central Catheters (FICCs) are a secondary option compared to CICCs, since in most newborns the femoral venipuncture is more difficult than the puncture of the brachio-cephalic vein (especially because of the caliber of the two veins: the femoral vein is always much smaller). If the caliber of the femoral vein is 3 mm or more, a 3Fr power injectable polyurethane catheter can be inserted. In smaller veins (2 mm) it is possible to use 2Fr catheters, although currently this caliber is only available for limited lengths (6 cm). Insertion must be performed according to the SICA-Ped protocol developed by GAVeCeLT: ultrasound evaluation of the groin veins using the RaFeVA protocol (Rapid Femoral Vein Assessment); maximum barrier precautions; skin antisepsis with chlorhexidine 2% in alcohol; ultrasound-guided venipuncture; tip navigation using ultrasound; tip location using intracavitary ECG technique and/or echocardiography; sutureless securement; coverage of the emergency site with cyanoacrylate glue and transparent semi-permeable dressing with high transpirability. It is possible (and desirable) to tunnel the catheter downwards to the mid-thigh, so as to obtain an exit site far from the inguinal fold. It is important to distinguish between two types of FICC: (a) those with the tip in the inferior vena cava (as verified by ultrasound), usable for infusions of any type and for blood sampling; (b) those with the tip in the right atrium tip (as verified with intracavitary ECG or echocardiography), which can be used not only for infusion and sampling, but also for hemodynamic monitoring. For best tunneling, we recommend the off-label use of central catheters marketed as PICC (3Fr single lumen or 4Fr bi-lumen): these catheters are in power injectable polyurethane, high flow, and they are inserted by modified Seldinger technique (which makes the tunneling easier).

Surgical insertion of central venous access devices by venous cutdown have been used in the past, before the introduction of ultrasound in the practice of venous access, but today it should be abandoned. The surgical preparation of the vein and its direct cannulation is associated with an increased costs and increased risks of infection, local hemorrhage, and venous thrombosis. Furthermore, repeated maneuvers of venous cutdown are inevitably associated with a progressive depletion of the venous patrimony of the child, both directly (sacrifice of the vein) and indirectly (local complications such as thrombosis, which may limit the future incannulation of local veins).

1.2 Venous Access in Neonates: Indications

The choice of venous access in the newborn depends on many factors, including: the time in which the need for venous access is identified (at birth vs. after birth); the clinical conditions of the newborn (stable vs. unstable or critically ill): the expected duration of intravenous treatment; the type of solutions to be infused.

1.2.1 Venous Access at Birth

In some full-term, non-acute ill neonates, venous access at birth may be indicated, even if there is no indication to UVC: in this case, the first-choice device is a short peripheral cannula. If the expected intravenous treatment is less than a week, the placement of a short peripheral cannula in a superficial vein will be sufficient. If venous access is required up to 2 weeks, an ECC can be used, inserted into the superficial veins. In infants with exhaustion of superficial veins or in newborns in which—although there are superficial peripheral veins available—the insertion of an ECC encounters repeated difficulties in positioning the tip, the positioning of a CICC or FICC will be indicated. In the case of intravenous therapy for duration of more than 14 days, it is advisable to resort directly to ultrasound-guided central venous access by puncture/cannulation of the brachio-cephalic vein (CICC) or of the femoral vein (FICC).

The umbilical venous catheter (UVC) plays a major role in the neonate that requires a venous access soon after birth or in the first day of life. The indication to UVC is linked to criteria of severity and gestational age. Typical indications are the following: newborn with severe asphyxia; gestational age equal to or less than 28 weeks; gestational age equal to or greater than 29 weeks, but with the need for assisted ventilation via orotracheal intubation, or hemodynamic instability, or the need for CPAP with $FiO2 > 40\%$, or difficulty in finding peripheral venous access.

In the stable preterm newborn, a single lumen umbilical venous catheter (UVC) can be positioned at birth for intravenous hydration and parenteral nutrition; after the first few days, it will be necessary to assess whether the venous access is needed for a limited period (< 14 days) or longer (> 14 days). In the first case, it will be sufficient to plan the positioning of an ECC; in the second case, it will be appropriate to insert an ultrasound-guided central venous access (CICC or FICC).

In the acutely ill newborn with a severe pathology already evident at birth, a double-lumen UVC is usually recommended; after few days, the UVC will be removed and replaced with an ultrasound guided central venous access (CICC or FICC).

In the severe, critically ill newborn, after the first days of intravenous treatment through the UVC, it is necessary to plan the placement of a CVC appropriate not only for standard infusions but also for high flow infusions, blood sampling, and possibly also hemodynamic monitoring. This can be achieved by ultrasound-guided insertion of power injectable polyurethane catheter—3Fr or larger—either in the brachio-cephalic vein (CICC) or in the femoral vein (FICC).

Examples of indications to placement of a CICC or a FICC are the following: need for central access for rapid fluid repletion (in emergency and/or during major surgery); hemodynamic instability and need for monitoring of CVP and O2 saturation in mixed venous blood, at any age of life (in the impossibility of positioning a UVC or in the case of malpositioned UVC); major malformation pathologies requiring surgery (e.g., esophageal atresia, omphalocele, gastroschisis, etc.); infants with severe type 2 bronchodysplasia (need for mechanical ventilation at 36 weeks of postconceptional age) and need for intravenous therapy. In the critically ill newborn, CICC or FICC should also be immediately placed when there are difficulties in positioning the UVC or in case of UVC-related complications (malposition, infection, thrombosis).

1.2.2 Venous Access >24 Hrs. After Birth

When the need for venous access arises days after birth, obviously the placement of a UVC is no longer possible. In these cases, the choice of the device depends on the clinical conditions of the newborn and the expected duration of the treatment.

In the full-term stable neonate who needs a venous access, the choice of the device depends on the expected duration of treatment. If the expected intravenous treatment is less than a week, the placement of a short peripheral cannula in a superficial vein will be sufficient. If venous access is required for less than 2 weeks, an ECC can be used, inserted into the superficial veins. In case of failure of the positioning of the ECC (lack of suitable peripheral veins, repeated malpositions, repeated ineffective attempts, etc.), a FICC or a CICC should be used.

In the premature newborn in stable conditions, in which a UVC has not been placed at birth, the choice of the device depends on the expected duration of treatment. If the expected intravenous treatment is less than a week, the placement of a short peripheral cannula in a superficial vein will be sufficient. If venous access is required for less than 2 weeks, an ECC can be used. In case of failure of the positioning of the ECC, or in case of intravenous treatment planned for more than 14 days, it is recommended to resort directly to a CICC or a FICC.

Critically ill neonates require a central access adequate not only for infusion of any type of solutions, even at high flow, but also for blood sampling and for hemodynamic monitoring. Ultrasound-guided placement of a power injectable polyurethane catheter, either single lumen (3Fr) or double lumen (4Fr), in the brachio-cephalic vein (CICC) or in the femoral vein (FICC) will be the first choice in this situation. Examples of indications to placement of a CICC or a FICC: need for central access for rapid fluid repletion (in emergency and/or during major surgery); hemodynamic instability and the need for monitoring of CVP and O2 saturation in mixed venous blood, at any age of life; major malformation pathologies requiring surgery (e.g., esophageal atresia, omphalocele, gastroschisis, etc.); infants with severe type 2 bronchodysplasia (need for mechanical ventilation at 36 weeks of postconceptional age) and need for intravenous therapy.

1.3 Other Vascular Access in Neonates

Other vascular access in neonates include arterial lines, double lumen catheters for hemodialysis and intraosseous devices.

The most frequently used arterial lines are the umbilical arterial catheters, inserted soon after birth or in the first hours of life. Main indication for the umbilical arterial catheterization is the need for repeated blood sampling in critically ill neonates. Peripheral arterial catheters may be also needed in selected acutely ill neonates for blood sampling and arterial gas analysis: the arteries most frequently accessed are the radial artery and the femoral artery. Peripheral arterial catheters are available of different calibers and lengths, either in polyurethane or in PEBA (polyether-block-amide) and should be inserted by ultrasound guidance. Access to the radial artery requires very small catheters (24G) and may not always be feasible, depending on the size and age of the newborn.

Dialysis catheters are double lumen polyurethane catheters available in different size and length. Considering the sizes appropriate for newborns, only non-cuffed dialysis catheters are available. The insertion of a dialysis catheter in a child with less than 30 days of age is a rather exceptional event, and requires a proper evaluation of venous access (the only veins usually adequate are the right brachio-cephalic vein and the femoral veins); as the availability of these catheters is very limited, it may be necessary to consider the 'off-label' use of double lumen power injectable catheters (for instance, 5Fr or 6Fr) originally marketed as PICCs.

The intraosseous route is currently considered as a very particular type of intravascular access, since it allows infusion of fluids and peripherally compatible solutions, even if at a very slow rate and for a brief period of time. In neonates, an intraosseous access may be required in severely hypovolemic patients, when all veins are collapsed and hard to puncture even using ultrasound, or in patients with cardiac arrest, when this access may be the only one feasible very rapidly. Intraosseous access is usually an emergency solution to be regarded as a temporary measure, while planning a more reliable venous access.

1.4 Venous Access in Infants and Children: Classification

The classification of venous access devices in infants and children is the same as in adults, the main differentiation being between central devices (tip in the superior vena cava, right atrium or inferior vena cava) vs. peripheral devices (tip in any other location). As in neonates, other criteria of classification include (a) the technique of insertion (i.e., percutaneous venous access, either 'blind' or ultrasound-guided or guided by Near-Infra-Red technology; direct insertion in a patent vein, as it occurs with umbilical venous catheters; etc.); (b) the vein utilized as entrance in the vasculature (i.e., a superficial vs. a deep vein; a vein located in the upper limb, in the lower limb or at the scalp; etc.); (c) the location of the exit site of the catheter, in case of external devices, or of the percutaneous access, in case of totally implantable devices (i.e., the chest area, or the groin, or mid-arm, or mid-thigh, etc.). Last but not least, venous access devices may be further classified according to specific structural features regarding their design or the material they are made of.

VADs can be furtherly classified as short term, if they are appropriate exclusively for an intra-hospital use, or medium term, if they are appropriate both for an intra-hospital use and for an extra-hospital use for a limited period of time (months). Long term VADs are appropriate for extra-hospital use for an unlimited period of time (months or years).

1.4.1 Peripheral Venous Access Devices

Peripheral VADs are currently classified according to their catheter length. Short venous cannulas are less than 6 cm long; long peripheral catheters (also sometimes named 'short midlines' or 'mini-midlines') are long 6–15 cm; midline catheters (also sometimes named 'midclavicular') are longer than 15 cm. Short cannulas and long peripheral catheters are usually considered short term VADs. Midline catheters are regarded as medium term VADs.

The substantial differences between these short cannulas and long peripheral catheters (mini-midlines) are in terms of duration (the life expectancy of an ultrasound-guided short cannula is 24–48 hours, while a mini-midline can remain in place even for three or four weeks) and in terms of material (short cannulas are in polytetrafluoroethylene or in polyurethane; mini-midlines are in polyurethane or polyethylene or polyether –block-amide, PEBA) and in term of costs (higher for mini-midline).

In the child, the caliber of a mini-midline should be 3Fr (which corresponds approximately to 20G).

Some mini-midlines are designed to be positioned with simple Seldinger technique (needle puncture—insertion of the metal guidewire into the needle—needle removal—catheter insertion above the guide), while others have a more complex design, in which needle, cannula and metal guide are assembled in an all-in-one coaxial device. At present there is no evidence to recommend the latter type of mini-midline, characterized by a higher cost and less ease of use.

1.4.2 Central Venous Access Devices

Central venous catheters (CVCs) can be inserted with different approaches in terms of the cannulated vein. According to the new terminology suggested by WoCoVA Foundation, we can differentiate: PICCs = Peripherally Inserted Central Catheters, or CVC inserted in the deep veins of the arm (axillary, brachial, basilica); CICCs = Centrally Inserted Central Catheters, or CVC inserted in the supra-clavicular veins (internal jugular, external jugular, subclavian, brachio-cephalic) or infra-clavicular (axillary, cephalic); FICCs = Femorally Inserted Central Catheters, or CVC inserted in the veins of the inguinal region (common femoral, superficial femoral, saphenous).

PICCs, CICCs and FICCs allow the infusion of solutions of any kind, even incompatible with the peripheral route; all three devices allow repeated and frequent blood sampling; hemodynamic monitoring is possible only for those CVCs (PICC, CICC or FICC) whose tip has been placed in the right atrium.

Any central venous access in the pediatric patient (as in adults) must be placed using ultrasound. The 'blind' puncture of the subclavian or internal jugular vein is now considered a senseless, dangerous, ethically questionable and legally prosecutable practice. The positioning of central accesses by venous cutdown—used in the twentieth century—is now completely obsolete, since it is associated with a greater risk of complications (infectious, thrombotic, hemorrhagic, etc.), longer times, and higher costs.

Short term central VADs include non-tunneled CICCs and non-tunneled FICCs. PICCs are regarded as medium term central VADs, regardless if they are tunneled or not; tunneled CICCs and tunneled FICCs are also considered medium term venous access devices. Central VADs are considered long term when there is some specific feature potentially associated with 'long-term' stabilization; therefore, the list of long term central VADs include central catheters connected with a subcutaneous reservoir (totally implantable devices), tunneled-cuffed catheters, and tunneled non-cuffed catheters secured by subcutaneous anchorage.

1.5 Venous Access in Infants and Children: Indications

The choice of the most appropriate venous access device in infants and children depends whether the line is needed in an emergency situation or its insertion is planned as a non-emergency.

1.5.1 Emergency Venous Access

The VADs appropriate in emergency in the pediatric patient are substantially all short-term, either peripheral (short cannulas and long peripheral catheters) or central (non-tunneled CICCs and FICCs). In emergency, neither the PICCs nor the traditional midlines nor the tunneled catheters nor the devices for long-term venous access have a role, as a rule.

It is important to consider that with the term 'emergency' we also refer to peripheral and central venous access devices positioned in an unplanned way in the operating room, before an urgent or non-urgent surgical procedure. These VADs should be preferentially removed within 24–48 hours; in fact, emergency positioning (or in any case in a hurried and unscheduled manner) is not usually compatible with an appropriate adherence to international recommendations for infection prevention.

In case of urgent need for venous access (in the emergency room, in the operating room, in emergency wards, etc.) it is necessary to distinguish between children with easy peripheral access (i.e., well palpable/visible superficial veins in the upper limbs) vs. children with 'difficult' veins.

Though the child 'without veins' obviously does not exist, in many situations (in approximately 24% of pediatric patients who arrive in the emergency room) the superficial veins of the upper limbs may be hardly visible and/or palpable. This category of pediatric patients has recently been classified with the English acronym 'DIVA' (Difficult Intra-Venous Access), normally referring to the difficulty of accessing the superficial veins of the upper limbs (i.e. located less than 6–7 mm deep).

In the presence of visible/palpable superficial veins of the upper limbs, the insertion of a short cannula is usually feasible, and constitutes the first choice. In case of difficulty in accessing the superficial veins of the upper limbs, it is also possible to place a short cannula in superficial veins of the neck (external jugular vein in the cervical tract) or of the lower limbs: though, these accesses should be removed within 24 hours, due to the high risk of dislocation (external jugular vein) or venous thrombosis (veins of the lower limbs).

In emergency, it is advisable to use low-cost short-term cannulas (in polytetrafluoroethylene; with or without out wing; without preassembled extension), to be removed within 24–48 hours. In the child, the caliber should be 22G or 20G: in the hypovolemic child, in whom rapid infusion of fluids is expected, or in the child who needs transfusion, 20G cannulas should be used. Wherever possible, within the limits compatible with the emergency situation, it is advisable that any insertion should follow the recommendations of the INS and EPIC guidelines (insertion site away from flexion zones; hygiene of the operator's hands and clean gloves; skin antisepsis with 2% chlorhexidine in alcohol; cover and securement with transparent semipermeable dressing).

The presence of 'difficult' superficial veins (DIVA) is an indication to resort to an appropriate technology that helps in the identification and cannulation of the veins. An example is the NIR technology, which exploiting the properties of wavelengths in the near-infrared spectrum (NIR = Near Infra-Red) allows a better visualization of the superficial veins (i.e. located less than 6–7 mm deep).

In the absence of instruments based on this technology, it is necessary to resort to cannulation of deep veins (i.e., located more than 6–7 mm deep), using ultrasound guidance. In most cases, it is advisable to prefer an ultrasound-guided peripheral rather than central VAD. In fact, the majority of the therapies to be infused in emergency can be infused peripherally without risk; on the other hand, a peripheral VAD will be associated with less risk of complications (greater safety) and at a lower cost (greater cost effectiveness) if compared to a central VAD.

The ultrasound-guided technique allows to insert (into the deep veins of the arm) not only short cannulas, but also long peripheral devices, such as mini-midlines (6–15 cm) or traditional midlines (15–25 cm). While midlines have little role in the emergency setting, mini-midlines, although having an expectation of shorter duration (few weeks) compared to midlines, are ideal in the emergency/urgency setting since they are rapid and easy to insert (simple Seldinger's technique) and inexpensive.

The opportunity to remove emergency mini-midlines within 24–48 hours is controversial: removal is mandatory if the precautions recommended by the infection prevention guidelines have not been adopted. On the other hand, a mini-midline inserted with an appropriate technique (skin antisepsis with chlorhexidine 2% in alcohol, maximum barrier precautions, sutureless securement, cover with transparent dressing) can be left over 48 hours. Mini-midlines can be made of different materials; in the case of expected long duration, polyurethane rather than polyethylene mini-midlines is preferred (the latter being associated with greater risk of thrombosis). The difference in material obviously has little relevance if the mini-midline is to be removed within 48 hours.

In some emergency-urgency situations, an ultrasound-guided peripheral venous access may not be feasible or not sufficient or not advisable. In these cases, an ultrasound-guided central venous access is adopted, i.e., the ultrasound-guided placement of a catheter whose tip arrives in the superior vena cava or in the inferior vena cava or in the right atrium.

All current guidelines strongly recommend the use of ultrasound even in emergency-urgency. It has been demonstrated that ultrasound-guided venipuncture reduces times and risks—if compared to 'blind' maneuvers—also in the emergency setting.

The placement of a peripherally inserted central catheter (PICC) is almost never indicated in emergency, because of the longer time required for the maneuver and for the reduced cost-effectiveness (emergency catheters must be removed within 24–48 hours). Thus, we should choose between a centrally inserted central catheter (CICC) and a femorally inserted central catheter (FICC); this choice depends on several factors: the presence of local pathological issues that can hinder or make difficult the maneuver (i.e.: cervico-thoracic trauma),the more or less adequate ultrasound visualization of the veins above/below the clavicle (internal jugular, subclavian, brachio-cephalic, axillary) compared to the visualization of the femoral vein, the presence of hypovolemia (in the hypovolemic patient the femoral venipuncture will be simpler), or the opportunity to leave the facial-cervical area clear for any resuscitation maneuvers. ATLS (Advanced Trauma Life Support) recommends the placement of a FICC in the polytrauma patient: the potential higher incidence of FICC-related infections and thrombosis will not be a problem, as these emergency catheters must be removed within 24–48 hours.

The emergency FICC will usually have the tip in the inferior vena cava (ideal position: above the bifurcation of the iliac veins, under the bifurcations of the renal veins—the surface landmark being the navel): as such, it will be usable for infusions of any type and for blood sampling, but not for hemodynamic monitoring.

The ultrasound-guided positioning of a CICC in emergency implies the puncture and cannulation of deep veins of the supra/infra-clavicular area. In the supraclavicular area, we can approach the internal jugular vein (preferably, visualization in short axis and 'in plane' puncture), the subclavian vein (visualization in long axis and 'in plane' puncture) or the brachio-cephalic vein (visualization in long axis and 'in plane' puncture). In the infra-clavicular area, the only approach is usually to the axillary vein (visualization in oblique/long axis and 'in plane' puncture; or visualization in short axis and 'out of plane' puncture).

The choice of the vein should be based on the RaCeVA protocol (Rapid Central Vein Assessment), i.e. the rapid and systematic examination of the main deep veins of the area above/below the clavicle, so to identify the vein that appears to be the easiest to puncture (and therefore the safest for the patient). In the hypovolemic child, the internal jugular and axillary veins are often collapsed and more difficult to cannulate.

The ease of the venous approach also depends on the age of the child: in the infant the easiest and safest veins will be the brachio-cephalic and the internal jugular vein. The CICC used in emergency are made of low-cost polyurethane, and they are usually inserted by simple Seldinger technique. The number of lumens will be determined by clinical needs. They should preferably be removed within 24–48 hours.

The emergency FICC will be placed by ultrasound-guided puncture and cannulation of the common or superficial femoral vein (visualization on a short axis, 'out of plane' puncture) by simple Seldinger technique. Low-cost polyurethane catheters are used, of sufficient length to ensure that the catheter tip is actually in a central position (i.e., in the inferior vena cava). An approximate evaluation of this distance can be obtained by measuring the distance between the puncture site in the groin and the navel.

In infants and younger children, the femoral vein can sometimes be very difficult to puncture due to its small size. This also limits the caliber of the catheter to be positioned. The number of lumens will be dictated by clinical needs. Emergency FICC must be removed within 24–48 hours.

In emergency, an alternative option to the use of ultrasound-guided VADs is constituted by the intraosseous access, which can be utilized—but a limited time (12-24 hrs). This access allows to obtain rapidly a route that can be used as a peripheral venous route (i.e.: fluid therapy, blood transfusions, and infusions of peripherally compatible solutions).

The advantages of intraosseous access are its reliability, the extreme rapidity, and the possibility of a successful insertion even in the hands of a clinician with minimal training.

Its disadvantages are the high cost, the short duration of the line, the limited availability of the device, and the lack of confidence of the operator in the installation maneuver, which is perceived as traumatic or dangerous.

The ideal indication of intraosseous access—in terms of safety and cost-effectiveness—is certainly within the sphere of extra-hospital pediatric emergencies. There are still no convincing studies that demonstrate its superiority over other methods (such as ultrasound-guided venous access) in the pediatric intra-hospital setting or in the pediatric emergency room, with the obvious exception being the simultaneous arrival of numerous children serious or traumatized ('mass casualties').

1.5.2 Intra-Hospital Venous Access

Traditionally, a distinction is made between VADs appropriate only for intrahospital use (short-term devices) and VADs suitable only for non-hospital use (long-term devices). Medium-term devices are used both within and outside the hospital.

As already mentioned, any VAD whose tip is placed in the superior vena cava, or in the right atrium, or in the inferior vena cava is defined as 'central'. Any other device whose tip is in another venous district is classified as 'peripheral'.

The choice between central venous access and peripheral venous access depends on the type of use. The common indications to central VAD in the hospitalized child are:

1. need for intravenous infusion of drugs and solutions not compatible with the peripheral route because potentially associated with endothelial damage: this category include vesicant drugs, drugs with pH higher than 9 or less than 5, markedly hyperosmolar solutions (above 800–850 mOsm/liter) and many other drugs that with different mechanisms, even independent of pH and osmolarity, are able to cause irritation and/or damage to the endothelium; lists of peripherally compatible and incompatible drugs can be found on the web (e.g. on the website **www.gavecelt.info**) or in textbooks (such as in the "GAVeCeLT Manual of PICCs and Midlines").
2. need for hemodialysis procedures (for which dedicated devices are required).
3. need for repeated and frequent blood sampling.
4. need for hemodynamic monitoring (oxygen saturation in mixed venous blood; measurement of central venous pressure; use for thermodilution technique for cardiac output); this use is possible only with those central venous catheters whose tip is in the right atrium.

<u>Peripheral venous access</u>. In the hospitalized child, if a peripheral VAD is appropriate (i.e., if the VAD is required only for infusion of solutions compatible with the peripheral veins), the choice can fall on different types of devices, depending on the expected duration of treatment. Also, the strategy changes depending on the presence or absence of visible/palpable superficial veins of the upper limb, which may classify the child as DIVA (Difficult Intra-Venous Access) or not.

If the superficial veins of the upper limb are visible and/or palpable, for an expected duration of 24–48 hours (for example, for a radiological exam, for a surgical procedure, for a bolus infusion of a one-time drug) the obvious choice is a short cannula. In the child, 24G—22G cannulas should be used. 20G cannulas are preferably used only in case of expected infusion of contrast medium for radiological exams or in case of expected blood transfusion or infusion of blood products. For such short duration of treatment, it will be sufficient to resort to low-cost short cannulas (in polytetrafluoroethylene, with or without wing, without preassembled extension), leaving the 'integrated' short cannulas of greater performance (in polyurethane, provided with large wing, preassembled extension and preassembled needle-free connector) to clinical situation in which a peripheral access is required for several days (2–7 days). These 'integrated' short cannulas are associated with a prolonged duration (up to a week) only if positioned and managed according to the recommendations of the INS and EPIC guidelines (insertion site far from flexion zones; skin antisepsis with chlorhexidine 2% in alcohol; coverage with transparent bordered dressing; flushing with normal saline—preferably using pre-filled syringes—before and after each infusion; exclusive use for infusion of peripherally compatible solutions).

Even if placed and managed with the greatest care, it is rare that short peripheral cannulas positioned in superficial veins of the arm can—'integrated' or not—may last for more than a week. It is more likely that they will face different complications (dislocation, phlebitis, thrombosis, occlusion, and extravasation) that will eventually be configured as 'catheter failure' and the need to remove the device.

On the contrary, the ultrasound-guided insertion of a long peripheral catheter in the deep veins of the upper limb will allow a peripheral access for periods longer than one week (up to a month).

Therefore, the most suitable device for ultrasound-guided peripheral access for intravenous treatment scheduled for more than a week in an intra-hospital setting will certainly be the mini-midline.

In fact, ultrasound-guided short cannulas have a very short duration (24–48 hours) and traditional midlines are indicated mainly in the extra-hospital setting.

Central venous access. In the case of indication to a central venous access in an intra-hospital setting, the choice is between PICC, CICC and FICC. When the deep veins of the arm are available at ultrasound examination (at least on one side), the preferable central VAD is the PICC, in children as in adults. This access is in fact particularly free from risks of significant complications to the insertion, it can be implanted even in very fragile children from the cardiorespiratory or coagulative point of view, and it implies an exit site (at mid-arm) particularly favorable both for the low bacterial contamination of the skin both for its easy dressing. Furthermore, the placement of PICCs in pediatric age has the additional advantage of being associated with less need for sedation/anesthesia, compared to the placement of a CICC.

As in adults, also in children the main contraindications to the placement of a PICC are the presence of a chronic renal failure of grade 3b –4—5 (i.e., likely current or future need for chronic hemodialysis treatment) or the bilateral presence of various types of pathologies of the upper limb, vascular (previous or current venous thrombosis), lymphatic (previous axillary lymphadenectomy), neuromuscular (chronic paresis), cutaneous (burns or other skin lesions, infectious or dystrophic), osteo-articular (ankyloses, fractures, etc.).

The ultrasound-guided insertion of a PICC involves the ultrasound identification of a vein (a) of adequate internal caliber (at least three times the external diameter of the catheter), (b) of not excessive depth (not more than 2.5–3 cm from the skin surface), (c) preferably located in the middle third of the arm (Dawson's green zone).

The arm (from the elbow to the axillary cavity) can be divided into three bands of similar size, corresponding to the proximal third (yellow area of Dawson), the middle third (Dawson's green zone) and the distal third (Dawson's red zone).

Guidelines recommend locating the exit site of the PICC in Dawson's green zone, most appropriate both in terms of stability and in terms of risk of bacterial contamination. If in the green zone there is no adequate vein in terms of caliber and depth, it is possible, however, to puncture and cannulate a vein of the yellow zone (probably with a larger diameter since it is more proximal) and tunnel the catheter until it exits the green zone.

The location of the exit site in the green zone in fact allows a better clinical result in terms of dressing stability and infectious risk. If a vein of appropriate depth and caliber is visualized in Dawson's green zone, it is not necessary to tunnel and the PICC can be implanted with the traditional method: i.e., the venipuncture site will coincide with the emergency site (non-tunneled PICC).

In the child, where the caliber of the veins is on average smaller than in the adult, the occurrence of having to puncture in the yellow zone (and therefore tunneling) is more frequent than in the adult patient. A tunneled PICC is defined as a PICC where the venipuncture site (typically in the yellow zone) does not coincide with the exit site (typically, in the green zone). It is possible to tunnel any PICC, or in anterograde fashion (if the catheter is designed for a distal 'trimming') or even retrograde (only for catheters that provide a proximal 'trimming'). The benefit of tunneling in terms of infective risk will be twofold: directly (for protection against extra luminal contamination, since tunneling moves the exit site far from the entrance of the catheter into the vein) but also indirectly (because it allows to plan the exit site to an area with less bacterial contamination).

In terms of safety and cost-effectiveness, we should always use power injectable PICCs, in latest-generation polyurethane, non-valved and open-ended. The most widely used PICCs in the pediatric age group are 3Fr single lumen, 4Fr single lumen and 4Fr double lumen.

When placement of a PICC is contraindicated due to unavailability of the veins of the arm of adequate caliber and/or due to the presence of chronic renal insufficiency of grade 3b—4—5 and/or for the presence of vascular, lymphatic, neuromuscular or osteo-articular to both arms, it will be necessary to resort to a CICC (that is, a central catheter inserted by ultrasound guided puncture and cannulation of a vein of the cervico-thoracic area or more precisely of the area above/below the clavicle).

The temporary immobility of the arms due to pharmacological effects (children under the effect of sedatives/muscle relaxants in intensive care unit) or the presence of acute renal failure (another frequent occurrence in intensive care unit) do not constitute a contraindication to PICCs. States of severe coagulation alteration do not constitute a contraindication to PICCs. There is no specific contraindication to the use of PICCs in children in intensive care, nor in the onco-hematologic patient: indeed, in these types of pediatric patients the PICC may have a specific indication compared to CICC, for example for the presence of tracheostomy or of abnormal coagulation.

An infra-clavicular approach is probably the best option for a non-tunneled CICC, on all occasions where central venous access is required for intra-hospital use in children with contraindication to the PICC. Ultrasound-guided approaches to veins of the infra-clavicular area are mostly approaches to the axillary vein, and not to the subclavian vein. According all anatomy texts, in fact, the transition between axillary vein and subclavian vein falls at the outer edge of the first rib. Since this rib is ultra sonographically inaccessible in most cases because hidden by the clavicle, the venous tract that is visualized in the infra-clavicular area is the axillary vein, and not the subclavian vein. The 'blind' infra-clavicular approach (as it was used in the twentieth century) was actually an approach to the subclavian vein, since the entrance of the needle into the vein occurred behind the clavicle: obviously this technique is absolutely proscribed today.

The advantage of the axillary approach is in its exit site, which is optimal in terms of reduction of the risks of dislocation and bacterial contamination (provided that there is no tracheostomy).

Unfortunately, in the pediatric age, the axillary vein is not always of suitable caliber for positioning of a CICC: it certainly is in the adolescent, but as one moves to lower age groups, the axillary vein becomes less and less accessible, until it is difficult to propose it in the toddler. In these cases, one will opt for a vein in the supra-clavicular area (brachio-cephalic, internal jugular, subclavian) and a 'non-optimal' emergency site, i.e. in the supra-clavicular area. The emergency site in the cervical area should nevertheless be avoided. Though, in children over the age of 7–8, a non-tunneled CICC inserted for example in the brachio-cephalic vein and with a supra-clavicular exit site may be an appropriate choice. By cannulating a vein in the supra-clavicular area (internal jugular, brachio-cephalic, subclavian), the exit site naturally falls in the supra-clavicular fossa (care should be taken to orient the catheter laterally, and not upward towards the neck).

In smaller children, however, it is necessary that the exit site is in the infra-clavicular area (a very favorable site in terms of controlling the risk of infection, thrombosis and dislocation); the catheter can then be tunneled downwards, below the clavicle. This occurs for example in the presence of a tracheostomy, where it is advisable to move the exit site caudally to at least 7–8 cm far from the ostomy, to minimize bacterial contamination via the extra luminal route.

Tunneling is always very appropriate in infants and very young children, wherever the management of the exit site in the supra-clavicular area may appear to be problematic.

As tunneled CICC, we recommend the off-label use of catheters marketed as PICCs, which have the advantage of considerable length (50 cm and more) and insertion with modified Seldinger technique (which simplifies the tunneling maneuver). The catheter will be placed in the best available central vein (the one whose puncture appears easier, and therefore safer) after an ultrasound evaluation of the region (RaCeVA), following a standardized implant protocol, such as the SICA-Ped protocol (Safe Insertion of Central Access in Pediatric patients) developed by GAVeCeLT.

In few selected cases, such as in the presence of an obstruction of the superior vena cava, insertion of a PICC or a CICC might be difficult or impossible. In these situations, central venous access can be achieved by placing a FICC. In contrast with the FICCs inserted in emergency, which may not be tunneled and have an exit site at the groin, any effort should be done to optimize the location of the exit site when the FICC is inserted in elective, non-emergency conditions. This goal can be reached by two different strategies: (a) the common femoral vein can be cannulated at the inguinal groove, but the catheter tunneled so to obtain an exit site far from the groin (either at mid-thigh, with caudad tunneling, or in the abdominal area, with cephalad tunneling); (b) in older children, the superficial femoral vein can be directly punctured and cannulated at mid-thigh.

Of course, all access to femoral veins must be achieved by ultrasound guidance. Depending on the purpose of the FICC, the tip will be placed either in the mid-portion of the inferior vena cava or—if hemodynamic monitoring is required—in the right atrium (this can be assessed using the intracavitary ECG method of tip location). For example, a FICC inserted for chemotherapy in a child with thoracic lymphoma may have the tip in the inferior vena cava; a FICC inserted in pediatric intensive care unit in a burned child will have its tip preferably in the right atrium, so to estimate the central venous pressure and/or measure the oxygen saturation in mixed venous blood.

1.5.3 Extra-Hospital Venous Access

It should be noted that discussing the extra-hospital context we refer not only to the VADs used in home care or in hospice, but also to devices used in children who are not hospitalized but followed as outpatients. In these patients, the main issue is to estimate the duration for which the device should be used. That is. It will be appropriate to choose between devices for medium-term venous access (< 4–6 months) and long-term venous access (> 4–6 months and/or indefinitely).

When venous access is required for few weeks or few months (medium term), a peripheral access is sometimes indicated, provided that the patient does not require repeated blood sampling or the infusion of solutions that are not peripherally compatible. An example of indication for medium-term peripheral venous access may be a patient in palliative care in which there is indication only to hydration and administration of analgesics; or a patient who needs periodic transfusions of blood or blood products (immunoglobulins, coagulation factors, etc.) at home; or a patient in OPAT (outpatient antimicrobial therapy) who receives antibiotics compatible with the peripheral route. In all other cases, if there is an indication for repeated daily blood sampling or infusion of solutions not compatible with the peripheral route (chemotherapy, strongly hyperosmolar parenteral nutrition, antibiotics irritating the endothelium, etc.) it will be appropriate to resort to a central venous catheter.

Midline catheters (according to European and Australian terminology) are peripheral venous access devices, inserted into the deep veins of the arm by ultrasound guidance, 15–25 cm long, whose tip is placed in the subclavian or axillary vein (hence also the name ‘midclavicular’). Fallen into disuse in the USA, they are widely used in Europe (Italy, Spain and UK), especially in palliative care. The duration of the midline is substantially linked to the appropriateness of use (i.e., exclusively for the infusion of solutions compatible with the peripheral route).

We recommend using polyurethane midlines: open-ended, non-valved, preferably power injectable. Silicon midlines are fragile, have low flow, and possible lumen occlusions are difficult to treat; they should be abandoned. Also, there are no advantages in using valved midlines—in fact there are specific disadvantages (such as an increased incidence of malfunctions and higher costs). The use of midlines is not widespread in the pediatric field and is usually reserved for older children in adolescence, where the calibers and lengths provided for in the adult can be used.

In the case of short chemotherapy, or temporary home parenteral nutrition, or where there is an indication for infusion of solutions that are not compatible with the peripheral route, it is advisable to insert a medium term central venous access. Although there is no consensus on the definition of the medium term, in most situations it is now understood that this is a period of around 4–6 months, to be interpreted flexibly.

Medium-term central VAD used in the pediatric patient include PICCs (non-tunneled or tunneled), tunneled CICCs and tunneled FICCs. In the past, a non-tunneled silicone CICC (Hohn catheter) had also been included in this category, but this device has now fallen into disuse because it is characterized by a high risk of accidental dislocation and breakage, because of the fragility and morbidity of the silicon.

The choice between PICCs, tunneled CICCs and tunneled FICCs is based on the availability of the child's venous heritage. We recommend using non-cuffed PICC, either tunneled or not, depending on the vein availability. The presence of a vein of adequate internal caliber (at least three times the external diameter of the catheter) located in Dawson's green area allows the placement of a non-tunneled PICC. Although non-tunneled PICCs are normally considered an appropriate access for duration of a few months, there are reports in the literature of non-tunneled PICCs left in place and functioning for two to three years.

The tunneling of PICCs is a very recent strategy (developed in the last few years). Its rationale can be twofold: (a) when no appropriate vein in terms of caliber and accessibility is visualized in Dawson's green zone, the clinician may choose to puncture a vein (basilica, axillary, etc.) located in the yellow zone. However, this area is not appropriate as an exit site, due to its proximity to the armpit. In this case, tunneling allows to have the ideal puncture site and simultaneously also the ideal exit site. In other words, Dawson's ZIM (Zone Insertion Method) helps to define when to tunnel (i.e.: when the ideal venipuncture site is in the yellow zone) but also how long should the tunnel be (i.e.: long enough to locate the exit site in the green zone); (b) tunneling, by moving the exit site far from the catheter entrance into the vein, also has a direct protective effect against the risk of extra luminal bacterial contamination. In selected cases, tunneling can be adopted programmatically to reduce infectious risk.

For both tunneled and non-tunneled PICCs, the insertion technique strictly implies the use of ultrasound guidance for venipuncture; though, ultrasound is very useful and cost-effective also for the 'tip navigation'; wherever possible, the 'tip location' should be performed with the intracavitary electrocardiographic method. Fluoroscopy should be avoided as 'tip location' method, since is less safe, less accurate and less cost-effective than intracavitary ECG or echocardiography. The principles of the insertion technique are those summarized in the SIP protocol (Safe Insertion of PICCs), developed by the GAVeCeLT.

It is always preferable to use pressure injectable PICCs, in latest-generation polyurethane, open-ended, non-valved. The evidence of the literature shows that the silicon PICCs have no advantage over those in polyurethane, but only disadvantages (greater incidence of dislocations and rupture). There is no evidence of any advantage in the use of valved PICCs (which in fact are associated with an increased risk of malfunctions and higher costs).

When a PICC is contraindicated, the best option as medium-term central VAD in a non-hospitalized child is a CICC placed via ultrasound-guided puncture and cannulation of a vein in the supra-clavicular area (internal jugular, brachio-cephalic, or subclavian vein) or in the infra-clavicular area (axillary vein). The younger the child, the more the choice of vein will be restricted to larger veins, such as the brachio-cephalic and the internal jugular. In infants, the easiest and safest vein will almost always be the brachio-cephalic.

The exit site should preferably be in the infra-clavicular area (a very favorable site in terms of risk of infection, thrombosis and dislocation); another fundamental issue is that the catheter must be tunneled. The international guidelines advise against the use of non-tunneled CICCs in the non-hospitalized patient, due to the high risk of dislocations and infections.

As tunneled non-cuffed CICCs, we recommend the off-label use of catheters marketed as PICCs, which have the advantage of considerable length (50 cm and more) and insertion with modified Seldinger technique (which simplifies the tunneling maneuver). The catheter will be placed in the best available central vein (the one whose puncture appears easier, and therefore safer) after an ultrasound evaluation of the region (RaCeVA), following a standardized implant protocol, such as the SICA-Ped protocol (Safe Insertion of Central Access in Pediatric patients) developed by GAVeCeLT.

In selected cases, tunneled, non-cuffed FICCs should also be considered as medium-term venous access, if the superior vena cava is thought to be obstructed or compressed.

In the case of long-term central venous access (or presumably intended for use for more than 4–6 months), the fundamental criteria for choosing the most appropriate system lies in the frequency with which the system will be used.

A frequent use of venous access (more than once a week, for example every day or every other day) yields a preferential indication to an external system. An infrequent use of venous access (less than once a week, for example every two or three weeks) places a preferential indication on a totally implanted system (port).

A tunneled catheter with a Dacron cuff can be used as long-term venous access, provided it is properly implanted (important point: the cuff must be at 2 cm or more from the exit site). Many pressure injectable cuffed catheters are available on the market: they are in latest-generation polyurethane, open-ended, non-valved (Power Hickman, Powerline, Proline). These catheters are associated with minimal risk of breakage and mechanical complications, and lower risk of malfunction if compared to silicon catheters. They are available in various sizes (5Fr, 6Fr, etc.), both single and double lumen. The silicon tunneled cuffed catheters used in the past (cuffed Groshong, Hickman, Broviac, Leonard) are now obsolete and should no longer be used: they have no advantage in terms of biocompatibility, but instead have many disadvantages (difficulty in securement, low flow, fragility, tendency to dislocation and tip migration, greater incidence of lumen occlusion, difficult dis-obstruction, impossibility of use at high pressures).

The Dacron cuff becomes efficient for stabilization purposes only two to three weeks after implantation (i.e., only after the development of adhesions between the cuff and the subcutaneous tissue); in this first period after implantation, the catheter must be temporarily stabilized with a sutureless system with skin adhesiveness (or even with a subcutaneous anchorage).

A tunneled CVC secured with a subcutaneously anchored system (SAS) can be used as long-term venous access. In most cases, the SAS will remain in place for many months, until the catheter is removed. In the pediatric patient, a device of this type has the great advantage of allowing an easy removal, that does not include either sedation or local anesthesia (as opposed to what necessary for removal of a cuffed catheter).

As tunneled non-cuffed catheters, we recommend using power injectable catheters, in latest-generation polyurethane, open ended, non-valved. These catheters are associated with minimal risk of rupture or mechanical complications, and lower risk of malfunction if compared to non-pressure injectable catheters. For this purpose, we recommend the off-label use of catheters marketed as PICCs, which have the advantage of considerable length (50 cm and more) and insertion with modified Seldinger technique (which simplifies the tunneling maneuver).

Ports are typically indicated for long-term venous access, when its use can be defined as 'infrequent'. Typical example of infrequent use (that is, less frequently than once a week) is the use of venous access for chemotherapy every two or three weeks. In most of these cases, the most appropriate choice will be that of a totally implantable central venous system, or a 'port'.

The choice of a port involves two conditions: (a) that venous access is to be used for prolonged periods (longer than 4–6 months), and (b) that access is infrequent. In this sense, the use of the port for home parenteral nutrition (HPN)—which implies a daily use of the device or in any case for several days a week—should be seen as an exception (usually linked to a strong and motivated preference of the patient). The daily use of a port for HPN is associated with an increased risk of local complications of the skin over the reservoir and an increased risk of lumen occlusions due to lipid precipitation; also, such occlusions will be more difficult to dis-obstruct if compared to an external system. The theoretical advantage of the port in terms of infection prevention is completely nullified when the port is used every day (see the INS guidelines).

In children, the advantages of the port must be carefully weighed against the inevitable disadvantage of having to access the system each time through a puncture for positioning the Huber, a sting that can be well tolerated in adults, but which is often poorly tolerated in the child (especially if preadolescent), despite the use of anesthetic creams.

All the ports available on the market are central venous ports (i.e. with a tip positioned in the superior vena cava, or in the right atrium, or in the inferior vena cava): there are no 'peripheral' venous ports. Central access is, however, obtainable by puncturing and cannulating different veins, in the cervico-thoracic region (chest port), at the arm (PICC-port), or—very rarely—in the groin area (femoral port). The choice will be guided above all by venous availability. In general, even in the pediatric age, if the veins of the arm are adequate, the first choice will be a PICC-port.

The port's reservoir can be made of completely radio-transparent material (plastic) or a mixture of plastic (resins of various types) and metal (usually, titanium); depending on the depth of the pocket, it is possible to choose between 'standard' (height about 12 mm) or 'low profile' (about 10 mm) or 'very low profile' (about 8 mm) reservoirs; for PICC ports, the reservoir is always 'very low profile'.

The catheter can be made of silicone or polyurethane, without significant difference in biocompatibility between the two materials. Evidence from the literature suggests avoiding valved catheters (greater risk of malfunction) and transparent silicone catheters (greater fragility). For PICC ports, polyurethane rather than silicon catheters should be preferred (easier to position). The diameter of the catheter (usually, 4–5 Fr for the PICC ports, 6–7 Fr for the thoracic ports) must be proportionate to the diameter of the vein.

1.6 Other Vascular Access in Infants and Children

Other vascular access in infants and children include arterial lines, accesses for hemodialysis and for apheresis, and intraosseous access.

Peripheral arterial catheters are typically used in pediatric intensive care unit, in critically ill children needing repeated blood sampling, arterial blood gas analysis and invasive monitoring of the blood pressure. The arteries most accessed are the radial artery, the common femoral artery and the pedidial artery. Placement of an arterial catheters will always require a careful choice of the caliber and the length, depending on the vessel to be cannulated. Arterial catheters are in polyurethane or in PEBA, and according to the current guidelines should be placed by ultrasound guidance.

Hemodialysis may be required in children as much as in adults, and it will be performed with the same accesses: arterio-venous fistula, arterio-venous graft, tunneled-cuffed catheters, and non-tunneled non-cuffed catheters. Dialysis catheters are double lumen, in polyurethane, and they are available in different calibers and lengths depending on the size of the vein and the age of the child. They must be inserted by ultrasound guidance. The veins more appropriate for dialysis catheters are the right brachio-cephalic vein, the right internal jugular vein, and the femoral veins. The same catheters used for dialysis may be also used for therapeutic apheresis.

Intraosseous access has its major role in the care on extra-hospital pediatric emergencies, where obtaining a rapid route for fluid infusion plays a vital role. In the intra hospital setting, intraosseous devices should be used in pediatric emergencies (shock, cardiac arrest) when it is impossible to insert a venous line within two minutes. The intraosseous access should always be regarded as a temporary solution, i.e., as a 'bridge' to a more permanent and reliable vascular access.

Bibliography

1. Cellini M, Bergadano A, Crocoli A, Badino C, Carraro F, Sidro L, Botta D, Pancaldi A, Rossetti F, Pitta F, Cesaro S. Guidelines of the Italian Association of Pediatric Hematology and Oncology for the management of the central venous access devices in pediatric patients with onco-hematological disease. J Vasc Access. 2020;10:1129729820969309. https://doi.org/10.1177/1129729820969309. Epub ahead of print
2. Barone G, D'Andrea V, Vento G, Pittiruti M. A systematic ultrasound evaluation of the diameter of deep veins in the Newborn: results and implications for clinical practice. Neonatology. 2019;115(4):335–40. https://doi.org/10.1159/000496848. Epub 2019 Mar 15
3. Barone G, Pittiruti M. Epicutaneo-caval catheters in neonates: new insights and new suggestions from the recent literature. J Vasc Access. 2020;21(6):805–9. https://doi.org/10.1177/1129729819891546. Epub 2019 Dec 5
4. Barone G, Pittiruti M, Ancora G, Vento G, Tota F, D'Andrea V. Centrally inserted central catheters in preterm neonates with weight below 1500 g by ultrasound-guided access to the brachiocephalic vein. J Vasc Access. 2021;22(3):344–52. https://doi.org/10.1177/1129729820940174. Epub 2020 Jul 10
5. Crocoli A, Cesaro S, Cellini M, Rossetti F, Sidro L, Pinelli F, Pittiruti M. In defense of the use of peripherally inserted central catheters in pediatric patients. J Vasc Access. 2021;22(3):333–6. https://doi.org/10.1177/1129729820936411. Epub 2020 Jun 27
6. Crocoli A, Tornesello A, Pittiruti M, Barone A, Muggeo P, Inserra A, Molinari AC, Grillenzoni V, Durante V, Cicalese MP, Zanazzo GA, Cesaro S. Central venous access devices in pediatric malignancies: a position paper of Italian Association of Pediatric Hematology and Oncology. J Vasc Access. 2015;16(2):130–6. https://doi.org/10.5301/jva.5000314. Epub 2014 Oct 14
7. Giovanni B, Miria N, Gina A. Off label use of PICC as umbilical arterial catheter: clinical case series. J Vasc Access. 2021;7:11297298211008089. https://doi.org/10.1177/11297298211008089. Epub ahead of print
8. Gorski L, Hadaway L, Hagle M, et al. Infusion therapy standards of practice. J Infus Nurs. 2021;44(1S Suppl 1):S1–S224.
9. Kolaček S, Puntis JWL, Hojsak I. ESPGHAN/ESPEN/ESPR/CSPEN working group on pediatric parenteral nutrition. ESPGHAN/ESPEN/ESPR/CSPEN guidelines on pediatric parenteral nutrition: venous access. Clin Nutr. 2018;37(6 Pt B):2379–91. https://doi.org/10.1016/j.clnu.2018.06.952. Epub 2018 Jun 18
10. Paladini A, Chiaretti A, Sellasie KW, Pittiruti M, Vento G. Ultrasound-guided placement of long peripheral cannulas in children over the age of 10 years admitted to the emergency department: a pilot study. BMJ Paediatr Open. 2018;2(1):e000244. https://doi.org/10.1136/bmjpo-2017-000244.
11. Spagnuolo F, Vacchiano T. Ultrasound-guided cannulation of the brachiocephalic vein in newborns: a novel approach with a supraclavicular view for tip navigation and tip location. J Vasc Access. 2021;16:11297298211001159. https://doi.org/10.1177/11297298211001159. Epub ahead of print
12. Ullman AJ, Bernstein SJ, Brown E, Aiyagari R, Doellman D, Faustino EVS, Gore B, Jacobs JP, Jaffray J, Kleidon T, Mahajan PV, McBride CA, Morton K, Pitts S, Prentice E, Rivard DC, Shaughnessy E, Stranz M, Wolf J, Cooper DS, Cooke M, Rickard CM, Chopra V. The Michigan appropriateness guide for intravenous catheters in Pediatrics: miniMAGIC. Pediatrics. 2020;145(Suppl 3):S269–84. https://doi.org/10.1542/peds.2019-3474I.

Chapter 2
Evidence Based Rationale for Ultrasound Guided Vascular Access in Children

Nicola Massimo Disma and Mauro Pittiruti

Ultrasound guidance is currently considered mandatory for central venous catherization. The only central venous access devices that do not require ultrasound for puncture and cannulation of the vein are the umbilical venous catheter (UVC) and the epicutaneo-cava catheters (ECC) in neonates. All other central lines used in neonates and in children (CICC, PICC, FICC, port) must be inserted by ultrasound guided cannulation of the vein.

Still, ultrasound has a 'global' role in central venous access, not limited to venous cannulation, but extended also to other maneuvers of great relevance during the procedure, such as the appropriate choice of the most appropriate vein, the early detection of puncture-related complications, the progression of the catheter in the proper direction (tip navigation), the appropriate location of the tip, and the early detection of late complications. From this point of view, any central venous access in neonates and children will benefit of ultrasound.

Tip navigation, tip location and detection of catheter-related complications will be addressed in dedicated chapters. Focusing on ultrasound guided venous cannulation, the impact of ultrasound is different in neonates vs. children.

In neonates, ultrasound guidance has been recently introduced in clinical practice for insertion of relatively large bore central venous catheters (i.e., 3 French) even in extremely preterm infants weighing well below 1 kg. It is usually achieved by puncture and cannulation of the brachio-cephalic vein or of the internal jugular vein (centrally inserted central catheters, CICCs) or of the femoral vein (femorally inserted central catheters, FICCs). As opposed to the peripherally inserted small-bore catheters (epicutaneo-cava catheters, ECC), 3 Fr power injectable CICCs and FICCs enable blood sampling, monitoring, and high flow infusions which may be

N. M. Disma
Anesthesia and Intensive Care, Pediatric Hospital 'G.Gaslini', Genova, Italy

M. Pittiruti (✉)
Department of Surgery, Catholic University Hospital, Rome, Italy

D. G. Biasucci et al. (eds.), *Vascular Access in Neonates and Children*,
https://doi.org/10.1007/978-3-030-94709-5_2

associated with a reduction of mortality and improved outcome. On the other hand, UVC and ECC will not require ultrasound for venous cannulation, though ultrasound may be previous for tip navigation and tip location.

In children, on the other hand, any central venous access should be placed by ultrasound guidance. As above mentioned, the 'blind' puncture of central veins based on surface landmarks and the surgical venous cutdown are not acceptable anymore from the clinical, ethical and legal point of view. Depending on the vein chosen for the procedure, pediatric central venous access devices can be classified as centrally inserted central catheters (CICC), peripherally inserted central catheters (PICC) and femorally inserted central catheters (FICC).

In small children, as regards the insertion of CICCs, the easiest approach is the cannulation of the internal jugular vein (IJV) or of the brachio-cephalic vein (BCV), which are large and easy to visualize. The IJV is visualized in short axis and should be preferably accessed in-plane. Due to its mobility and compressibility, the IJV may not always be a safe choice, because of the risk of passing the needle through the posterior wall of the vein, potentially injuring the underlying subclavian artery, particularly if adopting an out-of-plane approach. The BCVs are the ideal choice in small infants: these veins are large, stable, and relatively easy to access. The subclavian vein (SV) can be visualized in long axis in the supraclavicular region and punctured with the in-plane approach; still, there is some risk of inadvertent pleural injury if the tip of the needle is not consistently visualized during the maneuver. On the contrary, the approach to the BCV is quite safe: this vein is easily visualized in long axis with the ultrasound probe placed in the supraclavicular region. A supraclavicular in-plane cannulation technique from lateral to medial showing the advancement of the needle over the entire distance is the method of choice. According to some authors, it may be easier to cannulate the left over the right BCV due its horizontal course in small babies. On the other hand, pre-scanning of both BCVs will already predict the ease of the cannulation. The infraclavicular cannulation of the axillary vein at the chest has not been described in infants but it may be easy in older children. The axillary vein is small, compressible, and difficult to scan because it lies below the great pectoral muscle. Though this vein has not close contact with the pleura, when it is accessed by a short axis/out-of-plane approach, there is some risk of inadvertent passage through the intercostal space with eventual injury to the pleura.

The best strategy for choosing the best vein to access is to perform a RaCeVA (Rapid Central Vein Assessment) before the procedure, i.e., a systematic ultrasound scan for evaluating the morphologic characteristics of all the major veins in the supraclavicular area (IJV, BCV, SV and external jugular vein) and in the infraclavicular area (axillary vein and cephalic vein). There is no ideal vein to access in neonates, infants, and children: the most appropriate vein (the easiest to approach being also the safest) should be decided after appropriate ultrasound evaluation.

In bigger infants and in children, when the size of the deep veins of the arm reaches 3 mm, it is possible to insert PICCs. The difference between ECC and PICC has already been explained in the previous chapter. PICCs have a higher performance than ECC in any aspect; they are inserted in older infants and in children, while ECCs are inserted exclusively in neonates. All PICCs must be placed by ultrasound guidance, preferably after a systematic scan of the deep vein of the arms (RaPeVA—Rapid Peripheral Venous Assessment).

Femoral lines also play a role in infants and in children, usually as an alternative option when insertion of PICCs and CICCs is not considered feasible, or it is likely to be associated with late complications. FICCs must be inserted by ultrasound guidance, mostly in the common femoral vein; in older children, the superficial femoral vein may also be of appropriate caliber. The insertion of a FICC should always be performed after a systematic ultrasound study of the veins of the groin/thigh area (RaFeVA—Rapid Femoral Vein Assessment).

All the above techniques will be described in full detail in dedicated chapters. Blind percutaneous approaches (so called 'landmark-based' techniques) and surgical cutdown of the veins must be abandoned. All studies comparing the ultrasound-guided (USG) vs. 'blind' methods clearly favor ultrasound-guidance. Moreover, USG has opened the door to some approaches which were difficult or impossible in the past. For example, the BCV has become a suitable approach in neonates and small infants, though it was very rare in the pre-USG era. Additionally, the USG allowed comparison between different approaches of the same vein: the USG supraclavicular cannulation of the BCV is superior to the USG infraclavicular cannulation of the SBV. Obviously, comparison between US-guided and landmark-based approaches to the BCV will be never tested, as the BCV approach is exclusively ultrasound-guided.

Summarizing, USG introduced a significant increase of the success rate cannulation of many central veins, consistently reducing the time spent in achieving the successful cannulation and the number of punctures. However, what is far more important is that USG introduced the possibility of achieving a successful cannulation even in extremely low weight infants with a very low incidence of complications. Even if evidence cannot be offered for every single approach, USG should replace older techniques at all pediatric ages.

With the only exception of some central venous accesses in neonates (namely, umbilical venous catheters and epicutaneo-cava catheters), all the other central venous accesses in neonates, infants and children must be placed with ultrasound guidance.

Bibliography

1. Barone G, D'Andrea V, Vento G, Pittiruti M. A Systematic ultrasound evaluation of the diameter of deep veins in the newborn: results and implications for clinical practice. Neonatology. 2019;115(4):335–340. https://doi.org/10.1159/000496848. Epub 2019 Mar 15. PMID: 30878998.
2. Barone G, Pittiruti M, Ancora G, Vento G, Tota F, D'Andrea V. Centrally inserted central catheters in preterm neonates with weight below 1500 g by ultrasound-guided access to the brachio-cephalic vein. J Vasc Access. 2021 May;22(3):344–352. https://doi.org/10.1177/1129729820940174. Epub 2020 Jul 10. PMID: 32648811.

3. Biasucci DG. Ultrasound based innovations for interventional procedures: the paradigmatic case of central venous access. Minerva Anestesiol. 2020;86(2):121–3.
4. Bodenham A, Babu S, Bennett J, et al. Association of anaesthetists of Great Britain and Ireland: safe vascular access 2016. Anaesthesia. 2016;71(5):573–85.
5. Bouaziz H, Zetlaoui PJ, Pierre S, et al. Guidelines on the use of ultrasound guidance for vascular access. Anaesth Crit Care Pain Med. 2015;34(1):65–9.
6. Breschan C, Graf G, Jost R, Stettner H, Feigl G, Goessler A, Neuwersch S, Koestenberger M, Likar R. Ultrasound-guided supraclavicular cannulation of the right brachiocephalic vein in small infants: a consecutive, prospective case series. Pediatr Anesth. 2015;25:943–9.
7. Breschan C, Graf G, Jost R, Stettner H, Feigl G, Neuwersch S, Stadik C, Koestenberger M, Likar R. A retrospective analysis of the clinical effectiveness of supraclavicular, ultrasound-guided brachiocephalic vein cannulations in preterm infants. Anesthesiol. 2018;128:38–43.
8. Breschan C, Platzer M, Jost R, Stettner H, Beyer AS, Feigl G, Likar R. Consecutive, prospective case series of a new method for ultrasound-guided supraclavicular approach to the brachiocephalic vein in children. Br J Anaesth. 2011;106:732–7.
9. Breschan C, Platzer M, Jost R, Stettner H, Feigl G, Likar R. Pediatr Anesth Ultrasound-guided supraclavicular cannulation of the brachiocephalic vein in infants: a retrospective analysis of a case series. Pediatr Anesth. 2012;22:1062–7.
10. Brescia F, Pittiruti M, Ostroff M, Biasucci DG. Rapid Femoral Vein Assessment (RaFeVA): A systematic protocol for ultrasound evaluation of the veins of the lower limb, so to optimize the insertion of femorally inserted central catheters. J Vasc Access. 2020 Oct 16. https://doi.org/10.1177/1129729820965063. Epub ahead of print. PMID: 33063616.
11. Bruzoni M, Slater BJ, Wall J, St Peter SD, Dutta S. A prospective randomized trial of ultrasound- vs landmark-guided central venous access in the pediatric population. J Am J Coll Surg. 2013;216:939–43.
12. Byon HJ, Lee GW, Lee JH, Park YH, Kim HS, Kim CS, Kim JT. Comparison between ultrasound-guided supraclavicular and infraclavicular approaches for subclavian venous catheterization in children—a randomized trial. Br J Anaesth. 2013;111:788–92.
13. Cellini M, Bergadano A, Crocoli A, Badino C, Carraro F, Sidro L, Botta D, Pancaldi A, Rossetti F, Pitta F, Cesaro S. Guidelines of the Italian Association of Pediatric Hematology and Oncology for the management of the central venous access devices in pediatric patients with onco-hematological disease. J Vasc Access. 2020 Nov 10. https://doi.org/10.1177/1129729820969309. Epub ahead of print. PMID: 33169648.
14. Crocoli A, Tornesello A, Pittiruti M, Barone A, Muggeo P, Inserra A, Molinari AC, Grillenzoni V, Durante V, Cicalese MP, Zanazzo GA, Cesaro S. Central venous access devices in pediatric malignancies: a position paper of Italian Association of Pediatric Hematology and Oncology. J Vasc Access. 2015 Mar-Apr;16(2):130–6. https://doi.org/10.5301/jva.5000314. Epub 2014 Oct 14. PMID: 25362978.
15. Emoli A, Cappuccio S, Marche B, et al. The ISP (Safe Insertion of PICCs) protocol: a bundle of 8 recommendations to minimize the complications related to the peripherally inserted central venous catheters (PICC). Assist Inferm Ric. 2014;33(2):82–9.
16. Froehlich CD, Rigby MR, Rosenberg ES, Li R, Roerig PL, Easley KA, Stockwell JA. Ultrasound-guided central venous catheter placement decreases complications and decreases placement attempts compared with the landmark technique in patients in a pediatric intensive care unit. Crit Care Med. 2009;37:1090–6.
17. Habas F, Baleine J, Milesi C, Combes C, Didelot MN, Romano-Bertrand S, Grau D, Parer S, Baud C, Cambonie G. Supraclavicular catheterization of the brachiocephalic vein: a way to prevent or reduce catheter maintenance-related complications in children. Europ J Pediatr. 2018;177:451–9.
18. Lamperti M, Biasucci DG, Disma N, Pittiruti M, Breschan C, Vailati D, Subert M, Traškaitė V, Macas A, Estebe JP, Fuzier R, Boselli E, Hopkins P. European Society of Anaesthesiology guidelines on peri-operative use of ultrasound-guided for vascular access (PERSEUS vascular access). Eur J Anaesthesiol. 2020 May;37(5):344–376. https://doi.org/10.1097/

EJA.0000000000001180. Erratum in: Eur J Anaesthesiol. 2020 Jul;37(7):623. PMID: 32265391.
19. Leyvi G, Taylor DG, Reith E, Wasnick JD. Utility of ultrasound-guided central venous cannulation in pediatric surgical patients: a clinical series. Pediatr Anesth. 2005;15:953–8.
20. Montes-Tapia F, Rodríguez-Taméz A, Cura-Esquivel I, Barreto-Arroyo I, Hernández-Garduño A, Rodríguez-Balderrama I, Quero J, de la O-Cavazos M. Efficacy and safety of ultrasound-guided internal jugular vein catheterization in low birth weight newborn. J Pediatr Surg. 2016;51:1700–3.
21. Oulego-Erroz I, Muñoz-Lozón A, Alonso-Quintela P, Rodríguez-Nuñez A. Comparison of ultrasound guided brachiocephalic and internal jugular vein cannulation in critically ill children. J Crit Care. 2016;35:133–7.
22. Pirotte T, Veyckemans F. Ultrasound-guided subclavian vein cannulation in infants and children: a novel approach. Br J Anaesth. 2007;98:509–14.
23. Singh Y, Tissot C, Fraga MV, Yousef N, Cortes RG, Lopez J, Sanchez-de-Toledo J, Brierley J, Colunga JM, Raffaj D, Da Cruz E, Durand P, Kenderessy P, Lang HJ, Nishisaki A, Kneyber MC, Tissieres P, Conlon TW, De Luca D. International evidence-based guidelines on Point of Care Ultrasound (POCUS) for critically ill neonates and children issued by the POCUS Working Group of the European Society of Paediatric and Neonatal Intensive Care (ESPNIC). Crit Care. 2020 Feb 24;24(1):65. https://doi.org/10.1186/s13054-020-2787-9. PMID: 32093763; PMCID: PMC7041196.
24. Spagnuolo F, Vacchiano T. Ultrasound-guided cannulation of the brachiocephalic vein in newborns: A novel approach with a supraclavicular view for tip navigation and tip location. J Vasc Access. 2021 Mar 16. https://doi.org/10.1177/11297298211001159. Epub ahead of print. PMID: 33726580.
25. Spencer TR, Pittiruti M. Rapid Central Vein Assessment (RaCeVA): A systematic, standardized approach for ultrasound assessment before central venous catheterization. J Vasc Access. 2019;20(3):239–49.
26. Wu SY, Ling Q, Cao LH, et al. Real-time two-dimensional ultrasound guidance for central venous cannulation: a meta-analysis. Anesthesiology. 2013;118(2):361–75.

Chapter 3
Principles of Ultrasonography and Settings of Ultrasound Devices for Children

Gurinder Singh Malhi and James Bennett

Modern ultrasound scanners have become widely available; light-weight portable machines are commonly used to produce a rapidly updated two-dimensional gray-scale image that aids safe and successful vessel cannulation.

The term 'ultrasound' describes all sound waves of frequencies beyond the range of human hearing (>20 kHz). Ultrasound imaging utilizes a high range of sound waves frequencies (2–15 MHz) to localize and characterize different tissues.

The ultrasound transducer "probe" is a complex and sophisticated piece of electrical equipment, housing piezoelectric crystals, which vibrate to produce an ultrasound pulse when exposed to an electrical current. This phenomenon is named the piezoelectric effect. Hockey-stick linear probes have a small footprint making them ideal for neonatal and pediatric vascular access.

Artefacts describe a range of appearances in the displayed image that are not accurate to the original anatomical features being scanned. The presence of artefacts reduces image quality and leads to potential tissue damage, should images be misinterpreted during invasive procedures.

3.1 Introduction

In the United Kingdom, the use of ultrasound imaging for obtaining central venous access has become routine practice. A 2015 Cochrane review concluded a benefit in safety and quality using ultrasound over landmark technique for internal jugular

G. S. Malhi (✉) · J. Bennett
Anesthesia Department, Birmingham Children's Hospital, Birmingham, UK
e-mail: Gurinder.malhi@nhs.net; James.bennett11@nhs.net

D. G. Biasucci et al. (eds.), *Vascular Access in Neonates and Children*,
https://doi.org/10.1007/978-3-030-94709-5_3

vein cannulation. The Association of Anesthetists of Great Britain & Ireland (AAGBI) subsequently published recommendations in May 2016, stating ultrasound should be used routinely for internal jugular venous catheter insertion [1]. Furthermore, the AAGBI Working Party recommended its use for all other central venous access sites, and difficult arterial and peripheral venous cannulation.

Ultrasound imaging can provide useful information during vascular access procedures, including puncture site evaluation, identification of local pathology, guidance during needle puncture, verification of guidewire position and early recognition of complications.

This chapter will provide readers with a brief history of ultrasound, as well as an outline of the principles of ultrasonography, the methods for ideal probe selection and setting adjustments to improve image quality.

3.2 History of Medical Ultrasound

In 1794, an Italian priest (Lazzaro Spallanzani) deduced that bats use sound inaudible to humans to accurately navigate in complete darkness. His observation saw him become a pioneer, inspiring others to explore the use of sound waves to understand the environment.

By 1880, the Curie brothers had discovered the piezoelectric effect. They observed that the application of mechanical pressure to a quartz crystal produced an electric potential. They also described the reciprocal piezoelectric effect. The generation and reception of high frequency sound waves using crystals was a significant moment in the history of ultrasound and quartz crystals remain integral to modern day ultrasound scanners.

During World War I, ultrasound was used to aid submarine navigation with underwater SONAR (Sound Navigation and Ranging) systems and detect defects in metal constructions (the integrity of a ship's hull). The use of ultrasound in metal flaw detection alerted physicians to the possibilities within diagnostic medicine, with the first such application arriving when Karl Dussik, at the University of Vienna (1942) attempted to demonstrate changes in brain ventricle size secondary to tumor growth.

George Ludwig's 1949 experiments using industrial flaw detector equipment on animal tissues reported the mean velocity of sound transmission to be 1540 m/s. This value is still in use today.

Professor Ian Donald (University of Glasgow) explored the application of ultrasound in the field of obstetrics in the 1950s. He used the one-dimensional A-mode (amplitude mode) to measure the parietal diameter of the fetal head. Later he would help invent and construct the world's first two-dimensional compound B-mode scanner, enabling the operator to visualize the density of tissues.

Technological advances in electronics and piezoelectric materials are accredited for the subsequent developments in ultrasound application within medicine. Collectively these advances mean that ultrasound scanners have today become widely available light-weight portable machines capable of producing high quality real-time greyscale images.

As technology advances, the application of ultrasound expands. Current areas of development include portable wireless probes, three-dimensional images, elastography and contrast enhancement (microbubbles).

3.3 Ultrasound for Vascular Access

Ultrasound imaging utilizes high frequency sound waves to localize and characterize different tissues. With respect to pediatric vascular access, ultrasound technology can be used to produce a rapidly updated two-dimensional grayscale image that aids safe and successful vessel cannulation.

Ultrasound imaging lends itself to vascular access as it is portable and uses non-ionizing sound waves, with few (if any) contraindications. Real time images and Doppler mode help identify vessel type and patency.

The main disadvantages to its use are operator dependence, poor image quality beyond structures of high impedance, thermal or mechanical injury, and artefacts. The presence of artefacts is important as they reduce image quality and lead to potential tissue damage should images be misinterpreted during invasive procedures.

3.4 Principles of Ultrasonography

3.4.1 Physics

A sound wave is formed by the vibration of molecules in a medium, along a line of propagation in a series of compressions (areas of high pressure) and rarefactions (areas of low pressure).

Sound waves can be described by their frequency (f), wavelength (λ) or speed (ν) (Fig. 3.1).

$$n\left(m / s\right) = f\left(s^{-1}\right) x l\left(m\right)$$

The wavelength is the distance between two identical points on successive peaks or troughs. The number of waves passing a given point per second is the frequency. The speed of the sound wave is the product of the frequency and wavelength.

The term 'ultrasound' describes all sound waves of frequencies beyond the range of human hearing (>20 kHz). The ultrasound waves used in diagnostic medical imaging have a frequency of 2–15 MHz.

The speed of the sound wave in the human body varies depending on the tissue type through which the wave propagates (Table 3.1). The density and compressibility characteristics of different tissues (acoustic impedance) impact the speed at which the sound wave travels.

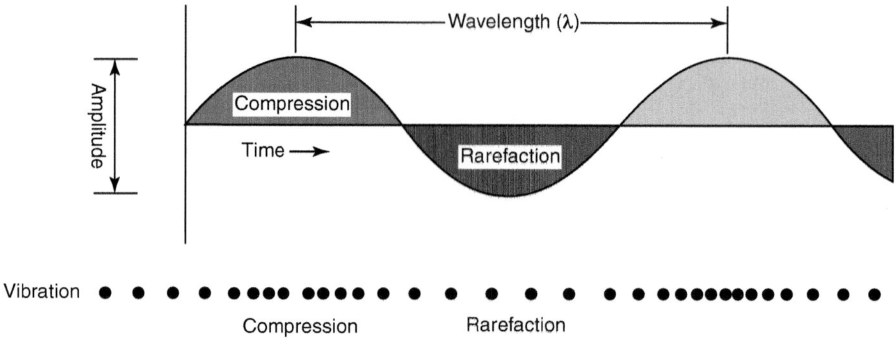

Fig. 3.1 Basic components of a sound wave

Table 3.1 The speed of sound in different tissue types

Tissue	Speed of sound through tissue (m/s) [2]
Air	330
Fat	1450
Water (37°)	1525
Blood	1560
Muscle	1600
Bone	3000

For the generation of a scan image an average speed in soft tissues is required for calculations.

The assumed average speed of ultrasound in soft tissue is 1540 m/s.

3.4.2 Ultrasound Wave Formation

The ultrasound transducer "probe" is a complex and sophisticated piece of electrical equipment, housing artificial polycrystalline ferroelectric materials (ceramics).

The piezoelectric crystals vibrate to produce an ultrasound pulse when exposed to an electrical current. This phenomenon is named the piezoelectric effect. Once a sound wave is produced, the crystals are dampened and switch to listening for the returning echoes. Modern ultrasound transducers oscillate between "emitting" and "listening" modes more than 7000 times a second (pulse echo principle).

The crystals convert the returning ultrasound echoes into an electrical impulse which is interpreted by the ultrasound machine to generate the displayed image.

The typical linear array probe has approximately 200 crystals along the flat surface of the transducer producing a rectangular field of view. Small subgroups of piezoelectric crystals are exposed to electric impulses in a coordinated and sequenced nature, to produce a narrow ultrasound beam that sweeps across the transducer surface (Fig. 3.2). Less than 0.1 s is required for all the crystals to emit their ultrasound waves, producing a high frame rate, allowing moving structures to be visualized in real time.

Each returning echo detected by the transducer is represented by a pixel on the screen, the brightness of which is directly proportional to the strength of the returning sound wave. Structures that strongly reflect ultrasound waves lead to the production of large electrical signal intensities, appearing white or hyperechoic on the final image.

The time from pulse generation to echo detection is used to determine the depth of the reflecting structure, which is represented by the pixel position on the display screen [3].

$$\text{Depth} = (\text{speed of sound} \times \text{time}) / 2$$

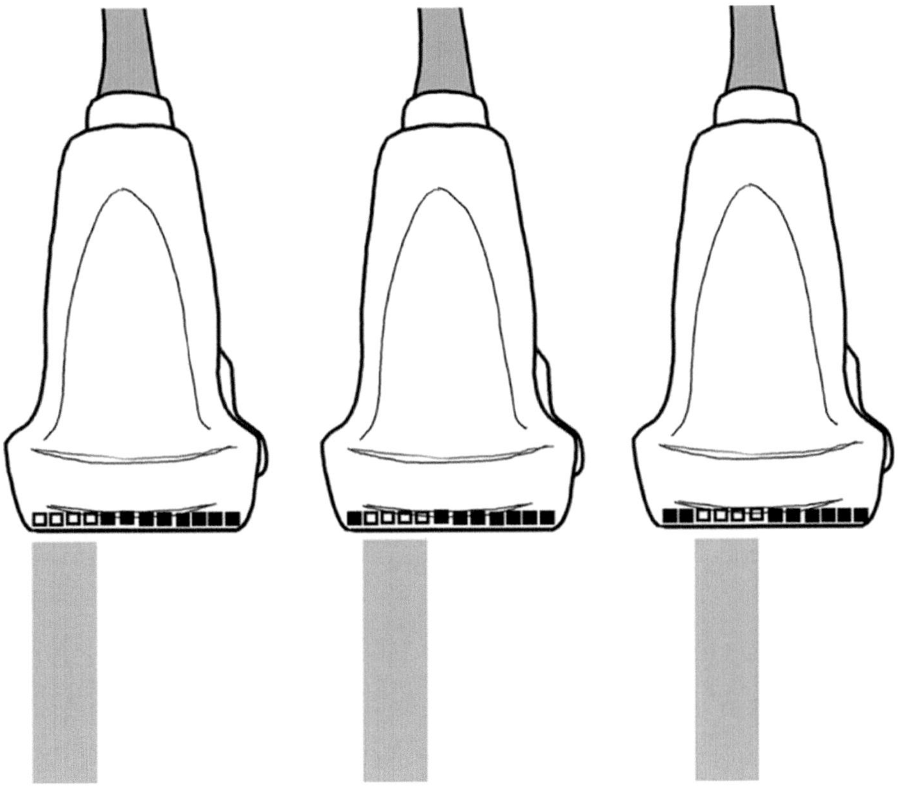

Fig. 3.2 Sequential and coordinated stimulation of piezoelectric crystal subgroups at the transducer surface [with permission from *Oxford Specialist Handbooks in Anaesthesia*]

Each small subgroup of crystals is responsible for the formation of a vertical line of pixels on the final ultrasound scan image. The brightness and depth of the pixels is dependent on the strength of the returning echo from each depth. As the vertical line of pixels from each crystal subset are compiled in series, a complete image of the tissue is produced.

A major problem with grey scale image production is that echoes reflected from deeper structures are characteristically weaker. As these sound waves have travelled further through tissues, they are subject to greater degrees of attenuation, which results in images becoming dimmer at greater depths. Ultrasound machines use "time gain compensation" to counter the effects of attenuation, by increasing signal amplitude at greater depths. This in theory should produce an image of uniform brightness when scanning homogenous tissue.

3.4.3 Resolution

Resolution is an important marker of image quality and refers to the machines ability to distinguish the structures we need to see. The three types of resolution include: spatial (axial and lateral), contrast and temporal.

Axial resolution describes the ability to differentiate two objects that both lie in the path of the ultrasound beam (one directly above the other) (Fig. 3.3). Good axial resolution is vital for pediatric vascular access and requires probes producing short pulses with short wavelengths (high frequency). Should the distance between the two objects be less than 1.5 × wavelength, the machine will not be able to differentiate the reflected echoes.

When the two objects are adjacent to each other (equal depth from probe face), the ability to differentiate them relies on the machine's lateral resolution (Fig. 3.4). Lateral resolution is always worse than axial and is improved with narrow and well-defined ultrasound beams (small subsets of crystals).

Temporal resolution is directly related to the frame rate and depends on the scanning rate (sweep speed) of the ultrasound machine. With relatively slow

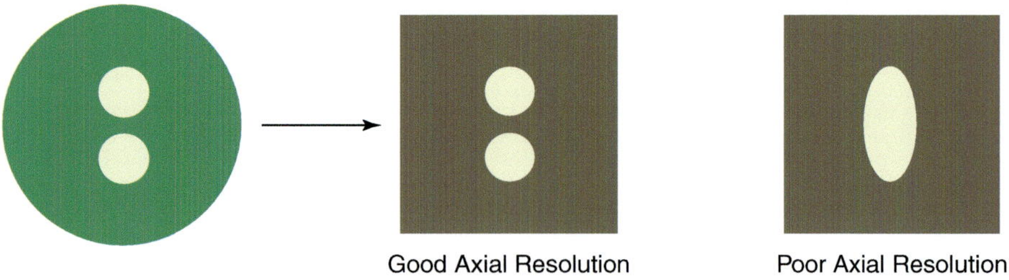

Fig. 3.3 Diagram to demonstrate differing axial resolution quality on final image production [with permission from SonoSite]

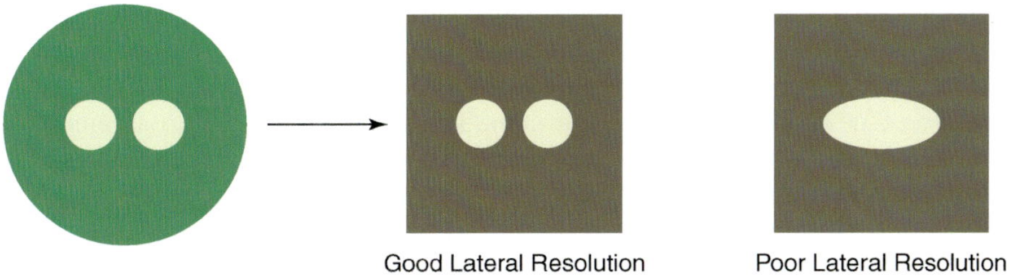

Fig. 3.4 Diagram to demonstrate differing lateral resolution quality on final image production [with permission from SonoSite]

Fig. 3.5 Demonstrates the use of a colour box, superimposed over the B-mode image to indicate directional blood flow [with permission from SonoSite]

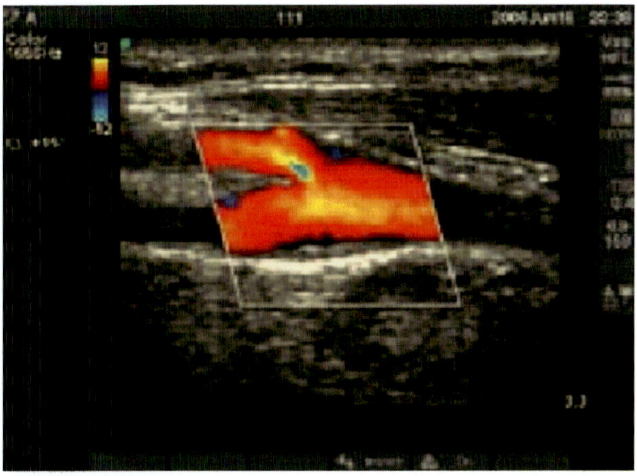

advancement of needles for regional or vascular access, this is rarely a major issue with modern machines.

Contrast resolution describes the ability to identify structures with different reflection characteristics, by subtle changes in their shade of grey on the image.

3.4.4 Doppler

Color Doppler ultrasound provides directional information about blood flow and can aid differentiation between veins and arteries. The "color map" is superimposed over the grayscale image (B-mode image), reducing the frame rate (Fig. 3.5).

The frequency of ultrasound echoes returning to the probe is dependent on the directional movement of the reflective source, relative to the probe. Should the scanned object be moving towards the transducer, the frequency of the ultrasound wave would increase. Such movement is best demonstrated at a vector 0° and completely absent at 90° (i.e., when flow is perpendicular to the probe).

For vascular access, Color Doppler ultrasound enables a color map to overlay the greyscale image. Flow towards the probe will be represented by colors from red to yellow dependent on calculated velocities. Flow away from the probe will be represented as blue through to green (Fig. 3.6). Therefore, it is wrong to assume that imaged blood flow highlighted as red is arterial or that blue would represent venous blood flow.

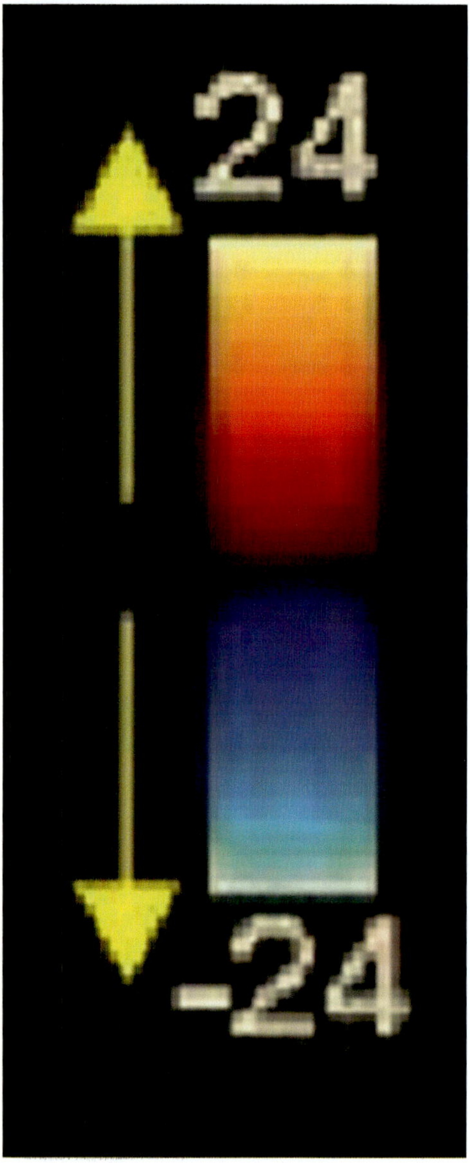

Fig. 3.6 Color bar used to indicate direction of flow [with permission from SonoSite [4]]

3.4.5 Artefact

Ultrasound machines rely on a number of assumptions to simplify the production of the displayed image, one of which is that the average speed of ultrasound in soft tissues at 1540 m/s. The net result of the assumptions is potential artefact generation.

Artefacts describe a range of appearances in the displayed image that are not accurate to the original anatomical features being scanned.

The false image can lead to misinterpretation and injury during invasive procedures. Therefore, structures in the displayed image should not be assumed to be real, until scanned in two planes (transverse and longitudinal).

It is not crucial to diagnose the artefacts affecting the image, but an understanding of why the artefacts occur may help in there eliminate or simply alert the operator to their existence.

3.4.6 Contact Artefacts

Images with shadowing or loss of image from the top are subject to contact artefact (Fig. 3.7). The use of smaller hockey stick ultrasound probes in pediatrics helps to avoid contact artefact. The most common reasons are poor skin contact with the probe, lack of gel, faulty transducers, or air interface.

3.4.7 Acoustic Shadowing

Bony structures reflect ultrasound waves extremely well (bone and calcification) and are said to be acoustically opaque. The lack of ultrasound penetration produces a dark shadow deep to the acoustically opaque structure on the display image. Vessel

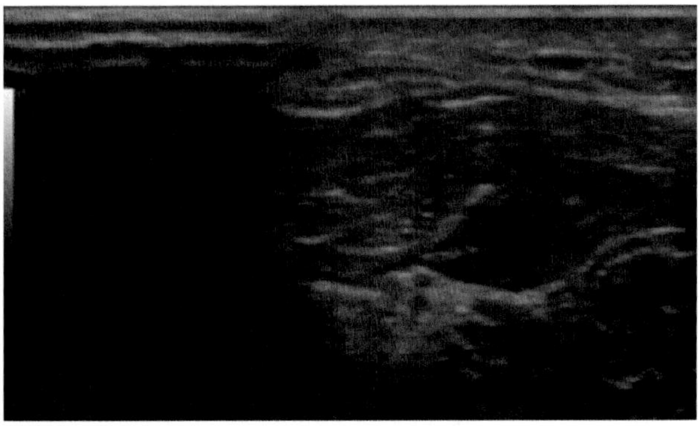

Fig. 3.7 Ultrasound image showing contact artefact

walls - when scanned in plane - exhibit the same acoustic shadowing, potentially complicating plane vessel cannulation.

3.4.8 Post-Cystic Enhancement

Echoes returning from deeper structures tend to be of lower signal strength because of attenuation. To produce an image with consistent brightness, the machine compensates by increasing the amplitude of echoes from deeper structures proportionally to their depth of origin (time gain compensation). However, fluid filled cysts have low echogenicity and the area distal to the cyst will have more gain applied, so appear (falsely) brighter; this artefact is often used to differentiate between solid and fluid filled cysts.

3.4.9 Reflection Artefact

Large smooth surfaces such as the pleura or diaphragm can act as mirror reflectors of the ultrasound beam. The resultant image will contain the true target structure, in addition to a false second reflected image. Good knowledge of anatomy will help differentiate between true and reflected images.

3.4.10 Reverberation

Multiple linear or hyperechoic areas distal to a reflective structure are observed when ultrasound waves reflect back and forth between two strongly reflecting structures (Fig. 3.8). Shallow or flat advancement of the cannulating needle during in plane vessel cannulation may be complicated by reverberation artefact. Increasing the angle of entry should reduce this.

Comet tail artefacts are a type of reverberation artefact. They are bright echoes that fade with depth, producing the characteristic comet tail appearance. They are often encountered during vascular access procedures, whilst scanning the needle tip out of plane.

3.4.11 Slice Thickness Artefact

This is a common artefact caused by structures outside the sector being scanned, producing echoes that affect the final displayed image. The curved nature of vessel walls means that when scanned in plane, echoes outside the image plane show up as in the vessel.

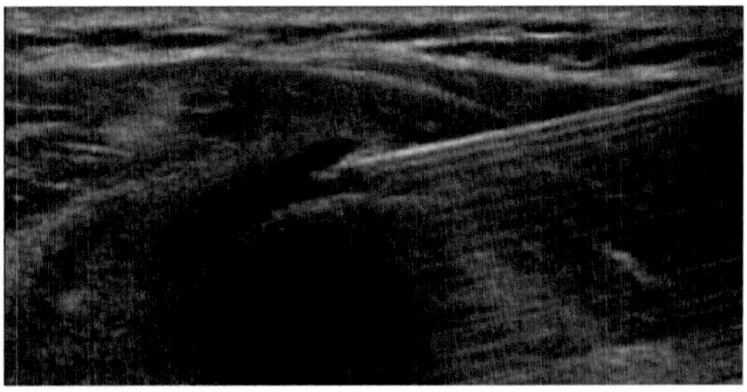

Fig. 3.8 Ultrasound image showing reverberation artefact

3.4.12 *Refraction Artefact*

As a needle passes through two tissues of different acoustic impedance, the final image may indicate a step deformity in the needle structure. This occurs as most scanners assume a fixed speed of sound in tissues, as previously discussed.

3.5 Transducer or "Probe" Selection

The part of the probe in contact with the patient is called the "face of the transducer" and it determines the probes' footprint. The common probes available are Linear, Curvilinear and Phased Array.

Each probe differs in their operating frequency, physical size, and footprint. Appropriate probe selection is critical in the production of high-quality images, so increasing the success rates of cannulation.

Inappropriate probe selection can make a difficult task even harder and potentially unsafe.

3.5.1 *Linear*

The piezoelectric crystals are arranged in a line across the flat transducer face, to produce a rectangular ultrasound image (Fig. 3.9). With operating frequencies between 5 and 18 MHz, they are ideal for older children, and will produce images with good resolution of detail at depths of 2–3 cm, ideal for vascular access.

3.5.2 *Hockey-Stick Linear*

These probes are small and can be held with a "fountain pen" grip (Fig. 3.10). With a small footprint, this subtype of linear probe is ideal for obtaining images from awkward areas. Enabling excellent skin contact, the probe is ideal for neonatal and pediatric vascular access.

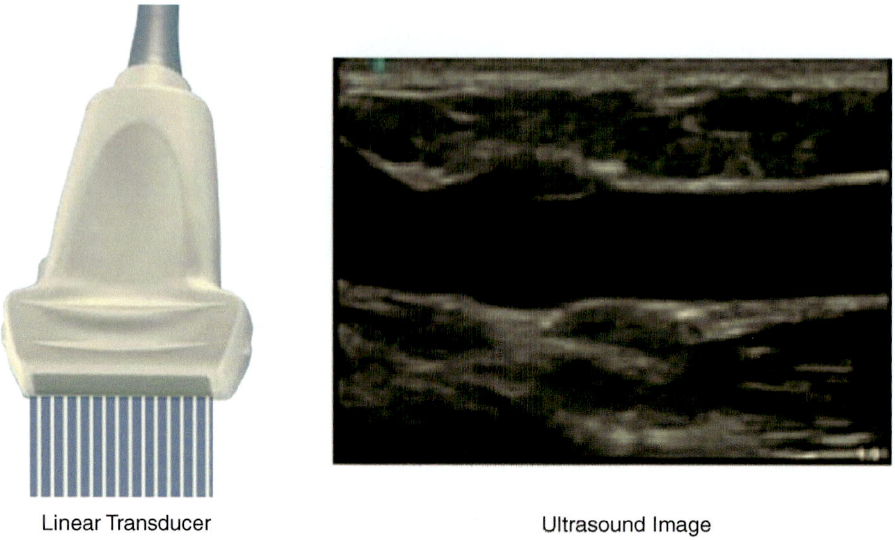

Fig. 3.9 A Linear probe accompanied by the typical rectangular image it produces [with permission from SonoSite]

Fig. 3.10 A "hockey stick" linear probe

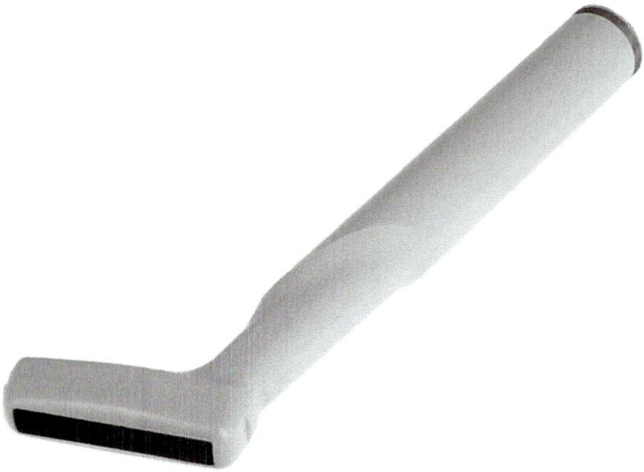

3.5.3 Curvilinear (Convex)

With their curved face, these probes produce a fan-shaped scan field, these probes operate at lower frequencies (2–5 MHz) and penetrate deeper structures (Fig. 3.11). They will produce images of structures up to 10 cm deep, albeit with coarse detail, ideal to examine the abdominal organs.

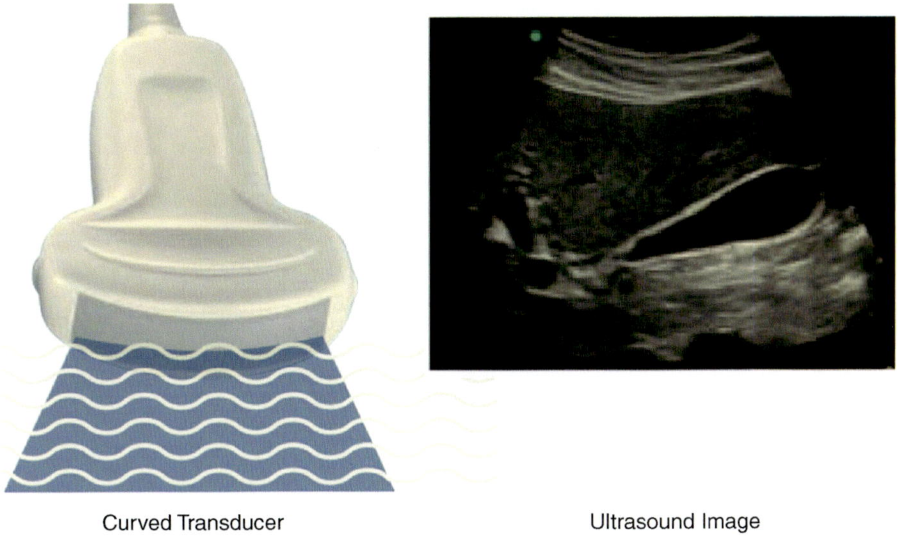

Fig. 3.11 A Curvilinear probe accompanied by the typical curved image it produces [with permission from SonoSite]

3.5.4 Phased Array (Sectorial)

The piezoelectric crystals produce ultrasound in phases resulting in a triangular image. They are frequently used for cardiac imaging.

Probes operating at a higher frequency, will produce images of higher resolution of detail. The draw back will be lack of depth. Therefore, appropriate probe and frequency selection is the first key step to achieving a quality image. Once this has been achieved, there are several further small adjustments that can be made to improve image quality to aid the operator.

3.6 Improving Images

3.6.1 Gain

The option of adjusting the overall gain allows the operator to control the brightness of the entire image (Fig. 3.12). Increasing the "receive" gain adjusts the amplitude of the ultrasound echoes and increases the "brightness" of the resultant image. As all pixels in the image are equally brightened, artefacts also appear brighter. Excessive gain is detrimental, as the image appears too bright, artefacts are enhanced, and subtle textural changes are obscured.

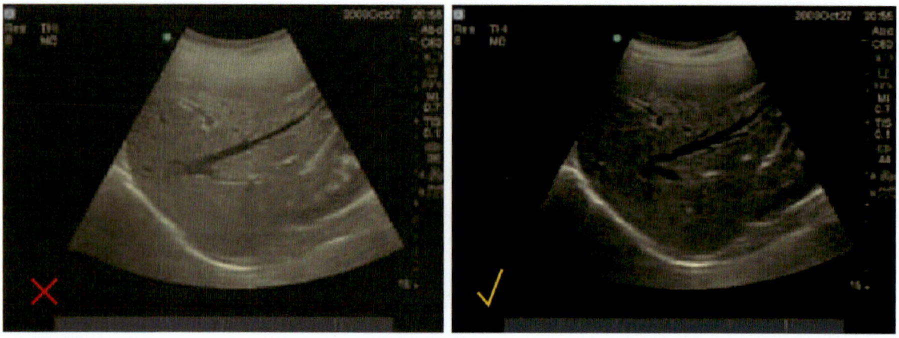

Fig. 3.12 Demonstrates the effect of overall gain adjustment on image quality [with permission from SonoSite]

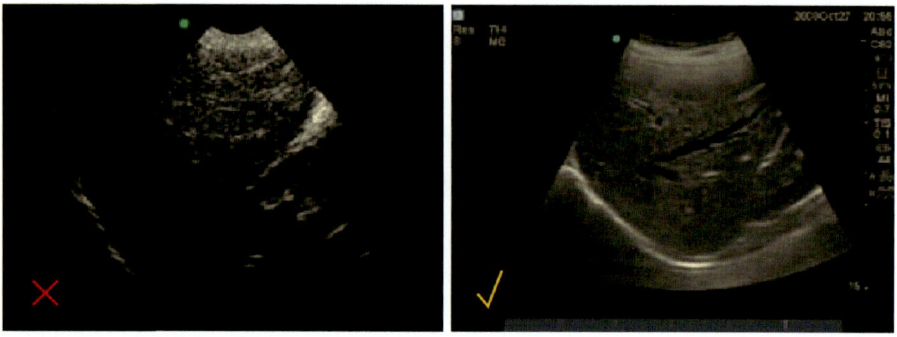

Fig. 3.13 Demonstrates the effect of TGC on image quality [with permission from SonoSite]

Time gain compensation (TGC) proportionally increases the amplitude of distant echoes to compensate for the effect of attenuation (Fig. 3.13). Without TGC, images would progressively become darker with depth. This compensation produces a more uniform image with regards to brightness. Sophisticated machines automatically increase the gain of echoes from deeper structures being imaged. Certain machines will allow the operator to control the level of gain by rotary control for "near gain" and "far gain", or slider controls.

3.6.2 Depth

The use of the depth control allows the target and other important structures to be appropriately placed on the display. Ideally the target area should be focused on the center of the screen, approximately two thirds of the total depth of the scan image.

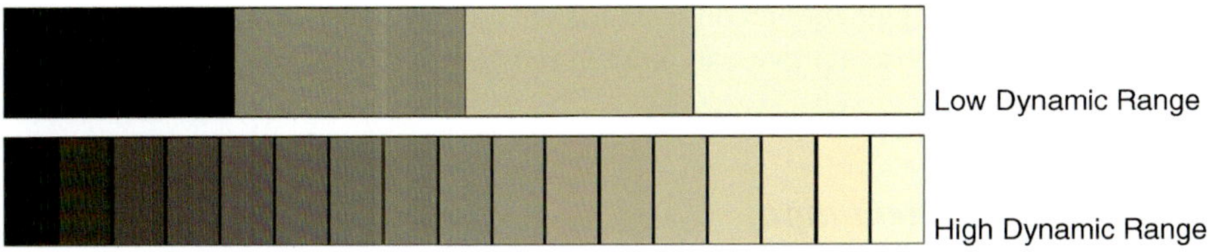

Fig. 3.14 Demonstrates the contrast between high and low dynamic range [with permission from SonoSite]

3.6.3 Focus

Most machines have a focus control that enables an area of the scan image to be enhanced, providing greater detail. For the best results, this should be set just deep to the target area.

3.6.4 Dynamic Range

This control adjusts the number of different shades of grey available for the image generation (Fig. 3.14). The lower the dynamic range, the greater the contrast and more "black and white" the ultrasound image. A low dynamic range is the ideal setting for vascular access.

With more shades of grey available, images using a high dynamic range show less contrast but subtler textural changes in the scan image. This setting would be ideal for imaging abdominal organs, especially the liver.

3.6.5 Zoom

The zoom feature enlarges an area of the image. There are two different types of zoom: the 'write zoom' increases the resolution of the selected area and the 'read zoom' simply magnifies the pixels.

3.7 Practical Tips

3.7.1 Tracking Structures

To aid understanding and image interpretation, target structures can be "tracked" from different locations where they are easier to identify. Tilting the probe in the longitudinal axis alters the angle of incidence at which the ultrasound wave strikes the target object. This phenomenon is called anisotropy and it can greatly improve image quality or expose a previously unseen target.

3.7.2 Probe Orientation

In-plane needling has the advantage of imaging much of the needle, thereby minimizing damage to adjacent structures. However, a pure in-plane technique requires considerable skill as the ultrasound beam may be only 0.2–3 mm thick. Complications can occur during advancement with a partial view of the needle shaft. The size of the neck in neonates can be so small that an in-plane technique is impractical due to significant loss of contact. Out-of-plane techniques are frequency used for this very reason. With an out-of-plane technique, the hyperechoic "dot" represents the needle crossing the ultrasound beam. To find the needle tip, the probe can be moved on the skin surface along the needle's axis until the "dot" disappears.

The more acute the angle of needle insertion, the poorer the ultrasound reflection from the needle surface. Therefore, insertion of the needle at less than 45 degrees to the ultrasound beam improves needle imaging.

Key Points

- Today, the use of ultrasound imaging for obtaining central venous access has become routine practice
- Ultrasound scanners have become widely available as light-weight portable machines capable of producing high quality real-time greyscale images
- The term ultrasound describes all sound waves of frequencies beyond the range of human hearing (>20 kHz)
- The ultrasound transducer "probe" is a complex and sophisticated piece of electrical equipment, housing piezoelectric crystals
- Ultrasound machines use "time gain compensation" to counter the effects of attenuation, by increasing signal amplitude at greater depths
- Artefacts describe a range of appearances in the displayed image that are not accurate to the original anatomical features being scanned
- Due to the occurrence of artefacts, structures in the displayed image should not be assumed as real, until scanned in two planes (transverse and longitudinal)
- Inappropriate probe selection can make a difficult task even harder and potentially unsafe.
- To aid understanding and image interpretation, target structures can be "tracked" from different locations where they are easier to identify.

Bibliography

1. Brass P, Hellmich M, Kolodziej L, Schnik G, Smith AF. Ultrasound guidance versus anatomical landmarks for internal jugular vein catheterization. Cochrane Database Syst Rev. 2015;1:CD006962.
2. Woo J. *A short history of the development of ultrasound in obstetrics and gynecology*. http://www.ob-ultrasound.net/history1.html. Accessed 10 Nov 2017.
3. SonoSite. *Physics of ultrasound notes*. http://cutsurgery.com/assets/physics_notes_v2.pdf. Accessed 12 Nov 2017.
4. Warman P, Nicholls B, Conn D, Wilkinson D, editors. Oxford specialist handbooks in anaesthesia: regional anaesthesia, stimulation, and ultrasound techniques. Oxford: Oxford University Press; 2014.
5. Association of Anaesthetists of Great Britain and Ireland. Safe vascular access 2016. Anaesthesia. 2016;71:573–85.
6. Kaproth-Joslin KA, Nicola R, Dogra VS. The history of US: From bats and boats to the bedside and beyond. *RadioGraphics*. 2015; 35 (3):960–970. https://pubs.rsna.org/doi/pdf/10.1148/rg.2015140300
7. Lin E, Gaur A, Jones M, Ahmed A. Sonoanatomy for anaesthetists. Cambridge: Cambridge University Press; 2012.
8. Smith T, Pinnock C, Lin T, editors. Fundamentals of anaesthesia. 3rd ed. Cambridge: Cambridge University Press; 2009.
9. Thoirs K. Physical and technical principles of sonography: a practical guide for non-sonographers. Journal of Medical Radiation Sciences. 2012;59(4):124–32. https://doi.org/10.1002/j.2051-3909.2012.tb00188.x.
10. Ziskin MC. Fundamental physics of ultrasound and its propagation in tissue. *RadioGraphics*. 1993; 13 (3):705–709. https://pubs.rsna.org/doi/pdf/10.1148/radiographics.13.3.8316679.

Chapter 4
Ultrasound Anatomy of Arterial and Deep Veins of the Limb and the Cervico-Thoracic Region in Children

Thierry Pirotte

Anatomy has always been important for physicians, especially if they are called to perform invasive techniques in fragile patients. Vascular access in children is one of these difficult tasks: small targets, frequent anatomical variations, major consequences in case of complications. It is there for not surprising that anesthesiologists, intensivists, surgeons, and pediatricians were so enthusiastic when the technological development of ultrasound started 15–20 years ago. It is almost unbelievable that we are now able to see and to target vessels as small as 1 mm with huge precision. But to do this, we had to learn another anatomy: the ultrasound anatomy. This grey-scale two-dimensional image that we had to correlate with the classical anatomy we knew. It all started in children with the ultrasound guided puncture of the internal jugular vein but, as I already wrote elsewhere 10 years ago, we are now far beyond the internal jugular vein. In this chapter, you will discover the ultrasound anatomy (applied to invasive puncture) of all major arteries and veins of the child's body: with more than 30 illustrations covering the upper limb, the lower limb, the neck region (with extension to supra- and retro-clavicular view), and the area under the clavicle.

T. Pirotte (✉)
Department of Anesthesia, Cliniques Universitaires Saint-Luc—Université Catholique de Louvain, Brussels, Belgium
e-mail: t.pirotte@uclouvain.be

D. G. Biasucci et al. (eds.), *Vascular Access in Neonates and Children*,
https://doi.org/10.1007/978-3-030-94709-5_4

4.1 Ultrasound Anatomy of the Arm

4.1.1 The Hand

Ultrasound (US) techniques are rarely performed at the level of the hand because veins at that level are extremely superficial and small. The largest vein among the dorsal venous network, is the origin of the basilic vein and can be found between the fourth and the fifth metacarpal bone (sometime between the third and the fourth one). The pressure caused by the US probe should be limited by using enough US gel between probe and skin (Fig. 4.1).

4.1.2 The Wrist

The cephalic vein (CV) is a relatively large vein that runs at the radial side of the wrist. Unfortunately, this vein is highly mobile in children and is therefore more difficult to puncture especially under US guidance (no possibility to stretch the skin because both hands are used). Some very tiny and superficial vein runs at the anterior aspect of the wrist but if imaging techniques are needed Near Infrared technologies will be more useful than US.

The radial artery (RA) runs above the lateral aspect of the distal radial bone (Fig. 4.2). In children younger than 2 years, its diameter is around 1.5 mm (0.8–2.3 mm). Extreme dorsiflexion of the hand should be avoided because it reduces the diameter of the RA even more. Zoom function and Doppler analysis are often necessary to offer a correct view (Fig. 4.3). The RA is usually surrounded by

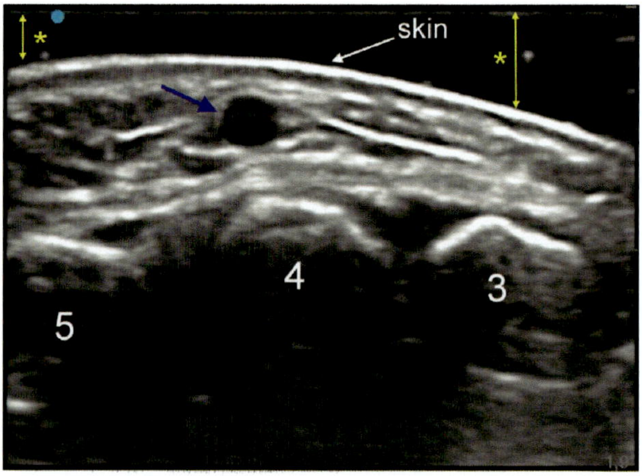

Fig. 4.1 Ultrasound anatomy of the dorsal side of the hand (6 years old). A large amount of US gel (*) is applied on the skin to limit the pressure on the subcutaneous tissues and to increase its echogenicity (acoustic enhancement). The largest vein, the origin of the basilic vein (blue arrow) is found above the fourth metacarpal bone (4). 3 and 5: Third and fifth metacarpal bone

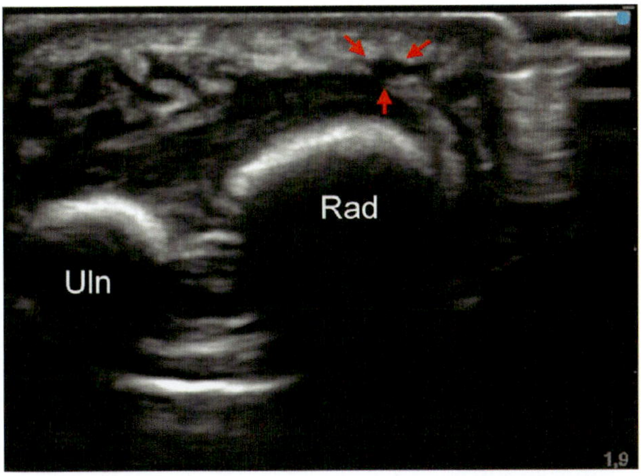

Fig. 4.2 Ultrasound anatomy at the palmar aspect of the wrist (infant). The complete wrist is seen despite the minimal depth used on the machine (1.9 cm). The radial artery (red arrow) is seen in short-axis view above the radial bone (Rad). Uln: ulnar bone

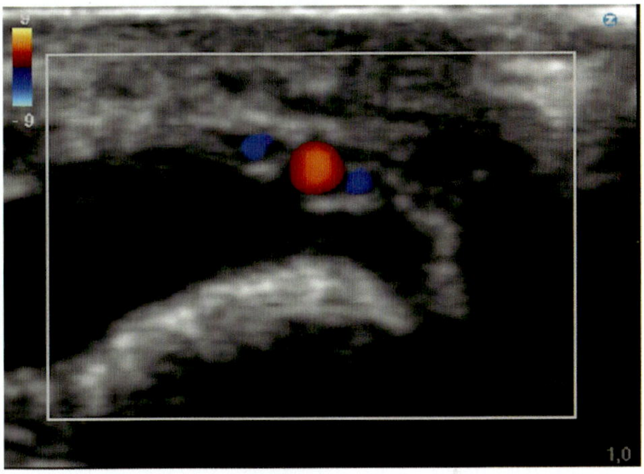

Fig. 4.3 Zoom and Doppler function prior radial artery puncture (infant). The diameter of the artery is approximatively 1 mm (full screen = 1 cm). The artery is surrounded by 2 small radial veins

two small vein visible only when the pressure of the US probe is minimal. In some case, the RA is absent and usually compensated be a medial interosseous artery (Fig. 4.4). Ultrasound screening can be used as a modern version of the Allen's test by analyzing the presence, the diameter, and the flow of the different arteries at the wrist.

The ulnar artery (UA), the other largest terminal branch of the brachial artery, runs above the distal ulnar bone side by side with the ulnar nerve (Fig. 4.5). In the adult population, the diameter of the UA is even slightly larger than the diameter of the RA.

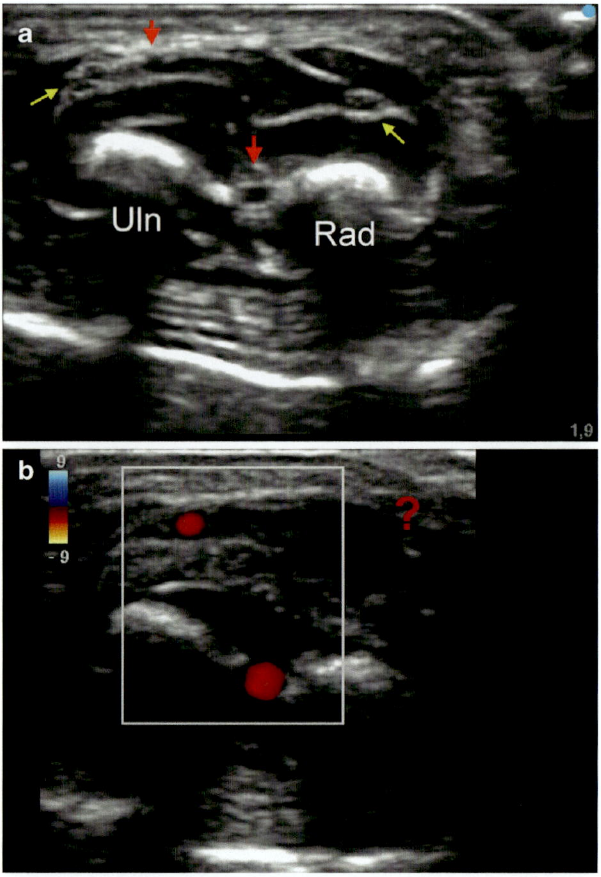

Fig. 4.4 Ultrasound anatomy at the wrist of a 2-day old syndromic infant. (**a**) 2-D image showing the absence of radial artery compensated by a large interosseous artery. *Red arrows* Ulnar and interosseous artery, *Yellow arrows* Ulnar nerve and displaced medial nerve, *Uln* ulnar bone, *Rad* radial bone. (**b**) Doppler analysis. No radial arterial flow detected. The largest artery is in this case the interosseous artery

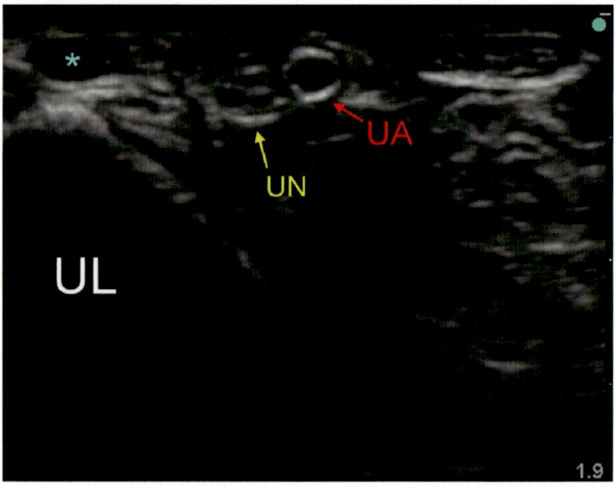

Fig. 4.5 Ultrasound anatomy of the ulnar artery at the wrist (6 years old). Ulnar artery (UA) and nerve (UN) side by side above the ulnar bone (UL). * Superficial vein

4.1.3 The Forearm

Different veins can be found along the ventral side of the forearm: the basilic and cephalic veins, the median basilic—cephalic (antecubital) and brachial veins, and perforating veins. US visualization of these veins and their bifurcations is possible when limited pressure is applied to the skin with the US probe (Fig. 4.6).

The RA (Fig. 4.6) can easily be followed from the wrist to the mid-forearm level. The depth increases progressively but remain limited is children allowing an easy access under US guidance.

The UA takes a medial course at the mid-forearm level leaving the ulnar nerve laterally (Fig. 4.7).

4.1.4 The Antecubital Fossa

Different superficial or deep veins can be visualized at the antecubital fossa: the basilic and cephalic veins, the median basilic vein (antecubital vein), and the two brachial veins (Fig. 4.8). These veins will fuse and bifurcate with a large variability among children. The brachial artery and veins are in contact with each other and with the medial nerve. During puncture, the correct probe position and needle direction must be chosen appropriately to avoid potential damage of surrounding structures.

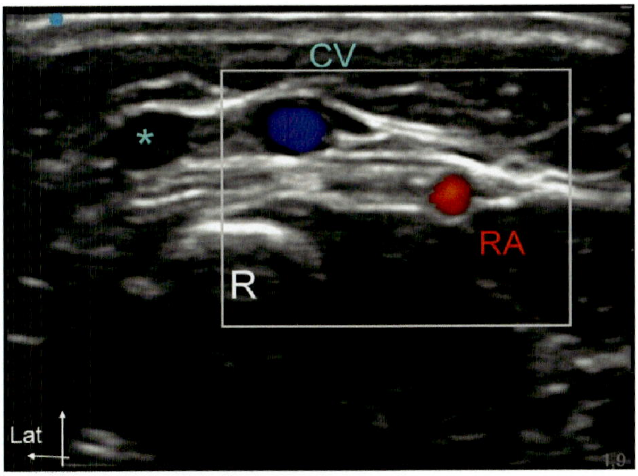

Fig. 4.6 Ultrasound anatomy of the vessels at the forearm (5 years old). The radial artery (RA) at mid-forearm level. Palpation is difficult due to the absence of posterior contact with the radial bone (R). US visualization and puncture is however possible. Different veins are also shown: the cephalic vein (CV) and probably the accessory cephalic vein (*)

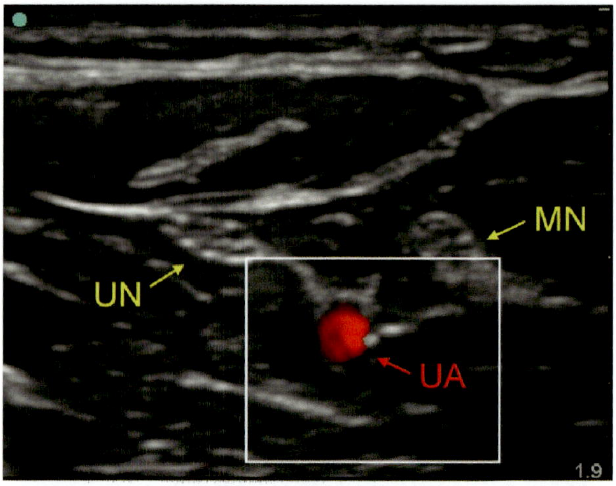

Fig. 4.7 Ultrasound anatomy of the ulnar artery at the mid-forearm level (6 years old). The ulnar artery (UA) comes from medial and reaches the ulnar side of the forearm to join the ulnar nerve (UN). *MN* medial nerve

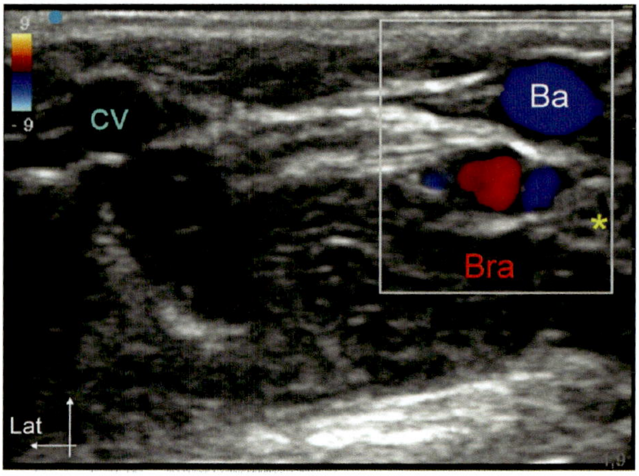

Fig. 4.8 Ultrasound anatomy of the antecubital fossa (5 years old). Different vessels and nerves are found close to each other. Precision is mandatory to target the chosen vessel. Large basilic vein (Ba) superficial to the brachial vessels. Medial nerve (*) medial to the brachial artery (Bra). Cephalic vein (CV) on the lateral side

4.1.5 The Arm

The mid-humeral level of the arm is the usual place to insert long peripheral cannulas, midline catheters or PICCs. At that level, different veins can be found (Figs. 4.9 and 4.10):

- the basilic vein (Fig. 4.11): a large vein located inside the groove between biceps muscle and humerus.
- the brachial veins: usually small veins running at both side of the brachial artery, though high variability in position and size should be expected. These vessels are often close to the median nerve. A correct choice in probe position and needle direction should be taken to avoid inadvertent nerve or artery damage while aiming for the vein.
- the cephalic vein (Fig. 4.12): a very superficial but relatively small vein running on the lateral border of the arm above the biceps muscle. Near the shoulder, this

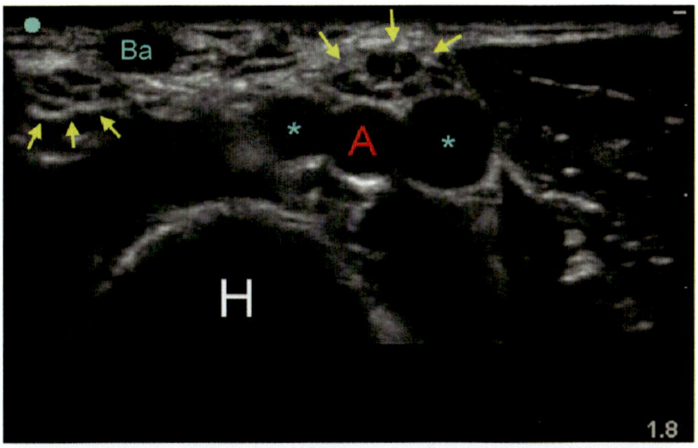

Fig. 4.9 Ultrasound anatomy of the arm at mid-humeral level (12 years old). Brachial vessels (A, *) and the medial nerve together above the humerus (H). Basilic vein (Ba) and the ulnar nerve at the ulnar side. *a* brachial artery; *: brachial veins; *yellow arrows* brachial and ulnar nerves

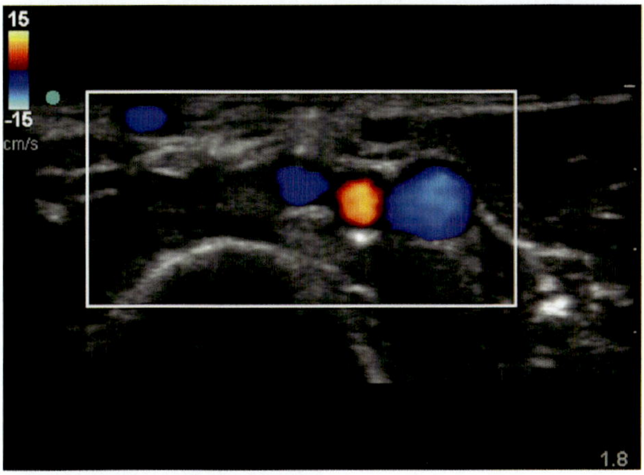

Fig. 4.10 Doppler analysis at mid-humeral level (12 years old). Tilting the probe the child's heart detect the red pulsating signal (flow to the transducer) of the brachial artery; squishing the forearm pushes blood in the different veins and gives a blue signal (flow away from the transducer)

vein passes between the deltoid and pectoralis major muscle (delto-pectoral groove), where it reaches the axillary vein (Figs. 4.33, 4.34 and 4.35).

4.2 Ultrasound Anatomy of the Leg

4.2.1 The Foot

Several small veins at the dorsum and lateral part of the foot can be cannulated: the lateral and medial marginal veins, the dorsal venous arch, and the short saphenous vein. US techniques are rarely performed at the level because of the superficiality and the very limited diameter of these veins.

The dorsalis pedis artery runs on the dorsal aspect of the foot, usually between the first two metatarsal bones (Fig. 4.13). US visualization is difficult even in case of a positive palpation. The diameter of this artery is smaller than the diameter of the radial artery without being more superficial, making US guided puncture difficult even in experienced hands.

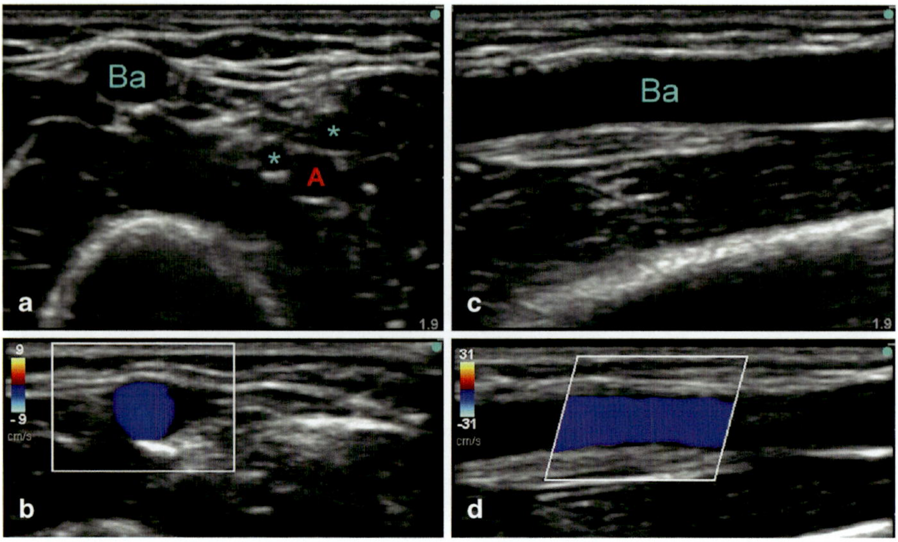

Fig. 4.11 Ultrasound anatomy of the basilic vein at the arm level (14 years). (**a**) Short-axis view of the basilica vein (Ba). (**c**) Long-axis view of the vein. (**b** and **d**) Doppler analysis. * brachial veins; (*a*) brachial artery

Fig. 4.12 Ultrasound anatomy of the cephalic vein at the arm level (14 years old). (**a**) Short-axis view of the cephalic vein (*arrow*). (**b**) Long-axis view with Doppler analysis. *BM* biceps muscle, *H* humerus

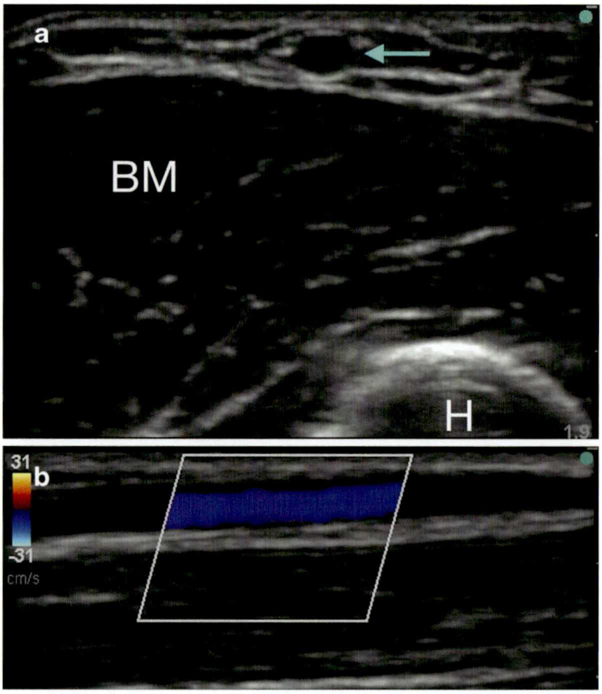

4.2.2 The Ankle

The internal or great saphenous vein runs at the anterior border of the medial malleolus and is rarely absent (Fig. 4.14). It is the longest vein in the body, running along the complete length of the lower limb from the ankle, leg, and thigh to the femoral vein (arch of the saphenous vein) (Fig. 4.18). Ultrasound guidance at the ankle is used in case of a negative palpation or to increase success rate. Under the knee, its visualization is used to identify and block the saphenous nerve.

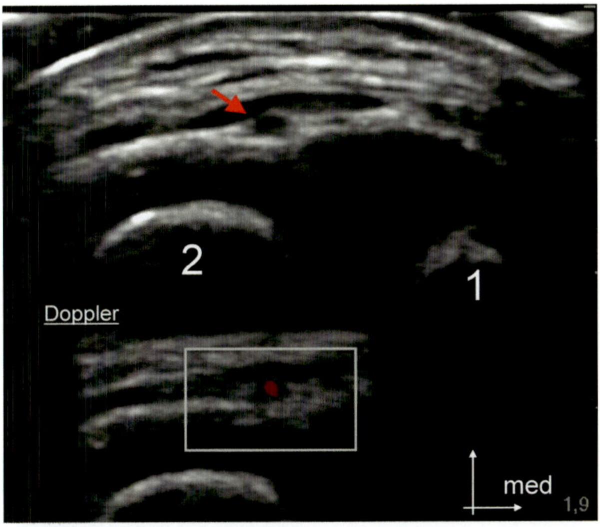

Fig. 4.13 Ultrasound anatomy of the dorsal pedis artery at the foot (3 years old). The dorsal pedis artery (arrow) is superficial and located between the first (1) and second (2) metatarsal bones. Doppler analysis gives only a weak signal but pulsation is usually visualized

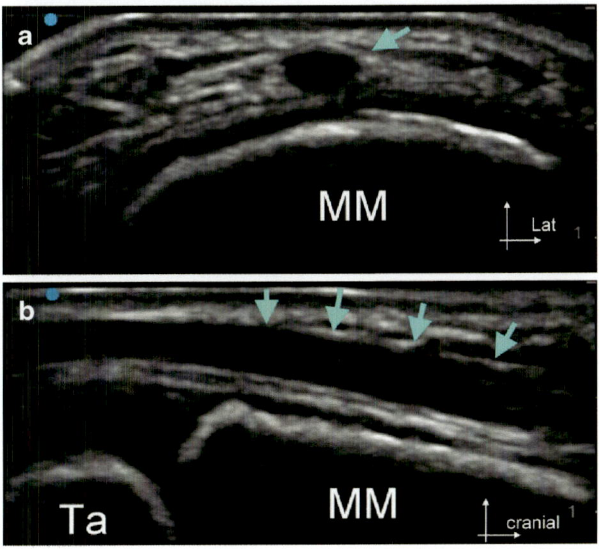

Fig. 4.14 Ultrasound anatomy of the great saphenous vein at the ankle (4 years old). Two different views of the great saphenous vein (arrows) just anterior to the medial malleolus (MM). (**a**) Short axis view. (**b**) long axis view. *Ta* talus

The posterior tibial artery (PTA) runs in the retro-malleolar grove posterior to the medial malleolus (Fig. 4.15). The PTA can be an alternative arterial cannulation site to the usual radial artery (RA) in young children. The diameter of the PTA is like the RA in children from 3 to 24 months.

4.2.3 The Popliteal Fossa

The popliteal fossa, well known for sciatic nerve block techniques, is not a usual place for vascular access. However, in extreme cases, during interventional radiology or potentially during anesthesia in prone position, the popliteal vein could be chosen as temporary central venous access. The popliteal vein is usually seen on top of the popliteal artery and under the medial part of the tibial nerve (Fig. 4.16). Experience in precise US guided punctures is mandatory.

4.2.4 The Inguinal Region

The common femoral vein (CFV) is located medially to the common femoral (CFA) at the level or just below the inguinal ligament (Fig. 4.17). The diameter of the CFV is around 4 mm at 1 year and 10 mm at the age of nine. This diameter of the vein can be increased by using either a reverse Trendelenburg position or a firm

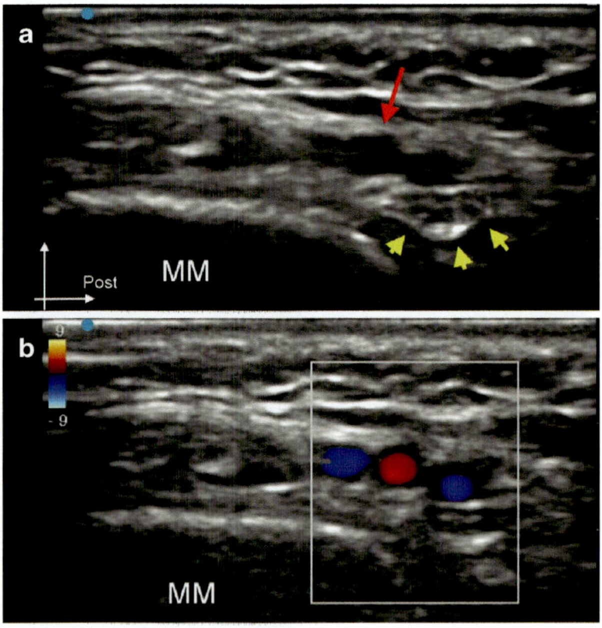

Fig. 4.15 Ultrasound anatomy of the posterior tibial artery at the ankle (5 years old). (**a**) The posterior tibial artery (*red arrow*) is situated just posterior to the medial malleolus (MM). (**b**) Doppler analysis. Small veins are usually seen at both side of the artery. The tibial nerve (*short yellow arrows*) runs just posterior to the vessels

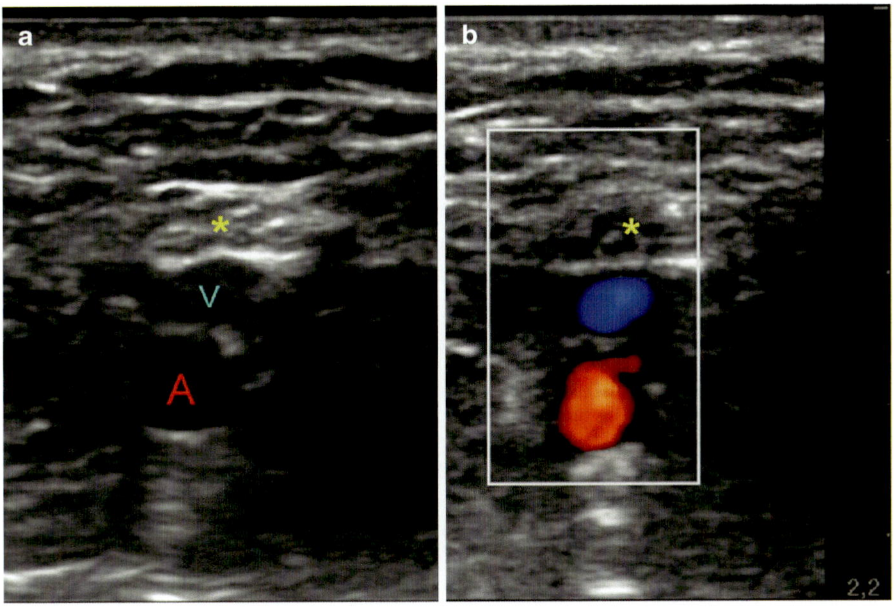

Fig. 4.16 Ultrasound anatomy of the popliteal fossa (4 years old). (**a**) Vertical alignment of the popliteal artery (*a*), the popliteal vein (*V*) and the tibial nerve (*). This US image is well-known in the field of locoregional anesthesia but could also be used by experienced physicians to find a venous access in extreme cases. (**b**) Doppler analysis

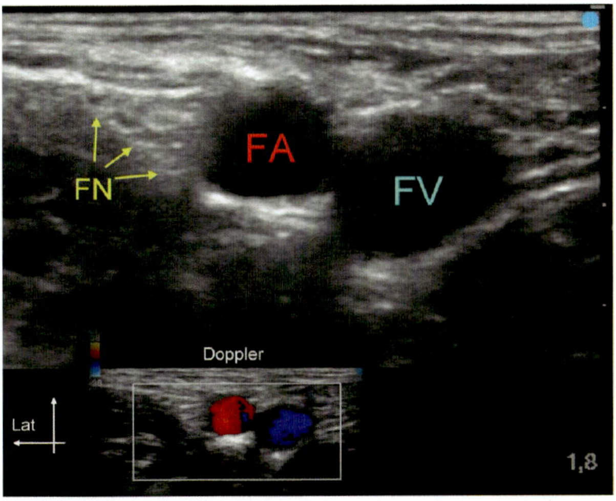

Fig. 4.17 Ultrasound anatomy of the right inguinal region (10 years old). Cranially, at the level of the common femoral artery (FA), the femoral vein (FV) is usually well positioned: medial to the artery. Doppler analysis at the bottom. *FN* femoral nerve

compression at the lower abdomen. These maneuvers are also used to check the patency of femoral and iliac veins. US examinations have shown high variability in the position of the CFV. Usually medial to the femoral artery (CFA), it can be found completely below the artery in some cases. Just below the inguinal ligament, the arch of the great saphenous vein is seen medially to the CFV giving the typical pattern of "Mickey Mouse" (Fig. 4.18). A few centimeters distal to the inguinal ligament, as the CFA bifurcates in deep (DFA) and superficial femoral artery (SFA), the incidence of overlapping increases from 5 to 60% (Fig. 4.19). More distally, after the bifurcation of the CFV into deep (DFV) and superficial femoral vein (SFV), the SFV is more consistently placed below the SFA. In children, the incidence of a CFV place below the CFA seems to be significantly lower at the left side compared to the right. External rotation of the hip (with or without leg abduction) will reduce this overlapping and bring the vein medial to the artery.

4.3 Ultrasound Anatomy above the Clavicle

The major vessels in the neck have a long way to travel from the submandibular area to the retrosternal fossa. High in the neck, the bifurcation of the common carotid artery (CA) in internal and external branches can be visualized (Fig. 4.20). In children where the internal jugular vein is absent or thrombosed, misinterpretation of this "double vessel" pattern carry the risk that one of the arteries is targeted and puncture.

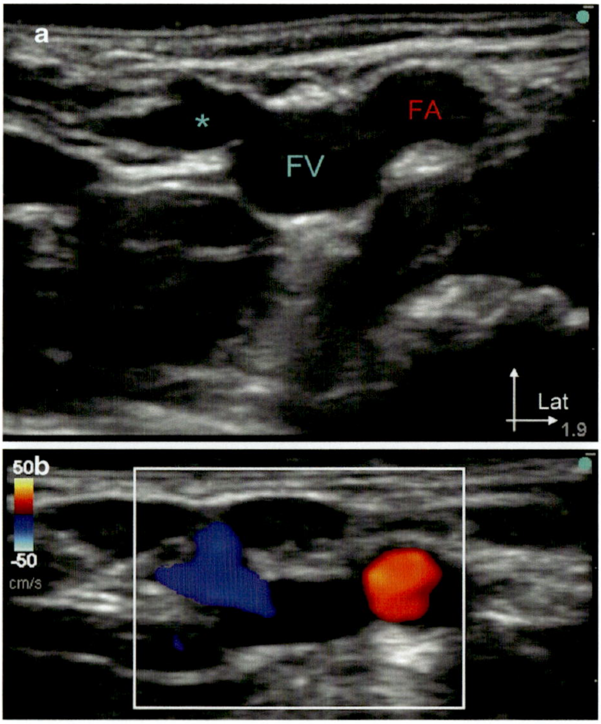

Fig. 4.18 Ultrasound anatomy of the arch of the great saphenous vein (*left leg*). (**a**) Typical "Mickey Mouse" pattern with the femoral vein (FV) representing the face, the arch of the saphenous vein (*) and the femoral artery (FA) the ears. (**b**) Doppler analysis

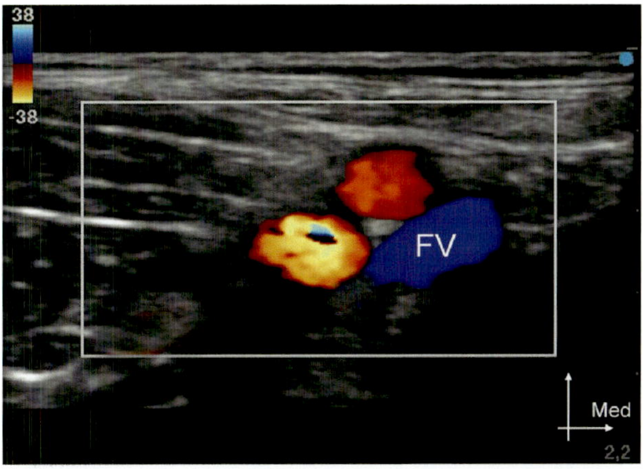

Fig. 4.19 Ultrasound anatomy lower in the right inguinal region (10 years old). Doppler analysis of the common femoral artery dividing in a superficial and a deep branch. The femoral vein (FV) is at that level often moving under the arteries

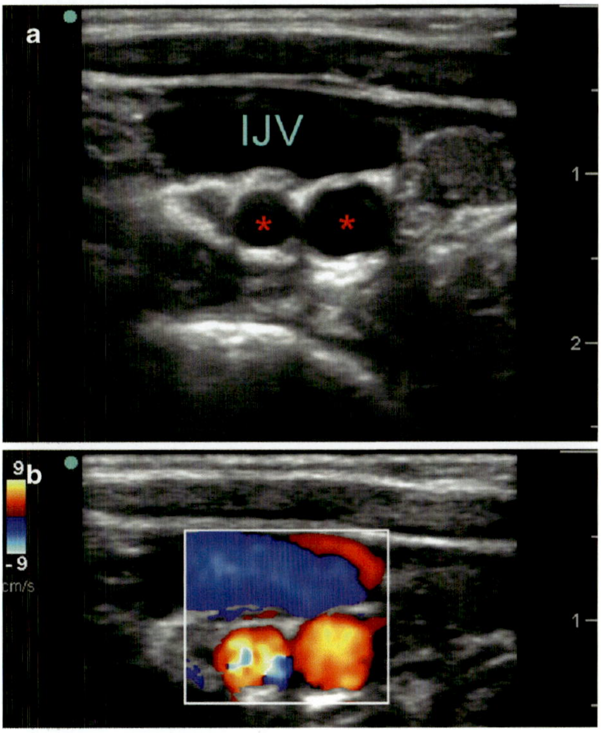

Fig. 4.20 Ultrasound anatomy high in the neck region (2 years old). (**a**) Visualization of the carotid artery bifurcation (*). *IJV* internal jugular vein. (**b**) Doppler analysis

For practical reason, the neck area will be divided in four levels: the level of the cricoid, the supraclavicular level, the retro-clavicular level, and the suprasternal view.

4.3.1 The Level of the Cricoid

The internal jugular vein (IJV) runs at the latero-vertebral site of the neck, alongside the common carotid artery (CA), usually in an antero-lateral position (Figs. 4.21 and 4.25).

US screening studies showed that at the level of the cricoid:

- the relationship between IJV and CA is highly variable and unpredictable.
- in neutral position, the IJV overlaps the CA in 25–44% of the cases and can be found medially in 6% of the cases.
- when the head is progressively turned away from the puncture site and up to 45°, the incidence of overlapping increases even more.
- the use of a laryngeal mask as airway management increases the IJV-CA overlapping when the head is in light rotation.

These data should however be read very carefully because the position of the probe on the neck is rarely well-defined and can have a major impact on the ultrasonographic findings, overestimating the real overlap (Fig. 4.22).

The diameter of the IJV can be increased by Valsalva maneuver, Trendelenburg position or liver compression. These effects are however limited in infants less than 1 year of age where the distance IJV—right atrium is short and the venous system highly compliant.

The lumen and patency of the IJV as well as the surrounding structures should to be carefully analyzed in sick children or children who had previous central catheters. Intraluminal thrombosis is detected by a hyperechoic signal into the lumen of a non-compressible vein (Fig. 4.23). Doppler analysis is useful to confirm the partial or complete nature of the thrombus. Cervical lymph nodes are frequent in children and sometimes massive in case of hematologic or oncologic pathologies (Fig. 4.24). Lymph nodes are echoic or anechoic structures than are not

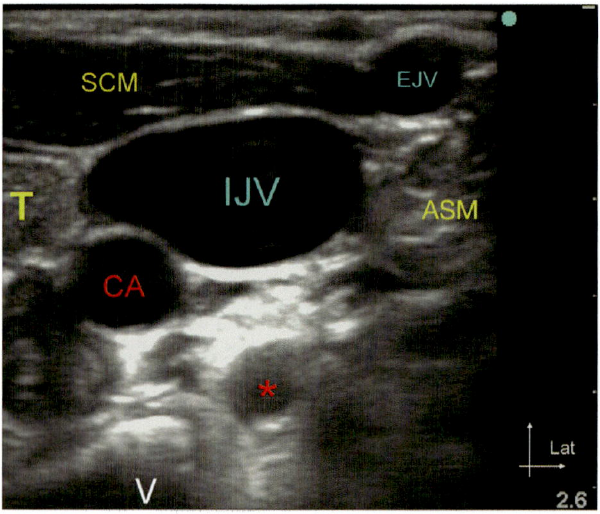

Fig. 4.21 Ultrasound anatomy of the neck at the thyroid level (4 years old). The internal jugular vein (IJV) is lateral and anterior to the common carotid artery (CA). The vertebral artery (*) is seen at the posterior aspect of the IJV. *SCM* sternocleidomastoid muscle, *ASM* anterior scalene muscle, *T* thyroid gland, *EJV* external jugular vein, *V* vertebra

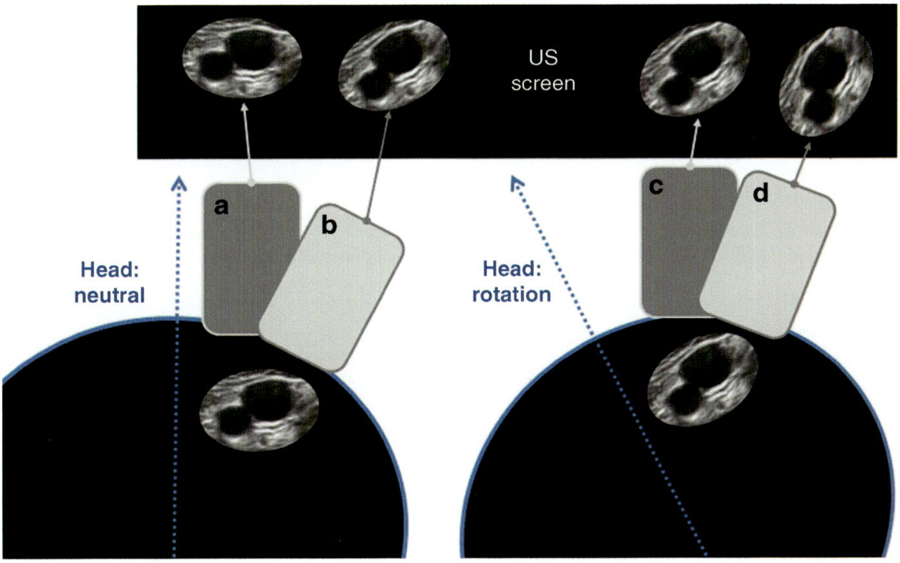

Fig. 4.22 Relationship between internal jugular vein and carotid artery. The observed relationship is highly dependent on the head rotation and the probe position. (*a*) When the head is hold in neutral position and the probe in a vertical way, the IJV is seen like on a CT scan and is often lateral to the CA. (*c*) Head rotation increase the IJV-CA overlap. For ergonomic reasons, the probe is usually moved laterally following the curve of the neck (*b*, *d*). It that configuration, the overlap increase (*b*) and the IJV can even be seen on top of the CA (*d*)

compressible and have no flow at the Doppler analysis. There limits are shown cranially and caudally by moving the US probe up and down on the neck.

The external jugular vein (EJV) is a more superficial and lateral vein that runs above the anterior scalene muscle. US can be used when clinical examination fails to detect it (Fig. 4.21). Lower in the neck, the EJV moves laterally above the clavicle before taking a sharp medial angle to run above and almost parallel to the end of the subclavian vein (Figs. 4.27 and 4.35). Due to these angulations, getting a central access by a EJV puncture is often difficult, unless the EJV is punctured directly in its last tract.

The vertebral artery (VA) is located between the major vessels and the vertebral body. In 60% of the cases, it is situated under the medial portion of the IJV (Fig. 4.21). In children, the VA is relatively larger (up to 50% of the CA) and located relatively closer (3–5 mm) to the IJV than in adults.

4.3.2 *The Supraclavicular Level*

By sliding the US probe on the skin from the cricoid level down to the clavicle, we notice the following changes:

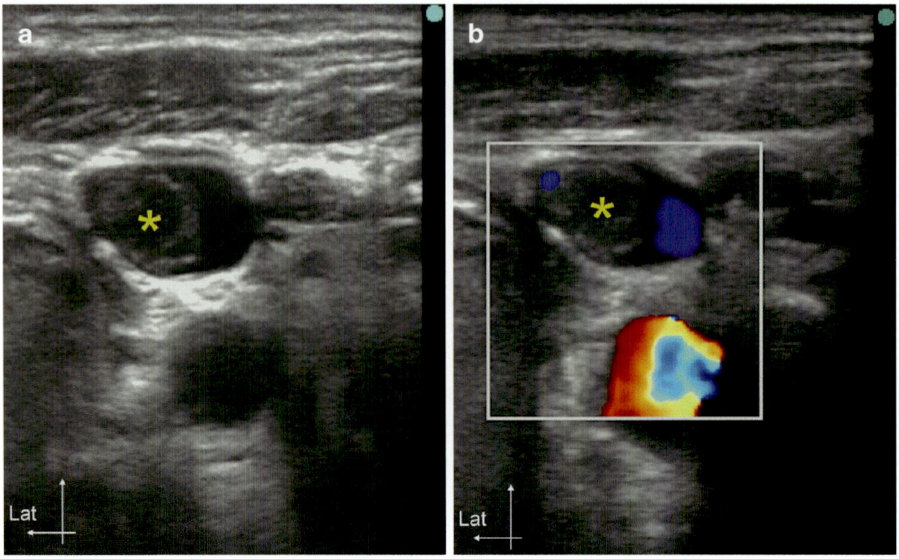

Fig. 4.23 Right internal jugular vein thrombosis (9 years old). (**a**) Echogenic structure within the IJV lumen. (**b**) Doppler analysis showing some residual flow. * partial thrombus

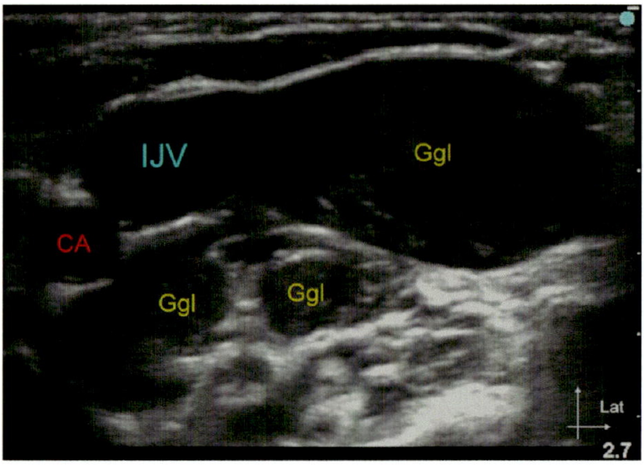

Fig. 4.24 Ultrasound of the left side neck region of a 12 years old child diagnosed with Hodgkin lymphoma. Presence of multiple large ganglions (Ggl). *CA* carotid artery, *IJV* internal jugular vein

- the diameter of the IJV increase
- a valve in the distal part of the IJV, just proximal to its confluence with the SCV, is commonly seen
- the distance between the CA and the IJV increase while the distance between the IJV and the VA decrease
- the overlap between the IJV and the VA increases from 50 to 75%
- the dome of the pleura is often already visible at that level, especially in young children.

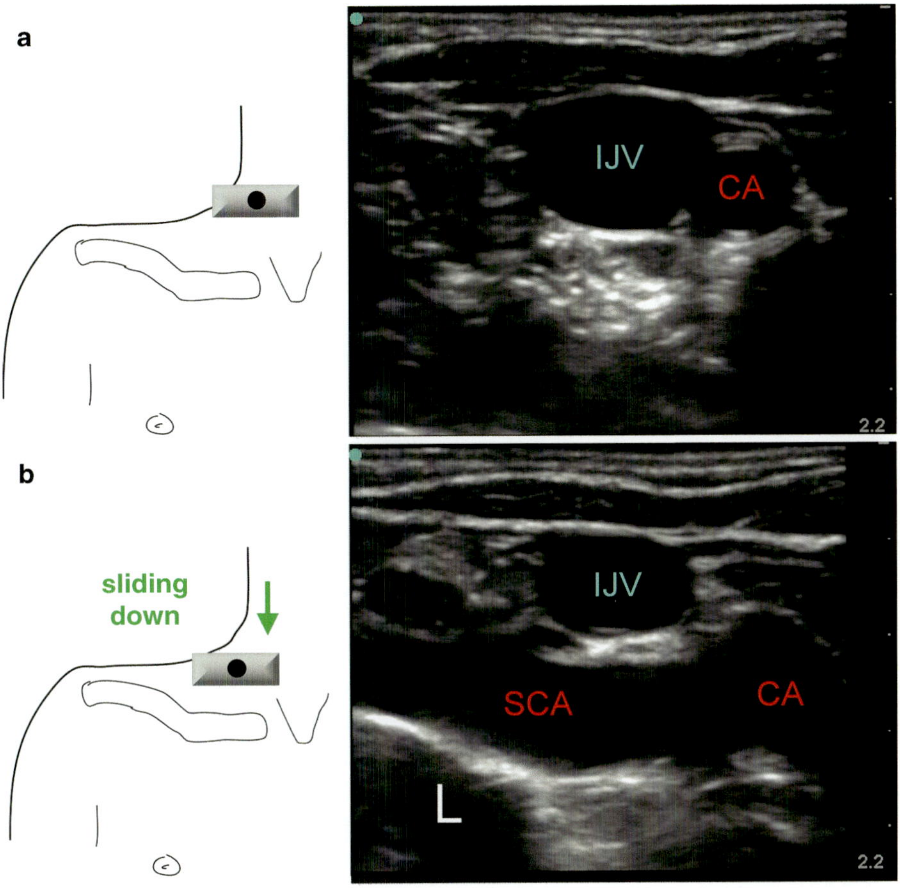

Fig. 4.25 From the internal jugular vein to the subclavian vein—Part 1. (**a**) US probe at the level of the cricoid. (**b**) by sliding the probe down (caudally), we have a longitudinal view of the subclavian artery (SCA) coming for lateral and reaching the carotid artery (CA). *IJV* internal jugular vein

- the subclavian artery (SCA) comes from lateral and reaches the common CA (with a fusion at the patient's right side). This large vessel is seen passing between the end of the IJV and the pleura (Fig. 4.25).

4.3.3 The Retroclavicular Level

Once the US probe meets the clavicle by its downwards sliding movement, the next step to have a look behind the clavicle is to tilt the probe cranially (Fig. 4.26). At first, the lower end of the IJV is seen at the medial side and a cross section of the SCA on the lateral side, both lying on top of the lung dome (Fig. 4.26). By

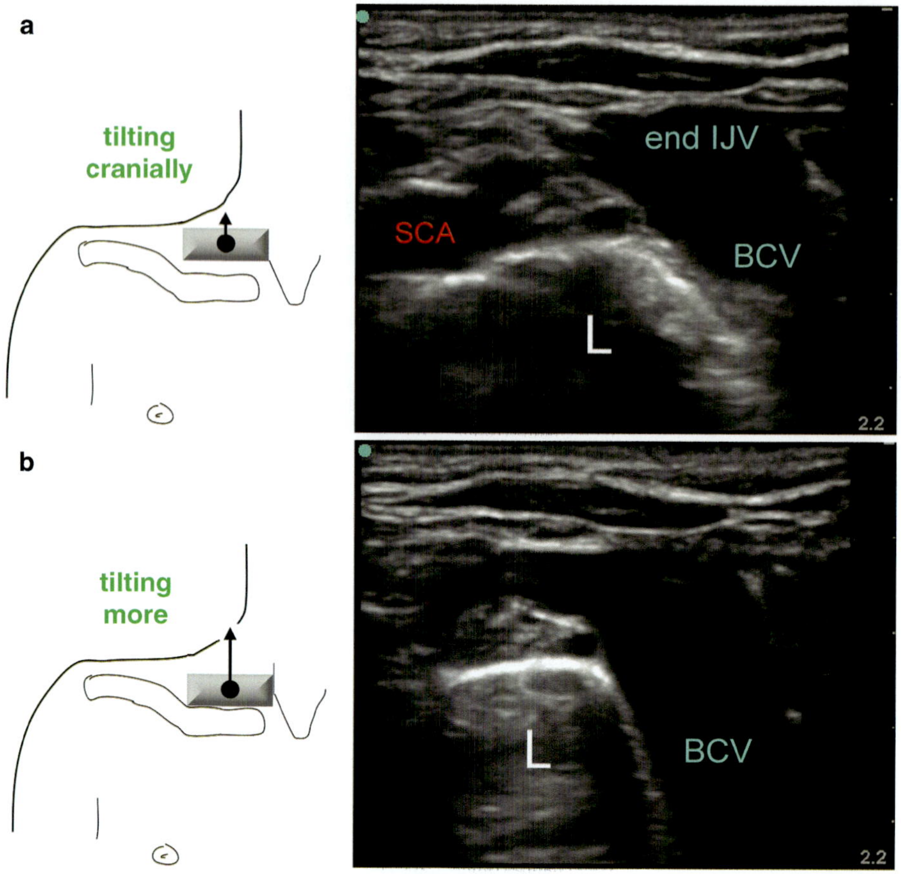

Fig. 4.26 From the internal jugular vein to the subclavian vein—Part 2. (**c**) The US probe being slidded down till the clavicle is now slightly tilted cranially (*short arrow*) to look behind the clavicle. (**d**) The tilting movement of the probe is accentuated (long arrow) to find the brachiocephalic vein (BCV). *SCA* subclavian artery, *IJV* internal jugular vein, *L* lung

increasing the tilt of the US probe, the brachiocephalic vein (BCV) is seen diving into the mediastinum just medial and in direct contact with the lung (Fig. 4.26). This view is used for in plane US guided supraclavicular puncture of the BCV. The degree of cranial tilting of the probe required is inversely proportional to the age of the child. The cranial position of the BCV in infants allow their visualization with a limited probe tilt compared to older children where the probe must be tilted a lot, often almost touching the child's chin.

The BCV diameter remains large regardless of the hemodynamic or respiratory status, even during hypovolemia, making its cannulation easier than other sites in critically ill children.

The presence of a floating thrombus (Fig. 4.28) or complete thrombosis of the BCV can be seen with this view.

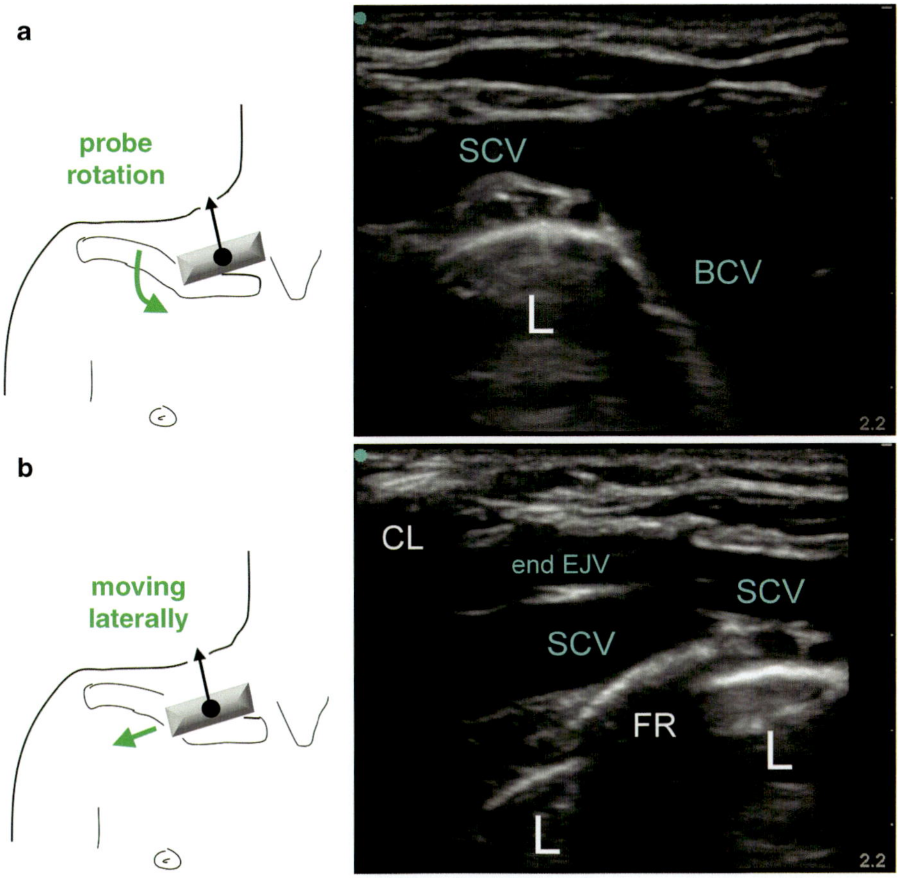

Fig. 4.27 From the internal jugular vein to the subclavian vein—Part 3. (**e**) While maintaining the probe tilted, its lateral part is rotated caudally to the axilla to find the subclavian vein (SCV). (**f**) The US probe is slightly moved laterally and brought on the clavicle to have a longer view of the SCV. *L* Lung top, *BCV* brachiocephalic vein, *CL* clavicle, *EJV* external jugular vein, *FR* first rib

To get a view of the subclavian vein (SCV), a last step must be performed: moving the lateral part of the US probe caudally by placing it on the clavicle in the direction of the axilla. By this way, the SCV is seen coming from lateral and joining the BVC medially (Fig. 4.27). The subclavian vein is thus much more caudal than the SCA, both vessels being separated by the anterior scalene muscle.

The SCV is a short vein (from 1 cm in neonates to 3–4 cm in adolescents) running from mid-clavicular to the distal end of the IJV behind to the sternoclavicular joint. Pulling the arm downwards flattens the clavicle and increase the visible length of the SCV.

Subclavian thrombosis can also be detected by this view, the thrombus being usually located above the first rib (Fig. 4.29).

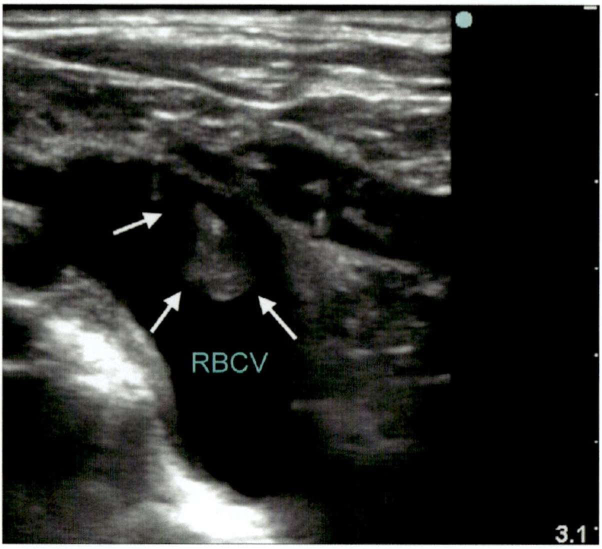

Fig. 4.28 Small floating thrombus visualized in the right brachiocephalic vein (2 years old having a previous central catheter). *Arrows* thrombus, *RBCV* right brachiocephalic vein

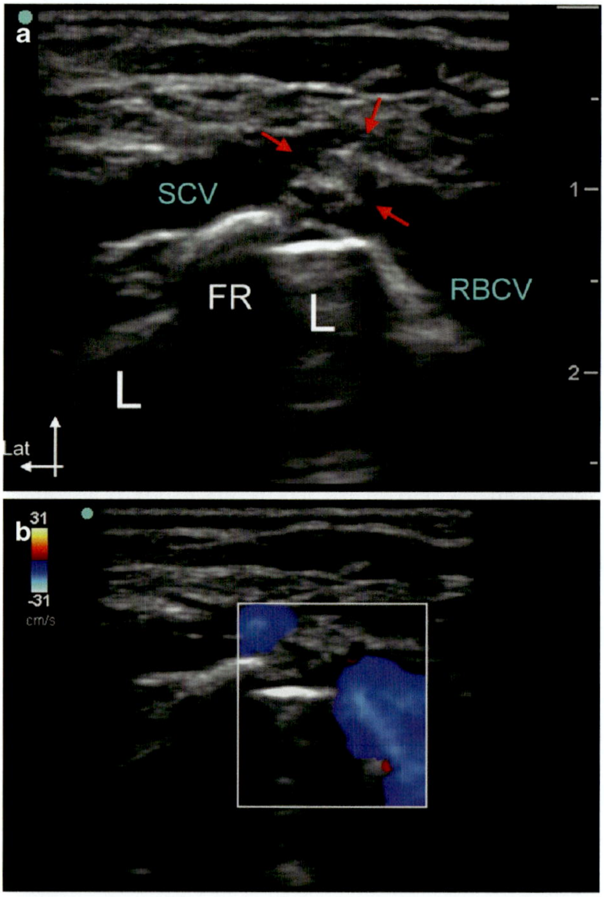

Fig. 4.29 Complete thrombosis of the right subclavian vein (4 years old). (**a**) Hyperechoic structure at the end of the subclavian vein (SCV). (**b**) Doppler analysis showing a complete interruption of the blood flow. *Arrows* thrombus, *RBCV* right brachiocephalic vein, *FR* first rib, *L* lung top

The diameter of the SCV is relatively unaffected by the hemodynamic status of the child. The vein is fixed at two level: laterally under the clavicle and medially at the jugular-subclavian confluence. Anterior wall compression cause by the approaching needle is therefore limited, even in newborns.

Lung deflation during the puncture seems not beneficial because it fails to increase both the diameter of the SCV and the distance from the pleura.

The direction taken by the SCV from mid-clavicular to its confluence with the IJV varies with age:

- in older children, the track is like in adults: retro-clavicular to the sternal notch. The US probe is above and parallel to the clavicle with an important tilting movement bringing the US probe often close to the chin of the child.
- in infants and up to 1 or 2 years of age, the track is different: from mid-clavicular to the cricoid. The need to tilt the US probe is limited leaving the probe in an oblique position from mid-clavicular to the cricoid level in the neck.

By moving the US probe slightly on the clavicle in the direction of the axilla, the initial portion of the SCV, passing between the clavicle and the first rib, can be seen. At that level, the end of the EJV is often seen coming from lateral and arriving above and parallel to the SCV reach it just before its junction with the IJV (Figs. 4.27 and 4.35).

The more cranial, almost extra-thoracic, track of the SCV and BCV in infants allows us to observe a panoramic view of this entire venous system from one clavicle to the other (Figs. 4.30 and 4.31). This shows us that the course of the left BCV to the SVC has a gentle curve above the aortic arch, whereas the right BCV makes a sharp angle to reach SCV.

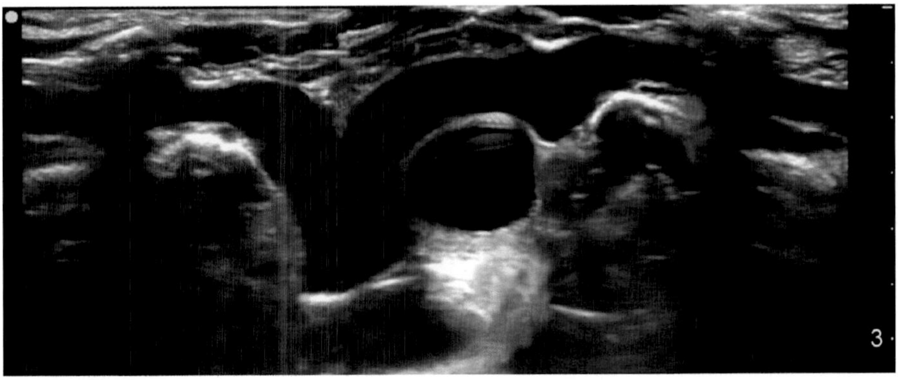

Fig. 4.30 Panoramic ultrasound view of the major thoracic vessels (infant)

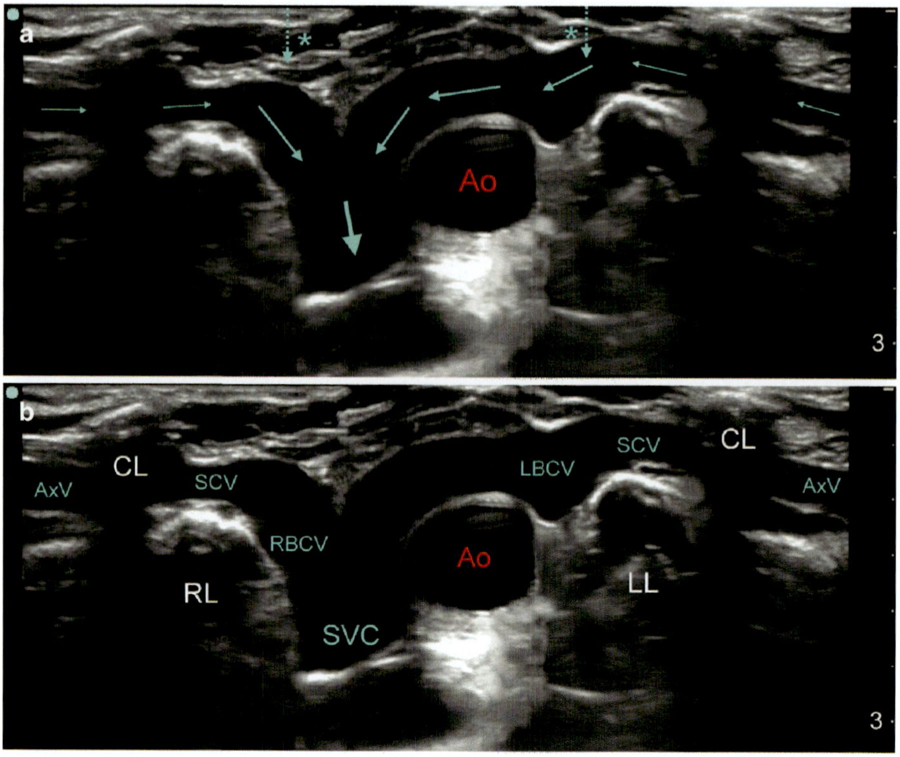

Fig. 4.31 Legends of the panoramic ultrasound view of the major thoracic vessels (infant). (**a**) Arrows showing the direction of the venous flow. Dashed arrows imaging the flow coming from the internal jugular veins (*). (**b**) Annotation of the major veins: axillary veins (AxV), subclavian vein (SCV), right (RBCV) and left (LBCV) brachiocephalic veins and the superior vena cava (SVC). *Ao* aorta, *CL* clavicle, *RL and LL* right and left lung top

4.3.4 The Suprasternal View

The US probe is placed in the suprasternal notch and tilted cranially to have a retrosternal view into the mediastinum. This view, also used by cardiologists, allows the visualization of the initial part of the superior vena cava (SVC), the largest central systemic vein in the mediastinum. Both right and left BCV join above the SVC making a typical "Y" pattern (Fig. 4.32).

Acquired (strictures, fibroblastic sleeve, thrombosis) and congenital (persistent left SVC) abnormalities can be detected. This can play a major role before choosing the best central venous catheter insertion site.

Once inserted, correct migration of guidewires or placement of catheters can be checked and corrected by maintaining this view.

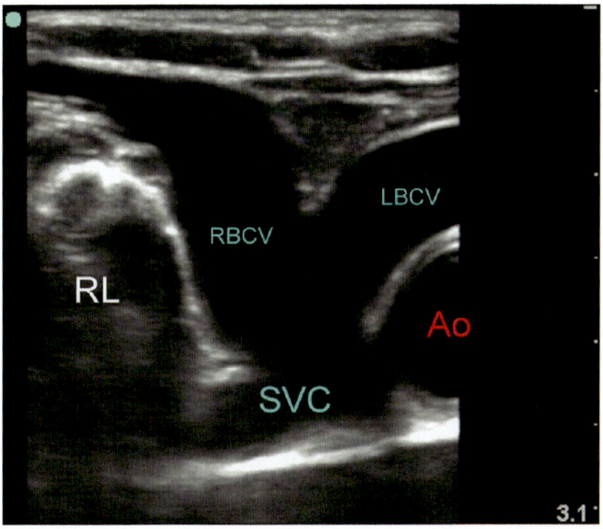

Fig. 4.32 Suprasternal visualization of the superior vena cava (infant). The typical “Y shape” pattern of the both right and left brachiocephalic veins (RBCV, LBCV). *SVC* superior vena cava, *Ao* aorta, *RL* right lung

4.4 Ultrasound Anatomy under the Clavicle

The name of the major vein coming from the upper limb changes from axillary vein to subclavian vein at the lateral border of the first rib, which usually corresponds to the area under the clavicle. This means that an infraclavicular position of the US probe will show the axillary vein (AxV) while the SCV is only show when the US probe has a supraclavicular position. The AxV and artery (AxA) are found close to each other in this infraclavicular region. The artery, surrounded cranially by the brachial plexus, is more cranial and deeper than the vein. The vessels pass deep under the pectoral muscles, above the pleura and crosses the clavicle at the mid-clavicular level. Two different US views can be useful under the clavicle:

4.4.1 The Sagittal Probe Position

By placing the US probe in a cranio-caudal position, we get a short-axis view of the vessels in a triangle pointing downwards and created by the pectoral muscles on top, the clavicle cranially and the pleura caudally (Fig. 4.33). Both axillary vessels can be visualized simultaneously with the artery being deeper and more cranial the vein. The AxV is quite deep, compressible and its diameter variates a lot with the respiration and the hemodynamic status (hypovolemia). Other vessels seen are:

– the cephalic vein (CV), more superficial and reaching the AxV just before it passes under the clavicle. The distal part of the AxV is the portion of the vein that

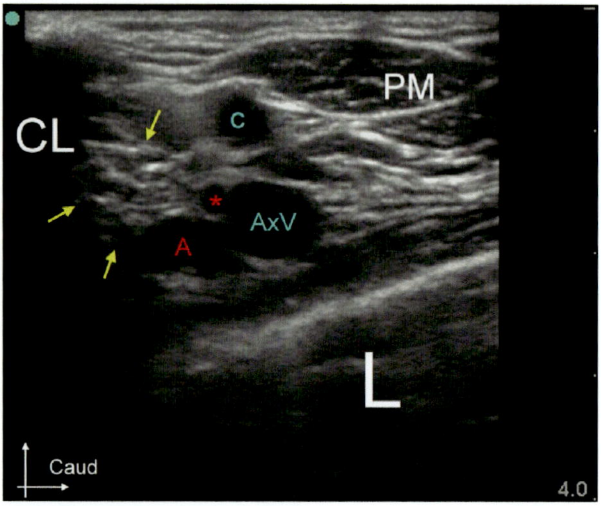

Fig. 4.33 Ultrasound anatomy of the infraclavicular area (13 years old)—the sagital view. Short axis view of the axillary vessels lying in a triangle formed by pectoral muscles (PM), the clavicle (CL) and the pleura. *A* axillary artery, *AxV* axillary vein, *C* cephalic vein, * thoracoacromial trunk, *L* lung

is usually targeted during punctures because its diameter is larger (due to the CV) and its compressibility reduced (due to its further fixation under the clavicle).

- the thoraco-acromial trunk (TAT), above the AxA and AXV. This artery comes from the AxA and gives four tortuous branches anteriorly: the pectoral, acromial, clavicular, and deltoid arteries.

The brachial plexus is seen at the cranial and posterior aspect of the AxA in the form of a unique grape or multiple cords.

4.4.2 The Oblique Axial Probe Position

By placing the US probe oblique from mid-clavicular to the axilla, we usually get a longitudinal view of the AxV (Fig. 4.34.). Both vessels, AxV and AxA, cannot be seen together on a unique view with this probe orientation because their run parallel to each other but in another plane. The AxV comes from the axilla, runs above the pleura, receives the flow from the CV and then passes under the clavicle. The AxA is deeper and more cranial. Both vessels shouldn't be confused. Therefore a few up and down sliding movements are performed to go from one vessel to the other. Here are some tips to distinguish them:

- the first vessels encountered by coming from caudal or medial is the AxV
- the AxA is more cranial and slightly deeper
- the CV always reaches the AxV
- the AxA is pulsative while the AxV size varies with breathing
- if you see a valve, it's a vein.

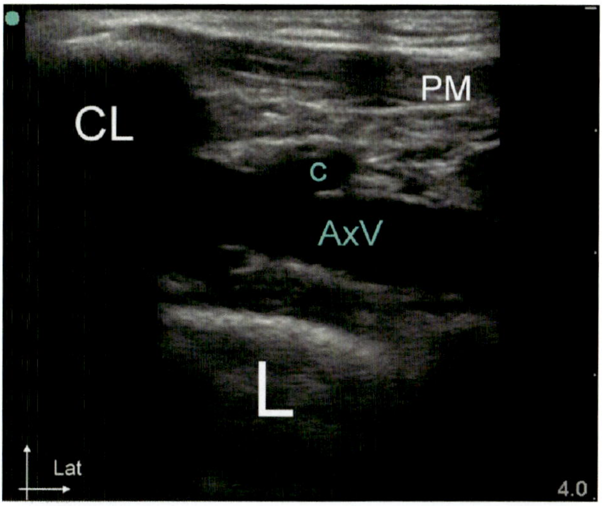

Fig. 4.34 Ultrasound anatomy of the infraclavicular area (13 years old)—the view from mid-clavicular to the axilla. Long-axis view of the axillary vein (AxV) and its fusion with the cephalic vein (C). *PM* pectoral muscles, *CL* clavicle, *L* lung

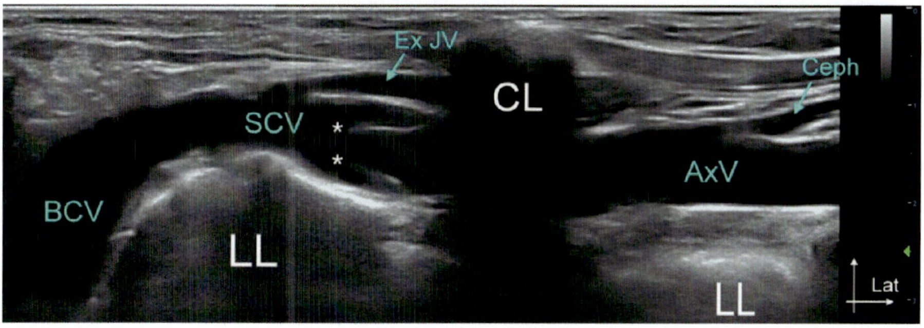

Fig. 4.35 Panoramic ultrasound view of the infra- and supra-clavicular areas (11 years old). The cephalic vein (Ceph) reach the axillary vein (AxV) just before they pass under the clavicle (CL). Valves (*) are often seen in the initial part of the subclavian vein (SCV). The end of the external jugular vein (ExJV) reach the SCV just above the clavicle. *BCV* brachiocephalic vein, *LL* left lung

In some cases, this longitudinal view of the veins can be maintained from the infraclavicular to the supraclavicular area passing over the clavicle. An example of this panoramic view is shown in Fig. 4.35.

Bibliography

1. Arai T, Matsuda Y, Koizuka K, et al. Rotation of the head might not be recommended for internal jugular puncture in infants and children. Pediatr Anesth. 2009;19:844–7.
2. Barone G, D'Andrea V, Vento G, Pittiruti M. A systematic ultrasound evaluation of the diameter of deep veins in the Newborn: results and implications for clinical practice. Neonatology. 2019;115(4):335–40. https://doi.org/10.1159/000496848.

3. Beniwal S, Bharqava K, Kausik S. Size of distal radial and ulnar arteries in adults of southern Rajasthan and their implications for percutaneous coronary interventions. Indian Heart J. 2014;66:506–9.
4. Bhatia N, Sivaprakasam J, Allford M, et al. The relative position of femoral artery and vein in children under general anesthesia—an ultrasound-guided observational study. Pediatr Anesth. 2014;24:1164–8.
5. Biasucci DG, La Greca A, Scoppettuolo G, Pittiruti M. Ultrasound-guided central venous catheterization: it is high time to use a correct terminology. Crit Care Med. 2015;43(9):e394–6.
6. Bream P, Gu E. Use of the popliteal vein as a guide for translumbar central venous access. J Vasc Interv Radiol. 2015;26:295–6.
7. Breschan C, Platzer M, Jost R, et al. Consecutive, prospective case series of a new method for ultrasound-guided supraclavicular approach to the brachiocephalic vein in children. Br J Anaesth. 2011;106:732–7.
8. Brescia F, Biasucci DG, Fabiani F, et al. A novel ultrasound-guided approach to the axillary vein: oblique-axis view combined with in-plane puncture. J Vasc Access. 2019;20(6):763–8.
9. Darge K, Brandis U, Zieger B, et al. Internal jugular venous valves in children: high-resolution US findings. Eur Radiol. 2001;11:655–8.
10. Hopkins J, Warkentine F, Gracely E, et al. The anatomic relationship between the common femoral artery and common femoral vein in frog leg position versus straight leg position in pediatric patients. Acad Emerg Med. 2009;16:579–84.
11. Jung C-W, Jalilov G, Song I-K, et al. Position and relative size of the vertebral artery according to age: implications for internal jugular vein access. Pediatr Anesth. 2017;27:997–1002.
12. Kai-Ming Y, En-Ci L, Ping L, et al. Anatomic variations of neck vessels and the course of pediatric internal jugular veins. Pediatr Anesth. 2017;27:1003–9.
13. Kim E-H, Lee J-H, Song I-K, et al. Posterior tibia artery as an alternative to radial artery for arterial cannulation site in small children. Anesthesiology. 2017;127:423–31.
14. Kim H, Kim J, Yim N, et al. Inferior vena cava filter insertion through the popliteal vein: enabling the percutaneous endovenous intervention of deep vein thrombosis with a single venous access approach in a single session. Diagn Interv Radiol. 2016;22:455–9.
15. Lim K, Kim J, Kim H, et al. The effect of lung deflation on the position and size of the subclavian vein in mechanically ventilated infants and children. Anesth Analg. 2011;112:1448–51.
16. Matsushita K, Yamaura K, Karashima Y, et al. Differences in anatomical relationship between vertebral artery and internal jugular vein in children and adults measured by ultrasonography. J Clin Monit Comput. 2016;30:221–5.
17. O'Leary R, Ahmed SM, McLure H, et al. Ultrasound-guided infraclavicular axillary vein cannulation: a useful alternative to the internal jugular vein. Br J Anaesth. 2012;109:762–8.
18. Ozbek S, Aydin B, Apiliogullari S, et al. Left femoral vein is a better choice for cannulation in children: a computed tomography study. Pediatr Anesth. 2013;23:524–8.
19. Ozcelik M, Guclu C, Meco B, et al. The airway device preference may affect the overlapping of the common carotid artery by the internal jugular vein. Pediatr Anesth. 2016;26:1148–56.
20. Pirotte T. Ultrasound-guided vascular access in adults and children: beyond the internal jugular vein. Acta Anaesth Belg. 2008;59:157–66.
21. Pirotte T, Veyckemans F. Ultrasound-guided subclavian vein cannulation in infants and children: a novel approach. Br J Anaesth. 2007;98:509–14.
22. Rhondali O, Attof R, Combet S, et al. Ultrasound-guided subclavian vein cannulation in infants: supraclavicular approach. Pediatr Anesth. 2011;21:1136–41.
23. Roth B, Marciniak B, Engelhardt T, et al. Anatomic relationship between the internal jugular vein and the carotid artery in preschool children: an ultrasonographic study. Pediatr Anesth. 2008;18:752–6.
24. Sonavane S, Milner D, Singh S, et al. Comprehensive imaging review of the superior vena cava. Radiographics. 2015;35:1873–92.
25. Suk E, Lee K, Kweon T, et al. Ultrasonographic evaluation of the femoral vein in anaesthetized infants and young children. Anesthesia. 2010;65:895–8.

26. Varga E, Candiotti A, Saltzman B, et al. Evaluation of distal radial artery cross-sectional internal diameter in pediatric patients using ultrasound. Pediatr Anesth. 2013;23:460–2.
27. Warkentine FH, Pierce MC, Lorenz D, et al. The anatomic relationship of femoral vein to femoral artery in euvolemic pediatric patients by ultrasonography: implication for pediatric femoral central venous access. Acad Emerg Med. 2008;15:426–30.

Chapter 5
Near-InfraRed Technology for Access to Superficial Veins: Evidence from the Literature and Indications for Pediatric Venous Access

Massimo Lamperti and Mauro Pittiruti

The use of near-infrared light imaging has been introduced to improve the number of visible veins in pediatric patients. This technology allows the visualization of small (0.2 mm) and superficial (up to 8 mm) veins. There are different devices based on a polarized infrared light or on low power lasers. The advantage of the NIR light devices is that they are portable and enhance the peripheral vein path when compared to naked-eyes visualization or palpation. There is currently not enough evidence to support the superiority of these devices in terms of first-time successful cannulation or reduced time to cannulation due to the heterogeneity of the studies conducted. The NIR light technology is still lacking information regarding the depth of field related to the position of the peripheral veins but with an appropriate training it could improve the success during peripheral IV cannulas in pediatric patients.

Peripheral venous cannulation and phlebotomy can be challenging in neonates and pediatric patients even in expert hands. For this purpose, different technologies have been investigated to evaluate their clinical feasibility and their advantage compared with the traditional palpation or landmarks methods.

The main research has been conducted on the use of ultrasound (US), trans-illumination and near-infrared (NIR) imaging technologies. Near-infrared has been investigated in neonates and pediatric patients; different devices have been marketed with different clinical specifications and outcomes.

M. Lamperti
Anesthesiology Institute, Cleveland Clinic, Abu Dhabi, UAE
e-mail: lamperm@clevelandclinicabudhabi.ae

M. Pittiruti (✉)
Department of Surgery, Catholic University Hospital, Rome, Italy

D. G. Biasucci et al. (eds.), *Vascular Access in Neonates and Children*,
https://doi.org/10.1007/978-3-030-94709-5_5

5.1 Near-Infrared Technology

NIR technology is not new in the medical-devices market, and it has been introduced as a method to measure cerebral blood flow and oxygenation non-invasively.

More recently, the use of NIR has been extended to allow vein visualization and phlebotomy in difficult cases where peripheral veins were difficult to either visualize directly or to palpate.

The main devices available in the market are the VeinViewer and the Accuvein but there are other new devices that have been used in the clinical setting such as the VascuLuminator (Netherlands), the 3-light-source method Total Reticular Vision (Mexico), VeinViewer Vision2, IRIS Vascular Viewer, and Veinsite.

5.1.1 How They Work

The VeinViewer (Christie Medical Holdings, Inc.) utilizes a 760-nm polarized near-infrared light to illuminate the patient's skin. The light source is from a ring of light illuminated diodes (LEDs). The NIR light can penetrate the skin at a right angle up to 10 mm of depth from around 60 cm. The skin and subcutaneous fat are not able to absorb this light properly, so they scatter the NIR light in all directions including back to a camera that is included in the device. Blood in the veins, however, absorbs or scatters forward the NIR light. A digital video camera picks up the NIR light reflection, the device then analyses and processes this information. Another LED is used to project back to the skin an enhanced real-time image over the position of existing vessels making the veins appear black on a greenish background (Fig. 5.1). The VeinViewer has two versions: the VeinViewer Flex is handheld, and the VeinViewer Vision 2 has an articulating arm and a flexible wrist joint making it easy to maneuver to better visualize the vessels.

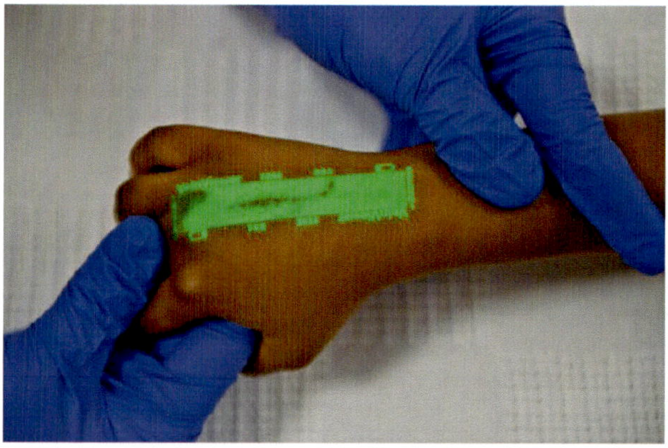

Fig. 5.1 Image of subcutaneous vessels obtained using the VeinViewer

The Accuvein (HF320; Avant Medical) uses NIR light from 2-low power lasers: a 642-nm wavelength red laser operating at 40 mW and a 785-nm wavelength IR laser at 25 mW. The resulting energy is reportedly 2.57 and 1.58 ohms, respectively. In this case, the resulting background on the skin is reddish and the veins will appear as black (Fig. 5.2).

The VascuLuminator (Quantivision) uses near-infrared light (~ 800 nm), which can penetrate up to several centimeters into tissue but is still absorbed by blood, which enables discrimination between blood vessels and surrounding tissues near the skin surface. Both reflected and trans illuminated NIR lights on the skin are imaged by a NIR sensitive digital camera and displayed on a LCD monitor in an ergonomic setting.

The IRIS Vascular Viewer includes the light or illumination source, the detector, and the display. The illumination source is a matrix of diodes emitting infrared light. The light source may be directed to the surface of the limb from a distance or applied directly. If applied directly, the light passes through the limb.

Veinsite (Vuetek, Grey, ME, USA), is the latest NIR vein visualizer introduced into the market. It uses a rechargeable battery and has an optional VGA cable for

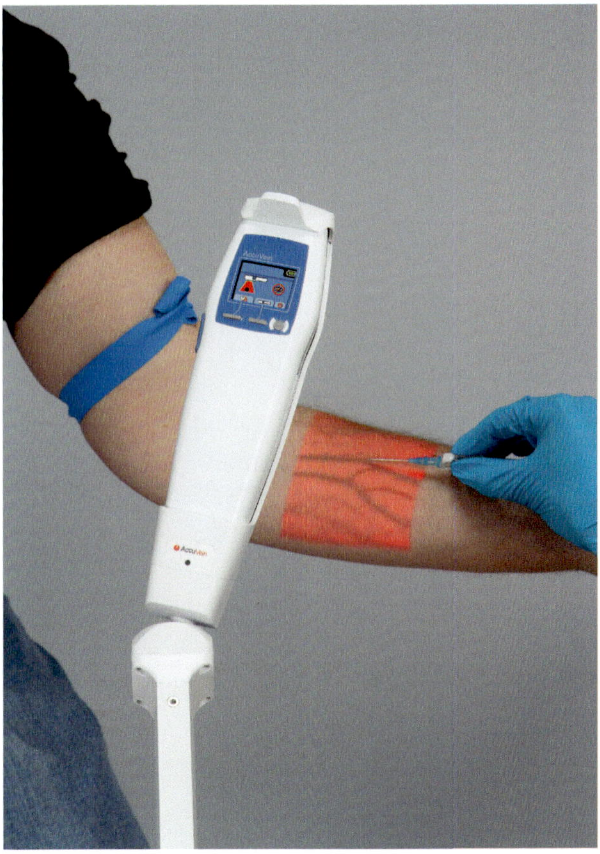

Fig. 5.2 Accuvein and visualization of peripheral veins

separate monitor display. The device allows for concurrent vein inspection with normal eyesight and operates independently of ambient light conditions. When powered on, it emits a NIR light (700–900 nm) that penetrates the skin. Upon contact with tissue, the NIR light (tissue absorption coefficient between 0.02 and 0.3 cm^{-1}) scatters, travelling a depth of <5 mm before deviating from its initial direction. Conversely, hemoglobin and other vascular fluids are highly absorptive. The Veinsite's electro-optical technology detects the absorption difference between vascular structures and surrounding tissue. After converting the raw image to greyscale, it then displays it on the headset's LCD screen (Figs. 5.3 and 5.4). In this way, the operator wearing the helmet can see the veins either by direct vision or through NIR-vision.

Fig. 5.3 Veinsite

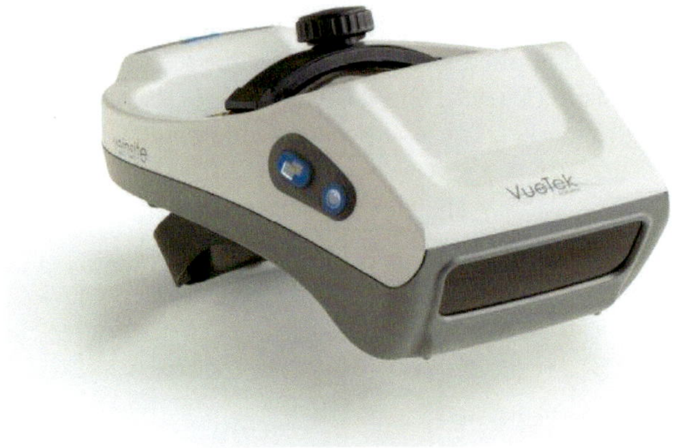

Fig. 5.4 View of veins as seen with the Veinsite

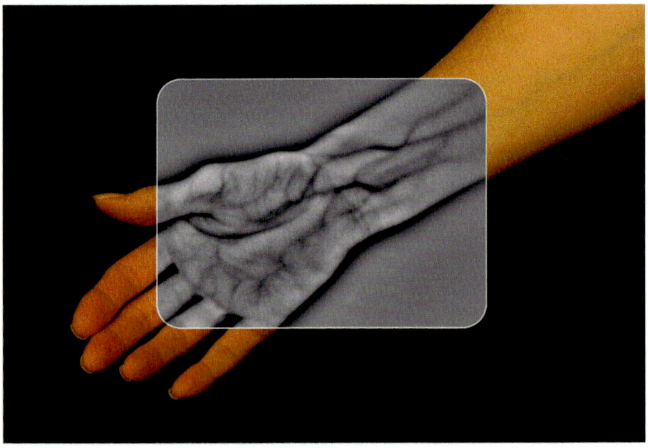

5.1.2 *Safety of the NIR Vein Visualizers*

NIR is a safe technology not harmful to patients as it does not produce ionizing radiation. The lasers emitted by Accuvein are classified as class 2 and considered safe as the blink reflex limits their exposure and prevents ocular damage. The manufacturers suggest that in cases where the blink reflex is altered, appropriate eye protection should be used.

5.2 When Should We Consider a Peripheral Venous Cannulation Difficult?

Peripheral venous cannulation can be particularly challenging in some patients when (a) the vein cannot be visualized with the naked eye and (b) the vein cannot be palpated where it should be according to the landmark anatomy. There are various patient factors making peripheral venous cannulation difficult such as darker skin, obesity, neonates and pediatric patients, previous chemotherapy, chronic illnesses, and multiple peripheral venous cannulation attempts.

A more objective peripheral venous cannulation scale has been proposed recently. Predictor variables from the DIVA (*Difficult Intra-Venous Access*) score are (1) visibility of vein after tourniquet placement, (2) palpability of vein after tourniquet placement, (3) age of the patient in months, and (4) history of prematurity. Skin shade is determined by using a Dermablend cosmetics card (Dermablend Inc., Ridgefield, NJ), which grades skin shade from 1 to 11, light to dark. For the purpose of analysis, it is dichotomized into two groups: light (shades 1, 2, 4, and 5) and dark (shade 3, and shades 6 through 11). A DIVA score greater than 4 has been recognized as the threshold to identify a patient as higher risk for predicted failure.

Table 5.1 summarizes the DIVA score.

Table 5.1 DIVA score. A score > 4 is the cut-off value for predicting peripheral venous cannulation failure

Predictor value	
Visibility	Visible = 0 Not visible = 2
Palpability	Palpable = 0 Not palpable = 2
Age	>36 months = 0 12–35 months = 1 < 12 Months = 3
Prematurity	Not premature = 0 Premature = 3
Skin shade	Light = 0 Dark = 1

5.3 Evidence from the Literature

5.3.1 NIR Light Devices' Ability to Visualize Peripheral Veins

Several studies have been conducted to study the ability of different NIR imaging devices in terms of improved visualization of peripheral veins not visible or not palpable in pediatric patients. Mihake and colleagues compared direct sight visualization with ultrasound and NIR imaging provided by a VeinViewer prototype. They found that NIR enhanced the visualization of peripheral veins by 67% compared to the naked eye alone. In the same study, NIR imaging was compared to ultrasound (by means of two different ultrasound machines: one portable and one high resolution). The authors noted that NIR can detect more superficial (up to 8.2 mm) and smaller vessels (0.2 mm) compared to ultrasound that was able to detect bigger and deeper vessels. The portable ultrasound was found to have an easier learning curve than the high resolution one.

Another paper was conducted by Chiao using the Veinsite to investigate the characteristic factors related to peripheral vein visualization on 384 subjects from different sub-cohorts including those more associated with decreased vein visibility. The study compared direct vision with NIR imaging. The authors found that an average of 3.3 additional suitable venous sites were found by using the Veinsite when compared with direct sight visualization. Veinsite increased the detection of possible peripheral venous cannulation sites in 97% of these difficult cases—including an additional 1.7 (89% increase) possible vein sites in infants and additional 3.7 (80% increase) possible vein sites in patients with dark skin. The visualization provided by NIR was also helpful in obese patients were the additional cannulations sites improved by 4.0 (82% increase) and in morbid obese patients where the visualization improved by 3 sites (83% increase).

The use of the VascuLuminator has been argued to increase the number of additional cannulation sites. The same authors conducted another study comparing VeinViewer, Accuvein and VascuLuminator in terms of visibility of suitable veins for cannulation and they found that VeinViewer was able to detect more veins suitable for cannulation (307/322 (95.3%)) than Accuvein (239/254 (94.1%)) while VascuLuminator had the lower visualization ability (229/257 (89.1%)) ($p = 0.03$).

5.3.2 Efficacy of NIR Light Devices in Successful Peripheral Vein Cannulation

A recent meta-analysis from Park and colleagues of 11 studies on pediatric patients analyzed 1994 patients in which NIR imaging was compared to a standard control group (eye alone) of 1577 patients. The failure rates were not different in the two groups: 31.9% (673/1994) in the NIR group compared to 30.9% (488/1577) in the control group. The authors of this meta-analysis concluded that the use of NIR light devices did not have any overall impact on failure of first attempt at peripheral vein cannulation (RR = 1.03, CI = 0.89–1.20, I2 = 48%) in a pediatric population. The study also concluded that there was no difference if the cannulation was performed in different settings (e.g., emergency department or operating theatres).

The synthesis of the included studies did not reveal a high heterogeneity. Different factors can contribute to an increased failure rate such as young age, the presence of dark skin color, weight less than 5 kg, obesity or increased subcutaneous fat, and previous chronic illness. A possible bias related to the non-inferiority of the NIR group compared to the traditional visualization/palpation technique can be found in the inclusion only of patients with an expected difficult peripheral venous cannulation as it happened in one study]. Other studies analyzed the results according to the operators' experience, but they were not able to find a difference related to this factor. The meta-analysis from Park found a significant positive effect of the use of NIR in terms of improved first-time successful cannulation when high power studies only were analyzed while another paper reported a higher risk of failure when NIR light devices were used even though their participants were all predicted to have difficult cannulation (DIVA score $\geq$ 4). In this study, the operators involved in the study belonged to an IV team to whom more than 1000 difficult cases per month were referred. Their proficiency without using cannulation assistance devices may have resulted in a higher failure risk in the NIR group; it was unknown what kind of training the operators received before starting to perform cannulation with the NIR light devices in patients.

5.3.3 *Time to Successful Peripheral Vein Cannulation for NIR Light Devices*

First-attempt success using a NIR light device has been considered as a secondary outcome in most of the studies conducted in this field, but it is important not to underestimate this factor, especially in emergency situations when a cannula is required for the administration of life-saving medications.

The data of first-attempt success with NIR light devices from different studies were too heterogenous and used different metrics and therefore, a meta-analysis could not be conducted. Most of the studies did not report any significant difference between the NIR light devices and the traditional methods in terms of time to obtain access while Sun et al. reported an increased time spent to insert a peripheral cannula in the NIR group. Other studies did not specifically address this aim in their analysis. This secondary aim seems to be highly related to the first-time success even if there is the need to have future studies in which the time to successful cannulation needs to be separated from the first-attempt success and it should be studied regarding the learning curve needed to obtain full competence in this technique.

5.4 How to Use NIR Light Devices in Peripheral Pediatric Venous Access

The various NIR light devices have specific characteristics that make their clinical use different.

The VeinViewer uses the reflection of the NIR light by light-emitting diodes to make sub-surface vessels visible. The veins are depicted as dark on a square green background projected on the patients' skin. The VeinViewer needs to be positioned approximately 30 cm above the puncture site until the focusing text is clearly visible. The operator can choose to adjust the size of the projection, to use the universal or fine mode, and to use normal (background green) or inverse mode (veins in green background black).

The Accuvein can be used with a second operator handling the device to optimize the veins' visualization or it can be mounted on a trolley a with a hands-free set. The AV300 is used at a height of 20–30 cm and perpendicular to the surface of the skin. The operator can freely cycle through the three different display settings (varying sensitivity) to define the best mode to locate the vein.

The VascuLuminator display/camera combination can be positioned approximately 20 cm above the puncture site, whilst NIR light source is placed underneath it. The operator can modify the focus and light intensity to optimize the image of the veins.

The Veinsite is a head-mounted system which includes a portable near-infrared (NIR) emitter, video acquisition, and display device. The device allows for concurrent vein inspection with normal eyesight and operates independently of ambient light conditions. The peripheral venous cannulation by using Veinsite can be divided in two phases: (1) visualization of the vein by NIR light and initial vein puncture, (2) once the vein is entered and flow-back flush is detected on the back of the peripheral IV cannula through direct sight the cannulation can be continued without NIR visualization. Once the cannula is in, the operator can check if there is extravasation by flushing the cannula with normal saline and with NIR visualization, assess if there is any sign of fluid outside the venous path.

5.5 Tips and Tricks

The NIR light devices can be useful as long as it is used for appropriately selected patients. First, all pediatric patients should be scored according to the DIVA score. Even in low-risk patients, the NIR devices can help in venous mapping and selecting the best vein site to be cannulated. Remember that all pediatric cannulations can be considered difficult "per se" because children are needle-phobic and require proper preparation with topical local anesthetics that. If the patient is a neonate or a toddler, it is important to involve the parents as they can help with reassuring the child and creating a calm environment.

The NIR devices should be part of the peripheral IV access tools as a dedicated peripheral IV set including tourniquet, swab gauzes, small IV cannulas (24G, 22G), needle-free connectors, and dressings.

As a rule of thumb, NIR light devices can detect peripheral veins up to 8 mm of depth. With deeper veins or those not visible even by using these devices, the next step should be to use an ultrasound device to detect bigger and deeper veins.

An important part regarding the use of NIR imaging devices is the training. There is currently no established training on how to use these devices and how steep the learning curve is. All the studies performed on these devices declared that the operators spent at least one month using the device, but it is not known when the full proficiency (100% successful cannulations) were obtained by a single operator.

The main limitation of the NIR light technology is the lack of depth perception. This can lead to puncturing the posterior wall of the vein causing extravasation once the cannula is inserted.

5.6 Conclusions

Pediatric patients are potentially at higher risk for difficult peripheral venous cannulation. A proper evaluation of potential sites and potential difficulty during the cannulation is mandatory. This procedure should be performed by expert operators and with specific tools including NIR light devices and ultrasound machines. The visualization of the veins by using NIR imaging is enhanced but the results related to first-time successful cannulation and time to cannulation are still not significantly different from the traditional palpation and direct visualization. Further studies are needed to understand if the lack of efficacy is due to technical reasons or by lack of training in these new devices.

Bibliography

1. Barone G, Pittiruti M. Epicutaneo-caval catheters in neonates: new insights and new suggestions from the recent literature. J Vasc Access 2020 Nov;21(6):805–809. https://doi.org/10.1177/1129729819891546. Epub 2019 Dec 5.
2. Black KJ, Pusic MV, Harmidy D, et al. Pediatric intravenous insertion in the emergency department: bevel up or bevel down? Pediatr Emerg Care. 2005;21:707–11.
3. Bustos LL, Fronek A, Lopez-Kapke L, et al. Nonvisible insufficient subcutaneous reticular venous plexus can be observed through the skin using a new illumination method. Dermatol Surg. 2010;36:1046–9.
4. Chapman LL, Sullivan B, Pacheco AL, et al. VeinViewer-assisted intravenous catheter placement in a pediatric emergency department. Acad Emerg Med. 2011;18:966–71.
5. Chiao FB, Resta-Flarer F, Lesser J, et al. Vein visualization: patient characteristic factors and efficacy of a new infrared vein finder technology. Br J Anaesth. 2013;110:966–71.
6. Cuper NJ, de Graaff JC, van Dijk AT, et al. Predictive factors for difficult intravenous cannulation in pediatric patients at a tertiary pediatric hospital. Pediatr Anaesth. 2011a;22:223–9.

7. Cuper NJ, Graaff JC, Verdaasdonk RM, et al. Nearinfrared imaging in intravenous cannulation in children: a cluster randomized clinical trial. Pediatrics. 2013;131:e191–7.
8. Cuper NJ, Verdaasdonk RM, de Roode R, et al. Visualizing veins with near-infrared light to facilitate blood withdrawal in children. Clin Pediatr. 2011b;50:508–12.
9. Curtis SJ, CraigWR LE, et al. Ultrasound or near-infrared vascular imaging to guide peripheral intravenous catheterization in children: a pragmatic randomized controlled trial. CMAJ. 2015;187:563–70.
10. De Graaf J, Cuper N, Mungra R, et al. Near-infrared light to aid peripheral intravenous cannulation in children: a cluster randomised clinical trial of three devices. Anaesthesia. 2013;68:835–45.
11. De Graaf J, Cuper N, van Dijk A, et al. Evaluating NIR vascular imaging to support intravenous cannulation in awake children difficult to cannulate; a randomized clinical trial. Pediatr Anesth. 2014;24:1174–9.
12. Goren A, Laufer J, Yativ N, et al. Transillumination of the palm for venipuncture in infants. Pediatr Emerg Care. 2001;17:130–1.
13. Haas NA. Clinical review: vascular access for fluid infusion in children. Crit Care. 2004;8:478–84.
14. Jacobson AF, Winslow EH. Variables influencing intravenous catheter insertion difficulty and failure: an analysis of 339 intravenous catheter insertions. Heart Lung. 2005;34:345–59.
15. Kaddoum RN, Anghelescu DL, Parish ME, et al. A randomized controlled trial comparing the AccuVein AV300 device to standard insertion technique for intravenous cannulation of anesthetized children. Paediatr Anaesth. 2012;22:884–9.
16. Katsogridakis YLM, Seshadri R, Sullivan C, et al. Veinlite transillumination in the pediatric emergency department: a therapeutic interventional trial. Pediatr Emerg Care. 2008;24:83–8.
17. Kim MJ, Park JM, Rhee N, et al. Efficacy of VeinViewer in pediatric peripheral intravenous access: a randomized controlled trial. Eur J Pediatr. 2012;171:1121–5.
18. Kuensting LL, DeBoer S, Holleran R, et al. Difficult venous access in children: taking control. J Emerg Nurs. 2009;35:419–24.
19. Park J, Kim M, Yim h et al. Utility of near-infrared light devices for pediatric peripheral intravenous cannulation: a systematic review and meta-analysis. Eur J Pediatr 2016; 175:1975–1988.
20. Perry AM, Caviness AC, Hsu DC. Efficacy of a near-infrared light device in pediatric intravenous cannulation: a randomized controlled trial. Pediatr Emerg Care. 2011;27:5–10.
21. Riker M, Kennedy C, Winfrey B, et al. Validation and refinement of the difficult intravenous access score: a clinical prediction rule for identifying children with difficult intravenous access. Academ Emerg Med. 2011;18:1129–34.
22. Simhi E, Kachko L, Bruckheimer E, et al. A vein entry indicator device for facilitating peripheral intravenous cannulation in children: a prospective, randomized, controlled trial. Anesth Analg. 2008;107:1531–5.
23. Stokowski G, Steele D, Wilson D. The use of ultrasound to improve practice and reduce complication rates in peripherally inserted central catheter insertions: final report of investigation. J Infus Nurs. 2009;32:145–55.
24. Sun CY, Lee KC, Lin IH, et al. Near-infrared light device can improve intravenous cannulation in critically ill children. Pediatr Neonatol. 2013;54:194–7.
25. Szmuk P, Steiner J, Pop RB, et al. The VeinViewer vascular imaging system worsens first attempt cannulation rate for experienced nurses in infants and children with anticipated difficult intravenous access. Anesth Analg. 2013;116:1087–92.
26. Woude OC, Cuper NJ, Getrouw C, et al. The effectiveness of a near-infrared vascular imaging device to support intravenous cannulation in children with dark skin color: a cluster randomized clinical trial. Anesth Analg. 2013;116:1266–71.
27. Wyatt JS, Cope M, Delpy D, et al. Quantification of cerebral oxygenation and haemodynamics in sick newborn infants by near infrared spectrophotometry. Lancet. 1986;2:1063–6.
28. Yen K, Riegert A, Gorelick MH. Derivation of the DIVA score: a clinical prediction rule for the identification of children with difficult intravenous access. Pediatr Emerg Care. 2008;24:143–7.

Chapter 6
Tip Navigation and Tip Location Methods

Mauro Pittiruti

The insertion of a central venous access is complex procedure that includes several phases: recognition of the need for a central line, ultrasound evaluation of the possible options in terms of venipuncture and location of the exit site, cannulation of the vein, intraprocedural ruling out of possible puncture-related complications, assessment of the proper direction of the catheter inside the vasculature, intraprocedural assessment of the final location of the tip of the catheter in a 'central' position, securement of the catheter and protection of the exit site.

The intraprocedural assessment of the direction of the catheter during its progression inside the vasculature is often called 'tip navigation', and it can be achieved either by ultrasound or by radiological methods (fluoroscopy).

On the other hand, the intraprocedural assessment of the final position of the tip is called 'tip location', and it may be performed either by ultrasound or by intracavitary electrocardiography or by radiological methods (fluoroscopy).

6.1 Tip Navigation

Tip navigation may not always be necessary, though it might be extremely important when placing central venous access devices with very long or difficult trajectory, as epicutaneo-cava catheters (ECC) and umbilical venous catheters (UVC) in neonates, or when placing catheters that may easily take a wrong direction during their progression inside the vasculature (FICCs and PICCs in children).

The only practical methods of tip navigation are ultrasound or fluoroscopy. Though, fluoroscopy is currently not recommended, for several reasons: (a) it is not

M. Pittiruti (✉)
Department of Surgery, Catholic University Hospital, Rome, Italy

D. G. Biasucci et al. (eds.), *Vascular Access in Neonates and Children*,
https://doi.org/10.1007/978-3-030-94709-5_6

safe, since it implies x-ray exposure, potentially dangerous both for the patient and for the operator; (b) it is not very accurate, since it allows to visualize clearly the guidewire or the catheter, but not the surrounding vasculature, which has to be guessed on the basis of radiological landmarks; (c) it is logistically difficult or impossible in intensive care unit, so that the neonate or child must be moved to a dedicated environment (operating room or radiological suite); (d) it is not cost-effective. In short, ultrasound-based tip navigation is the only option for neonatal and pediatric vascular access.

The use of ultrasound has several advantages: it is safe, easy, accurate, inexpensive, and cost-effective. The recent availability of portable wireless ultrasound probes has made the intraprocedural use of ultrasound even more simple. The only potential disadvantage is that ultrasound-based tip navigation requires some training, though the training required is variable depending on the type of central venous access, and such training is probably faster than the training required for the proper operation and interpretation of fluoroscopy.

Two recent papers have described in detail the method of ultrasound-based tip navigation in neonates and children. These two papers describe the so-called ECHOTIP protocol, which is a structured approach to the intraprocedural use of ultrasound during placement of any type of central venous access devices, both in neonates (Neo-ECHOTIP) and in children (ECHOTIP-Ped).

Tip navigation may be useful for any central venous access in the newborn: ECC, UVC, CICC. The ultrasound scan of the vasculature is particularly easy in neonates, as the tissues are all echogenic and even the bones allow the scan of the underlying veins.

According to the Neo-ECHOTIP protocol, the progression of the UVC is performed under direct ultrasound visualization, placing the probe in the epigastric area, between the umbilical cord and the xyphoid. Using a small sectorial probe 7–8 MHz, it will be possible to follow step by step the progression of the catheter inside the liver, until it reaches the junction between inferior vena cava and right atrium. A small pression with the probe may be helpful to direct the catheter to the target, avoiding misdirection inside the liver. Progression of a ECC inserted in the upper limbs or in a vein of the scalp is easily performed using a linear probe 10–14 Mhz in the supra-clavicular region. The same probe will be useful to follow the progression of a ECC inserted in the lower limbs through the femoral and iliac veins.

In children, the progression of PICCs, CICCs and FICCs into the vasculature can also be followed using a linear probe, according to the ECHOTIP-Ped protocol. When inserting a PICC or a CICC, a linear probe placed in the supraclavicular/suprasternal area (the same probe used for ultrasound-guided venipuncture) will allow to make sure that the guidewire or the catheter—either coming from the subclavian vein or from the internal jugular vein—are properly entering the brachiocephalic vein. When inserting a FICC, using the linear probe it will be possible to follow the guidewire or the catheter inside the common femoral vein and the external iliac vein.

6.2 Tip Location

While tip navigation may be not necessary in all cases, tip location is mandatory for any central venous access. In fact, the proper function of a central access with minimization of complications is based on the correct placement of the tip. A central venous access is defined by the location of the tip either in the superior vena cava or in the inferior vena cava or in the right atrium. When the tip has not been placed in this location, the device cannot be used for central purposes (infusion of parenteral nutrition and of any solution potentially associated with endothelial damage; hemodynamic monitoring; hemodialysis; repeated daily blood samples); if this happens, serious thrombotic complications may occur.

For ECC, CICC and PICC, the best location of the tip is in proximity of the junction between superior vena cava and right atrium; for UVC, the junction between inferior vena cava and right atrium; for FICC, either the inferior vena cava or the junction between inferior vena cava and right atrium (depending on the purpose of the FICC: if hemodynamic monitoring is required, the tip should be at the junction).

Therefore, tip location is mandatory and must be accurate. Most current guidelines recommend that tip location should also be intra-procedural, rather than post-procedural. The old method of checking the position of the tip by radiological methods (typically, chest x-ray) after the procedure is not recommended anymore. Post-procedural control by x-ray has several disadvantages: (a) it is less accurate than other intra-procedural methods; (b) it is not safe, as it is associated with x-ray exposure of the patient; (c) it implies a significant waste of time, with delayed start of treatment; (d) when the tip location is not correct, the procedure must be done again, with relevant waste of time and money.

At present, the intra-procedural methods for tip location currently available are fluoroscopy, trans-esophageal echocardiography (TEE), trans-thoracic/trans-abdominal echocardiography (TTE) and intracavitary electrocardiography (IC-ECG). Fluoroscopy is not recommended, for the same reasons explained above (it is inaccurate, unsafe, expensive, and logistically difficult), and should be avoided as much as possible in neonates and children. TEE is invasive, expensive, and logistically difficult. Thus, the only options for an appropriate tip location in neonatal and pediatric patients are IC-ECG and TTE.

6.2.1 Tip Location by Intracavitary ECG

Intracavitary ECG is the most recommended method for intraprocedural tip location, according to current guidelines. The IC-ECG method is more than 70 years old, but it has entered the clinical practice in Europe in the 90s and in USA a decade ago. Several clinical studies carried out in the first decade of this century have demonstrated that tip location by IC-ECG is more accurate than tip location by radiological methods, when the two methods are compared with the golden standard for tip location, TEE. This is no surprise, since IC-ECG very precisely detects the passage between the electrically inactive area (superior vena cava) and the electrically active area (right atrium), which morphologically corresponds to the cavo-atrial junction. On the contrary, radiological methods for tip location (chest x-ray, fluoroscopy, etc.) localize the tip of the catheter using uncertain radiological landmarks, largely based on statistical approximations.

The rationale of IC-ECG is based on the observation that when the tip of the catheter acts as a travelling electrode inside the vasculature, the cavo atrial junction can be detected as the position where a maximal P wave is seen on the intracavitary ECG, using a sort of intracavitary lead II (tip of the catheter vs. electrode on the left flank). The method is easy and expensive, since it can be carried out with a standard ECG monitor; the only device needed is a sterile cable connecting the column of saline contained inside the catheter with the electrode that usually is placed on the right shoulder. When the catheter is closed and filled with saline, the voltage inside the catheter will be equal to the voltage read in the only open hole of the catheter, i.e., the tip.

The technique is simple and fast. As the catheter is inserted, a sterile cable is connected to the central line: the simplest sterile cable consists of a saline adapter connected to the hub of the catheter (Fig. 6.1), while the other end is connected to the ECG monitor, either directly (Figs. 6.2 and 6.3) or indirectly, through a switchbox (Fig. 6.4). The line is flushed with saline, so to avoid the presence of air bubbles inside the catheter, since these may block the electric signal. The intracavitary ECG is read, focusing on the height and shape of the P-wave (Fig. 6.5). The maximal P-wave corresponds to the junction between SVC and right atrium (Fig. 6.6), while a diphasic or a negative P-wave (Figs. 6.7 and 6.8) corresponds to an intra-atrial position of the tip.

IC-ECG has been used for neonatal and pediatric central venous access since the 90s. Ten years ago, a multicenter study on more than 300 children has shown that IC-ECG matches 98% with the results of chest x-ray. Further studies have

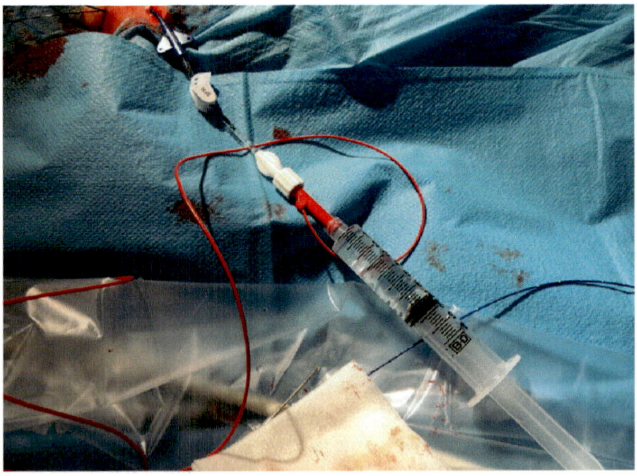

Fig. 6.1 Saline adapter connected to the catheter

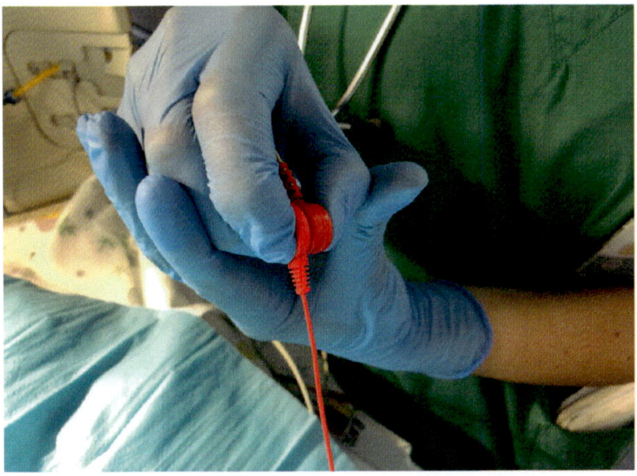

Fig. 6.2 Direct connection of the sterile cable with the ECG monitor

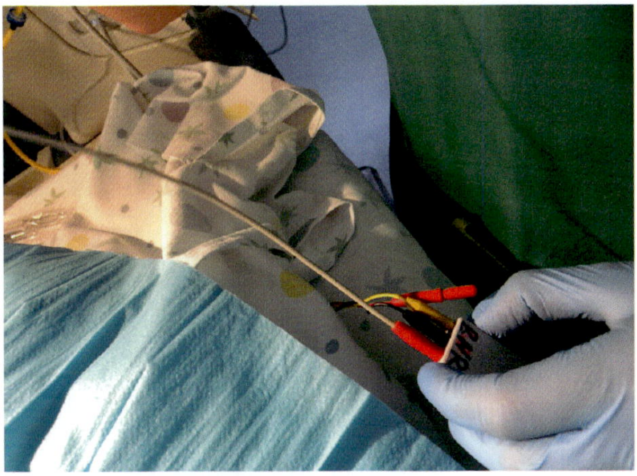

Fig. 6.3 Direct connection of the sterile cable with the ECG monitor (connection by jack)

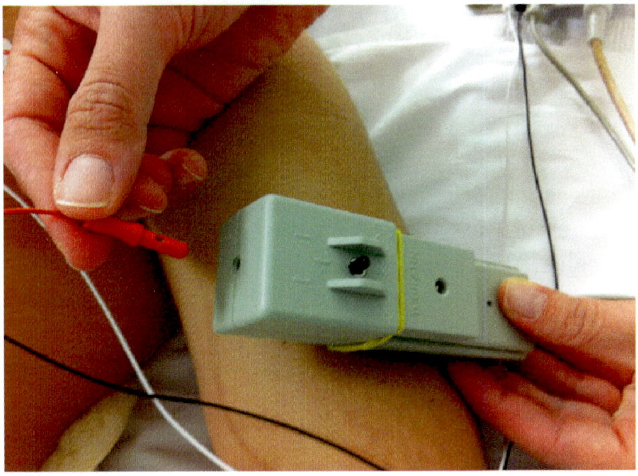

Fig. 6.4 Indirect connection of the sterile cable with the ECG monitor through a switchbox

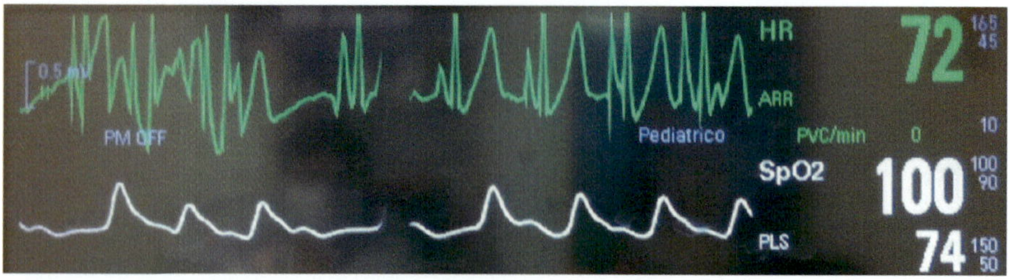

Fig. 6.5 Intracavitary ECG tracing with changing height and shape of the P wave

Fig. 6.6 Intracavitary ECG tracing: maximal P wave (tip at the junction between superior vena cava and right atrium)

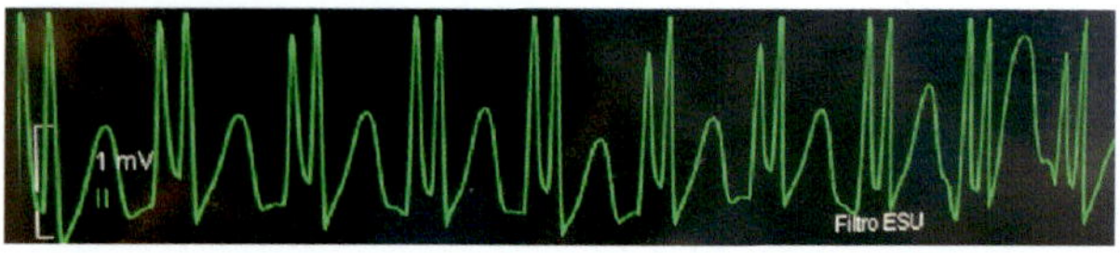

Fig. 6.7 Intracavitary ECG tracing: negative P wave (tip inside the right atrium)

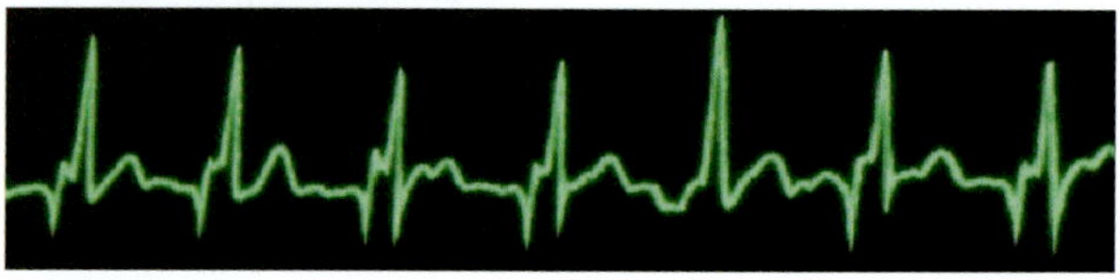

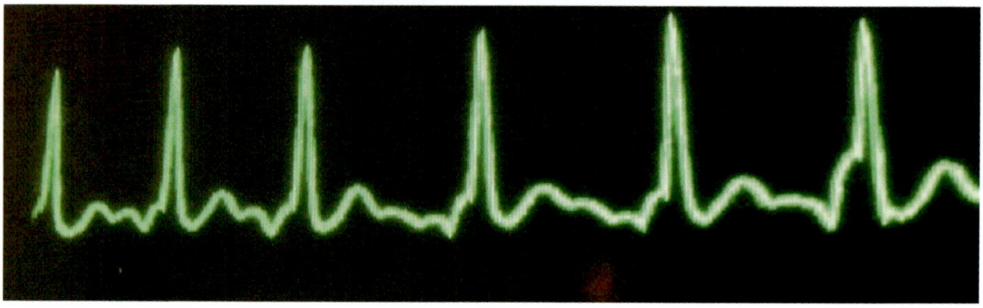

Fig. 6.8 Intracavitary ECG tracing: diphasic P wave (tip inside the right atrium)

demonstrated that this method of tip location is accurate, safe, and inexpensive in most central venous accesses in pediatric patients. Interestingly, the only limit of applicability of IC-ECG is the presence of atrial fibrillation, pacemaker, or severe arrhythmias, as in these situations the P wave is absent or difficult to identify; though, these cardiac abnormalities are extremely infrequent in the pediatric patient, so that applicability of IC-ECG is 100% in neonates and children.

Also, the IC-ECG is extremely easy to perform, easy to teach and easy to learn. Training is very fast (complete training is achieved within few procedures) and the learning curve quite steep.

In neonates, there might be some problems of feasibility of the IC-ECG when inserting ECCs. These catheters have and extremely narrow lumen, so that the column of saline contained inside the catheter may not be reliable in terms of conductivity. Though several interesting clinical studies have shown the possibility of using IC-ECG for ECCs, it seems reasonable that for this type of catheters ultrasound-based methods of tip location might be logistically easier and more cost effective.

Many clinical studies have shown that IC-ECG is applicable and feasible also during the insertion of UVC. Though, there are some considerations that suggest that ultrasound-based tip location might be preferable for UVC: (a) insertion of UVC requires ultrasound for tip navigation, so that it seems simpler and more logical to complete the maneuver using ultrasound also for tip location; (b) while the electrical correlate of the junction between superior vena cava and right atrium is very well define (maximal P wave), this is not true for the junction between inferior vena cava and right atrium, which is the ideal location for the tip of the UVC; (c) the clinical setting of UVC insertion (often in the delivery room, soon after birth) is compatible with use of bedside ultrasound (in particular if adopting wireless probes), while to perform an electrocardiogram as surface ECG and then intracavitary ECG may be logistically more complex.

Apart from these two exceptions (ECC, UVC), IC-ECG is certainly the tip location method to be preferred in all central lines (CICC, FICC, PICC, port) inserted in neonates, infants, and children, being characterized by 100% applicability, 100% feasibility, maximal accuracy (no false positives; false negatives only in untrained hands or when technical problems of the ECG monitor occur) and maximal safety.

6.2.2 Ultrasound Based Tip Location

Ultrasound has been thoroughly investigated as tip location method for central venous access in the last two decades. Not surprisingly, many studies have been carried out in pediatric patients, as this population is easier to explore with ultrasound if compared to adults. The term TTE (trans-thoracic echocardiography) may be slightly imprecise, since ultrasound-based tip location is preferably carried out placing the probe in the epigastric area (subcostal view), while actual trans-thoracic views (apical view, etc.) are used only as a second option.

Two documents have recently standardized ultrasound-based tip location in neonates (Neo-ECHOTIP) and in infants and children (ECHOTIP-Ped).

Ultrasound based tip location is carried out by visualization of the right atrium (with or without visualization of the last tract of the cava veins) using a microconvex probe or a sectorial probe ('phase array'). The best option is to locate the probe in the epigastric area, under the xyphoid process (so-called 'sub-xyphoid view'), directing the probe upward to diaphragm, so to visualize the liver and the heart. Two views are commonly used: the four-chamber subcostal view (transverse visualization of both atria and both ventricles) (Figs. 6.9 and 6.10) and the bi-caval subcostal view (oblique visualization of the right atrium, of the last tract of the superior vena cava and the last tract of the inferior vena cava) (Figs. 6.11 and 6.12).

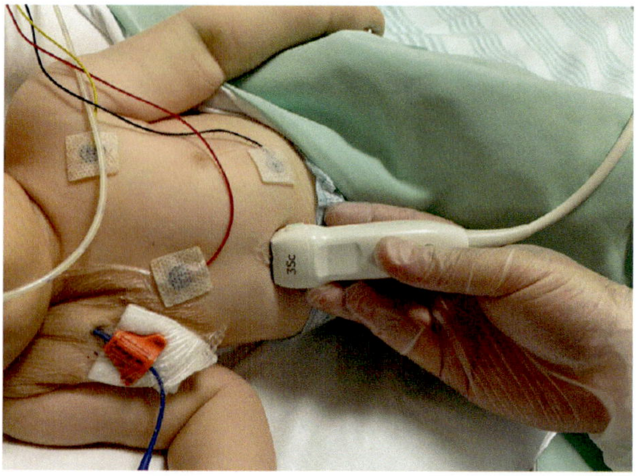

Fig. 6.9 Subcostal transverse view: position of the probe

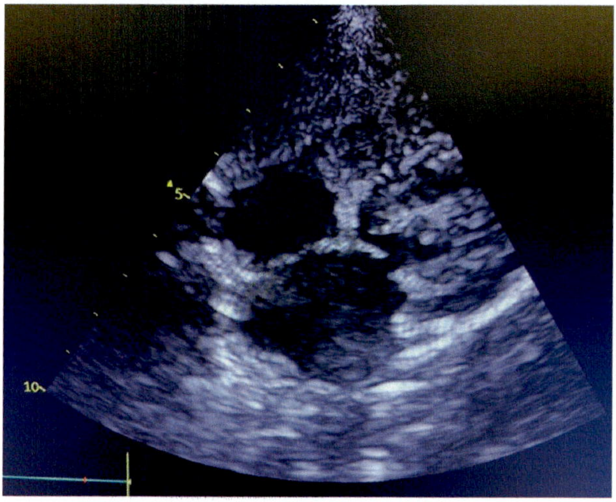

Fig. 6.10 Subcostal transverse view: four-chamber visualization

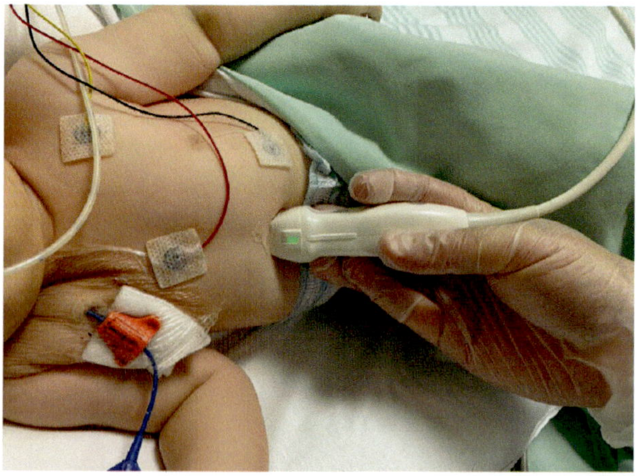

Fig. 6.11 Subcostal oblique 'bi-caval' view: position of the probe

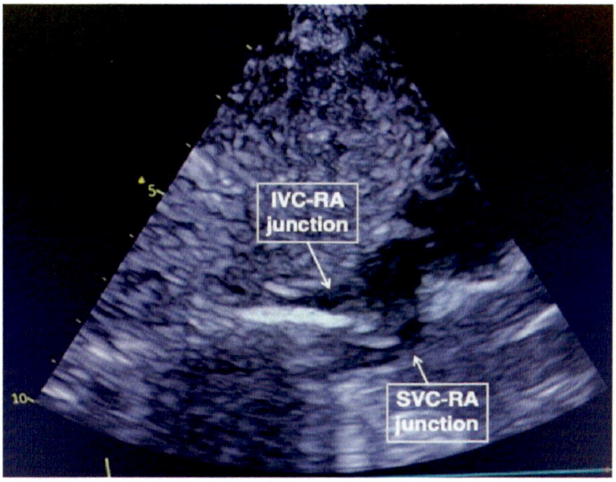

Fig. 6.12 Subcostal oblique 'bi-caval' view: visualization of right atrium, last tract of the superior vena cava and last tract of the inferior vena cava

When the subcostal views are difficult or nor feasible, the second option is to use a 'real' transthoracic view, such as the four-chamber apical view (visualization of both atria and both ventricles). In neonates, a trans-thoracic para-sternal view may be useful for visualization of the superior vena cava and of the right atrium.

The rationale of ultrasound-based tip location is either the direct visualization of the tip of the catheter or an indirect visualization of the tip by the so-called 'bubble test' (rapid injection of saline into the catheter, visualized as micro-bubbles in the right atrium).

When the tip of the CICC or PICC or FICC or ECC is in the right atrium, the catheter can be directly visualized by any type of subcostal view or trans-thoracic view; if the image is not clear, the 'bubble test' can improve the detection of the tip.

When the tip of the FICC or ECC or UVC is in the upper portion of the inferior vena cava, the tip can be easily seen by a subcostal 'bi-caval' view or even by the direct visualization of the inferior vena cava below the liver.

When the tip of the CICC or PICC or ECC is in the lower third of the superior vena cava, the tip can be directly visualized by a subcostal bi-caval view (or by a parasternal view in neonates); if the image is not clear, the 'bubble test' can improve the detection of the tip. Or, the position of the tip can be indirectly visualized with the bubble test, watching the delay in the appearance of micro-bubbles in the right atrium (using anyone of the views above described) after saline injection through the catheter. The immediate appearance of the bubbles after the injection (Fig. 6.13) confirms that the tip is very close to the right atrium, i.e., in the lower portion of the SVC or in the upper portion of the IVC.

In neonates, injection of 5 ml of standard saline is enough, as the ultrasound visualization of the bubbles is very easy. In children, it may be useful to use 10 ml of saline and 'shake' the saline in the syringe before injection. The infusion must be very rapid. If the delay in appearance of the micro-bubbles in the right atrium is one second or more, it is likely that the tip of the catheter is too high in the SVC (or even in the BCV) or too low in the IVC (or even in the iliac veins).

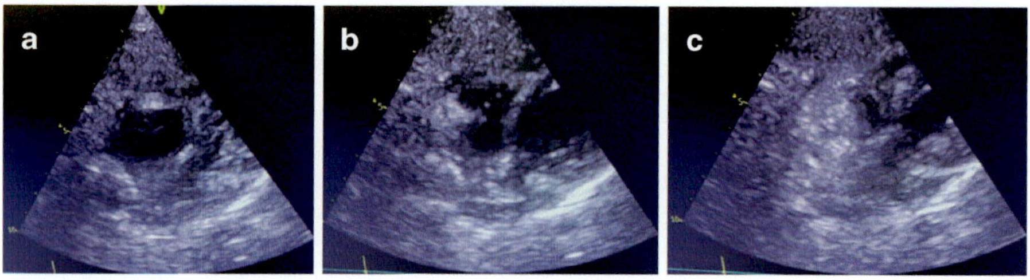

Fig. 6.13 From A to C: progressive visualization of 'micro-bubbles' inside the right atrium soon after saline injection through the catheter

In summary, ultrasound-based tip location has a 100% applicability. Feasibility may vary, depending on the training of the operator, on the type of view adopted and on the body size of the patient (neonates are much easier to explore by ultrasound if compared to children). The accuracy is 100% in neonates (no false positives; no false negatives, when training is appropriate) but somehow less in children, considering that the 'indirect' visualization of the tip is less precise than the direct visualization: the interpretation of the magnitude of the delay of appearance of the micro-bubbles may be quite subjective and affected by the technical performance of the ultrasound device.

In comparison with IC-ECG, ultrasound-based tip location (a) is logistically simpler (in particular if using wireless probes), (b) requires more training, (c) may be less accurate in older children.

Considering that both methods are 100% safe and quite cost-effective, it is reasonable to use them simultaneously, so to avoid the radiological methods in any central venous access in neonates, infants, and children. Ultrasound based tip location is expected to give the best results in neonates and infants, while IC-ECG is the method of choice in children of any age.

Bibliography

1. Barone G, Pittiruti M, Ancora G, Vento G, Tota F, D'Andrea V. Centrally inserted central catheters in preterm neonates with weight below 1500g by ultrasound-guided access to the brachio-cephalic vein. J Vasc Access 2021a May;22(3):344–352. https://doi.org/10.1177/1129729820940174. Epub 2020 Jul 10.
2. Barone G, Pittiruti M, Biasucci DG, Elisei D, Iacobone E, La Greca A, Zito Marinosci G, D'Andrea V. Neo-ECHOTIP: a structured protocol for ultrasound-based tip navigation and tip location during placement of central venous access devices in neonates. J Vasc Access 2021b Apr 5:11297298211007703. https://doi.org/10.1177/11297298211007703. Epub ahead of print. PMID: 33818191.
3. Capasso A, Mastroianni R, Passariello A, Palma M, Messina F, Ansalone A, Bernardo I, Brescia D, Crispino F, Grassia C, Romano A, Ausanio G. The intracavitary electrocardiography method for positioning the tip of epicutaneous cava catheter in neonates: pilot study. J Vasc Access 2018 Nov;19(6):542–547. https://doi.org/10.1177/1129729818761292. Epub 2018 Mar 18. PMID: 29552936.

4. Cellini M, Bergadano A, Crocoli A, Badino C, Carraro F, Sidro L, Botta D, Pancaldi A, Rossetti F, Pitta F, Cesaro S. Guidelines of the Italian Association of Pediatric Hematology and Oncology for the management of the central venous access devices in pediatric patients with onco-hematological disease. J Vasc Access 2020 Nov 10:1129729820969309. https://doi.org/10.1177/1129729820969309. Epub ahead of print. PMID: 33169648.
5. Crocoli A, Tornesello A, Pittiruti M, Barone A, Muggeo P, Inserra A, Molinari AC, Grillenzoni V, Durante V, Cicalese MP, Zanazzo GA, Cesaro S. Central venous access devices in pediatric malignancies: a position paper of Italian Association of Pediatric Hematology and Oncology. J Vasc Access 2015 Mar-Apr;16(2):130–136. https://doi.org/10.5301/jva.5000314. Epub 2014 Oct 14. PMID: 25362978.
6. Iacobone E, Elisei D, Gattari D, Carbone L, Capozzoli G. Transthoracic echocardiography as bedside technique to verify tip location of central venous catheters in patients with atrial arrhythmia. J Vasc Access 2020 Nov;21(6):861–867. https://doi.org/10.1177/1129729820905200. Epub 2020 Mar 4. PMID: 32126882.
7. Lamperti M, Biasucci DG, Disma N, Pittiruti M, Breschan C, Vailati D, Subert M, Traškaitė V, Macas A, Estebe JP, Fuzier R, Boselli E, Hopkins P. European Society of Anaesthesiology guidelines on peri-operative use of ultrasound-guided for vascular access (PERSEUS vascular access). Eur J Anaesthesiol. 2020 May;37(5):344–376. https://doi.org/10.1097/EJA.0000000000001180. Erratum in: Eur J Anaesthesiol. 2020 Jul;37(7):623. PMID: 32265391.
8. Mastroianni R, Capasso A, Ausanio G. The intracavitary electrocardiography method for tip location of jugular internal vein access device in infants of less than 5 kg: a pilot study. J Vasc Access 2018 Nov;19(6):639–643. https://doi.org/10.1177/1129729818769028. Epub 2018 Apr 13. PMID: 29651905.
9. Pittiruti M, Pelagatti F, Pinelli F. Intracavitary electrocardiography for tip location during central venous catheterization: a narrative review of 70 years of clinical studies. J Vasc Access 2020 Jun 24:1129729820929835. https://doi.org/10.1177/1129729820929835. Epub ahead of print. PMID: 32578489.
10. Raffaele A, Segal A, Romano P, Vatta F, Boghen S, Bonetti F, Parigi GB, Avolio L. Intracavitary electrocardiography-guided positioning of central vascular access device can spare unnecessary ionizing radiation exposure in pediatric patients. J Vasc Access 2021 Jan;22(1):64–68. https://doi.org/10.1177/1129729820923936. Epub 2020 May 26. PMID: 32452241.
11. Rossetti F, Pittiruti M, Lamperti M, Graziano U, Celentano D, Capozzoli G. The intracavitary ECG method for positioning the tip of central venous access devices in pediatric patients: results of an Italian multicenter study. J Vasc Access 2015 Mar-Apr;16(2):137–143. https://doi.org/10.5301/jva.5000281. Epub 2014 Sep 2. PMID: 25198817.
12. Singh Y, Tissot C, Fraga MV, Yousef N, Cortes RG, Lopez J, Sanchez-de-Toledo J, Brierley J, Colunga JM, Raffaj D, Da Cruz E, Durand P, Kenderessy P, Lang HJ, Nishisaki A, Kneyber MC, Tissieres P, Conlon TW, De Luca D. International evidence-based guidelines on point of care ultrasound (POCUS) for critically ill neonates and children issued by the POCUS working Group of the European Society of paediatric and neonatal intensive care (ESPNIC). Crit Care 2020;24(1):65. https://doi.org/10.1186/s13054-020-2787-9. PMID: 32093763; PMCID: PMC7041196.
13. Spagnuolo F, Vacchiano T. Ultrasound-guided cannulation of the brachiocephalic vein in newborns: a novel approach with a supraclavicular view for tip navigation and tip location. J Vasc Access 2021 Mar 16:11297298211001159. https://doi.org/10.1177/11297298211001159. Epub ahead of print. PMID: 33726580.
14. Weber MD, Himebauch AS, Conlon T. Use of intracavitary-ECG for tip location of femorally inserted central catheters. J Vasc Access 2020 Dec 25:1129729820982864. https://doi.org/10.1177/1129729820982864. Epub ahead of print. PMID: 33356809.

Chapter 7
Chest Ultrasound for Early Diagnosis of Complications

Daniele G. Biasucci

7.1 Introduction

Point-of-care Pleural and Lung Ultrasound (PLUS) is a non-ionizing, rapidly available at bedside and easily repeatable imaging technique which is already well-established for adult emergencies and critical care. In recent years, PLUS is rapidly growing also in the field of neonatal and pediatric care.

Furthermore, PLUS is a part of the so-called '*Global Use*' of ultrasound applied to the field of vascular access. In fact, the modern ultrasound application to this field is not only limited to ultrasound-guided venipuncture but it has been extended to assist all steps of central venous catheterization allowing rational choice of appropriate vein and proper approach, prevention of malposition and ruling-out of early and late complications. Possible respiratory complications after central venipuncture substantially consist in pneumothorax (PNX) or, less frequently, hemothorax. These conditions may be diagnosed or excluded at bedside using PLUS with both high specificity and sensitivity. Even brief training and a few supervised examinations have been shown to allow safe and reproducible recognition of these conditions. Moreover, recent data suggest that the use of PLUS, which is a radiation-free imaging technique, reduces both cumulative radiation and number of chest X-rays (CXR) in neonates and children.

The present chapter will focus on the basics of PLUS and how to perform and interpret a PLUS exam focused on the diagnosis of PNX or hemothorax. Then, all the published evidence supporting the use of PLUS to prevent and rule-out or, eventually, confirm respiratory complications will be reviewed. Finally, how to integrate PLUS during bedside procedure of central venous access will be discussed.

D. G. Biasucci (✉)
Intensive Care Unit, Department of Emergency, Anesthesiology and Intensive Care, Fondazione Policlinico Universitario "A. Gemelli" IRCCS, Rome, Italy
e-mail: danieleguerino.biasucci@policlinicogemelli.it

D. G. Biasucci et al. (eds.), *Vascular Access in Neonates and Children*,
https://doi.org/10.1007/978-3-030-94709-5_7

7.2 Fundamentals of Pleural and Lung Ultrasound

The lung has historically been considered unsuitable for ultrasound evaluation. In fact, being it an air-rich organ and because ultrasound energy is known to be rapidly dissipated by air, theoretically, ultrasound imaging might not be useful for the evaluation of the pulmonary parenchyma. On the other hand, exactly this limitation of ultrasound is paradoxically advantageous for lung assessment. In fact, PLUS basically relies on the analysis of ultrasound artifacts generated by the mismatch at the acoustic interface between air and surrounding tissues. The two prevalent artifacts consist in A-lines and B-lines whose dynamic changes are mostly related to the air–fluid ratio and lung density.

Pleura is the only detectable structure in a normally aerated lung. It is visualized as a hyperechoic horizontal line moving synchronously with respiration. A-lines are reverberation artifacts of the pleural line (Fig. 7.1A). The progressive loss of aeration determines the appearance of B-lines, vertical artifacts belonging to the family of the comet-tails, whose number increases along with decreasing air content and increasing in exudate or transudate in the interstitial or alveolar compartment (i.e. pulmonary edema, pneumonia, ARDS etc.) (Fig. 7.1B). Then, this phenomenon is followed by the development of pleural line abnormalities and thickening and subpleural consolidations (Fig. 7.1C). Finally, when the air content further decreases,

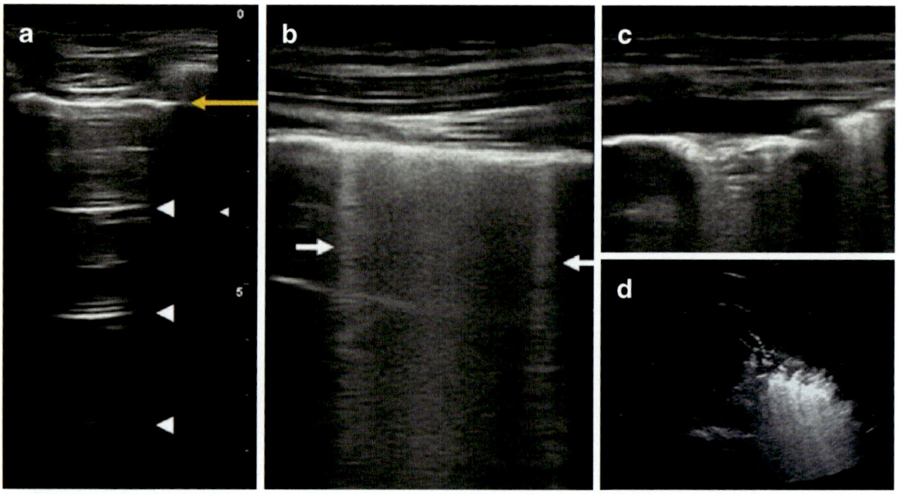

Fig. 7.1 **A.** In a normally aerated lung, the only detectable structure is the pleura, visualized as a hyperechoic horizontal line (yellow arrow). A-lines are hyperechoic horizontal lines deep to the pleural line, recurring at regular intervals (arrowheads). A-lines are reverberation artefacts of the pleural line. **B.** *B-lines.* B-lines are vertical hyperechoic lines, belonging to the family of the comet-tail artifacts, arising from pleural line, and extending downward to the edge of the screen (white arrows). **C.** Pleural line abnormalities and anterior subpleural consolidations. **D.** Lung consolidations: when the air content decreases—as in consolidations—the acoustic window on the lung becomes completely open and the lung may be directly visualized as a solid parenchyma

such as in lung consolidations (i.e., pneumonia, atelectasis etc.), the complete loss of aeration increases lung density lowering the acoustic mismatch between air and surrounding tissues, so the sonographic beam is partly reflected at deeper layers allowing the lung to be directly visualized with ultrasound as a solid parenchyma (Fig. 7.1D). In other words, PLUS acts as a sort of '*densitometer*' being sensitive to the variation of air–fluid ratio and lung density.

In a normal and physiologically aerated lung, PLUS allows to detect the regular rhythmic movement, synchronized with respiration, of the two pleural layers one over each other. This sonographic sign is called *lung sliding*. A further subtle rhythmic pleural line movement synchronized with cardiac beats can be detected with PLUS. This sign is called *lung pulse*. Lung sliding is determined by lung inflation and deflation during respiration, whilst lung pulse is caused by the transmission of the heart beats through the lung. All the above-mentioned signs can be evaluated using brightness mode (B-mode) and motion mode (M-mode). The latter can be used for objectifying and documenting lung sliding, generating the so-called *seashore sign*, and also the presence of lung pulse (Fig. 7.2). In the *seashore sign* the "sea" is represented by the chest wall, the "foam" is the pleural line and the "shore" is the granular pattern of the normal sliding of the two pleural layers.

The above-mentioned B-lines are often visualized also in the normal 'dry' lung, even if isolated in some specific areas of the chest. B-lines move synchronously with lung sliding and since such an artifact originates from the visceral pleura, its simple presence proves that the visceral pleura is opposing to the parietal one (Fig. 7.1B). Multiple B-lines are considered the sonographic sign of lung interstitial syndrome, and their number increases along with increasing in extravascular lung water.

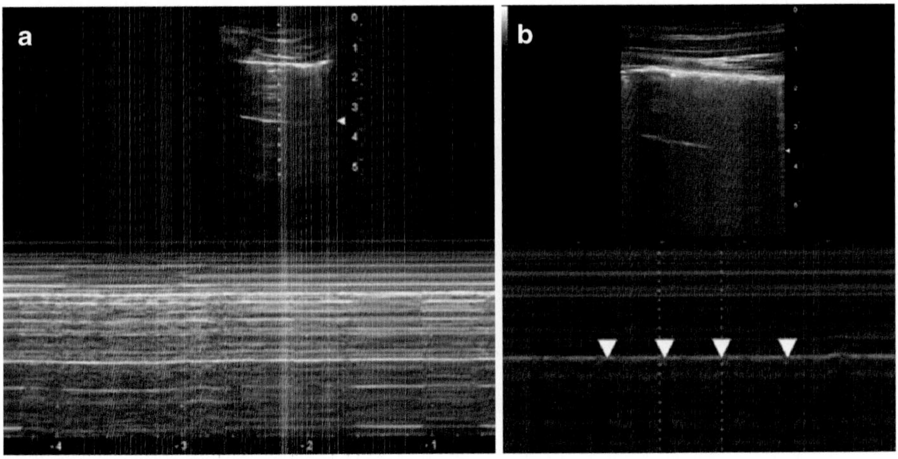

Fig. 7.2 **A.** For objectifying and documenting lung sliding, M-mode yields a simple pattern, the seashore sign: the 'sea' is the not moving chest wall, the 'foam' is the pleural line and the 'shore' is the granular pattern of the normal sliding lung. **B.** Lung pulse: the subtle rhythmic movement of the pleura, synchronous with cardiac beats (arrowheads)

7.3 How to Perform a Lung Ultrasound Exam

The use of linear probes in neonates and infants and micro-convex probes in older children is recommended. Linear probes are high frequency transducers (5–14 MHz), generally well suited for the analysis of the pleural line, which is superficial and easily visualized. Convex and micro-convex probes are lower frequencies transducers (2–5 MHz) useful to evaluate deeper artifacts and structures.

The probe can be positioned longitudinally, perpendicular to two or more consecutive ribs (Fig. 7.3A). This kind of approach allows visualization of the so-called '*bat-sign*', in which the upper and lower ribs are the wings of the bat and, a little deeper, the pleural line is the body of the bat (Fig. 7.3B). The probe can be positioned obliquely, along the intercostal spaces (Fig. 7.4A). This latter kind of approach allows visualizing a larger part of the pleural line not interrupted by the rib shadows (Fig. 7.4B).

PLUS examination has to be started placing the probe parallel to the long axis of the patient's body in the parasternal area so to visualize the above mentioned *bat sign* (Fig. 7.3). Beginning the procedure through this plane is important since it allows inexperienced operators to identify immediately pleural line. In fact, without a simultaneous visualization of ribs and pleura, the sonographer may inadvertently interpret the hyperechoic costal surface as the pleural line. Once the latter has been detected, the probe can be rotated to be aligned with the long axis of the intercostal

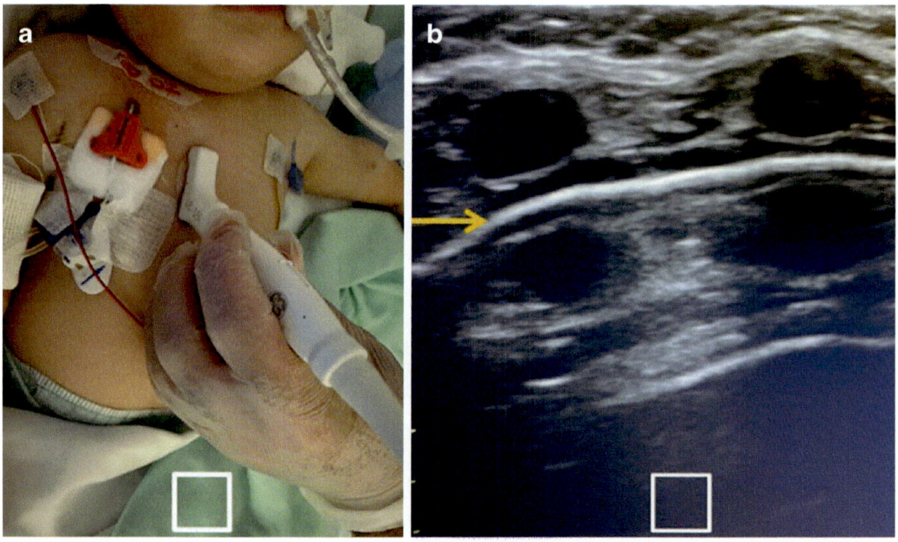

Fig. 7.3 **A.** The probe is positioned longitudinally, perpendicular to two (or more) consecutive ribs. **B.** The longitudinal approach allows visualization of the so-called "bat-sign": the upper and lower ribs are the wings of the bat and, a little deeper, the pleural line is the body of the bat (yellow arrow)

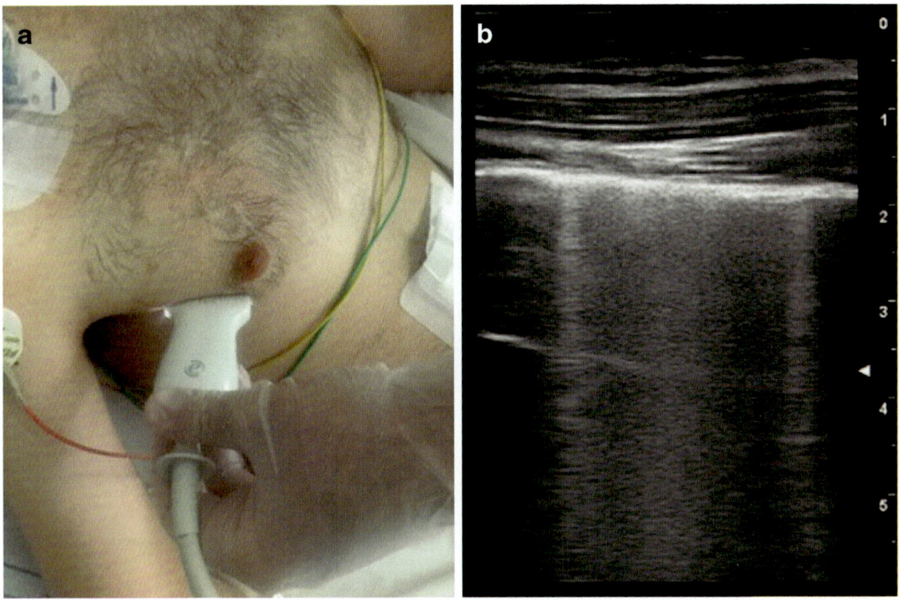

Fig. 7.4 **A.** The probe can also be positioned obliquely, along the intercostal space. **B.** The oblique approach allows visualizing a larger part of the pleural line not interrupted by the rib shadows

space. This oblique plane allows the visualization of a larger extension of the pleural line (Fig. 7.4).

PLUS exam must include the anterior, anterolateral and posterior-lateral portions of the chest wall evaluated in a clinically integrated goal-directed manner based on patient's clinical presentation. In fact, depending on several factors such as the diagnostic questions and clinical conditions, it is necessary to scan more intercostal spaces by moving the probe laterally and inferiorly.

The conventional B-mode imaging, often associated with M-mode, is adequate. Occasionally color Doppler may be helpful.

7.4 How to Diagnose or Rule-out Pneumothorax

PNX is a pathological condition characterized by the presence of air between the two pleural layers, causing a change of the sonographic dynamic image of the lung. In fact, the air below the parietal pleura does not allow to visualize the visceral pleura. In case of PNX the parietal pleura is the only detectable structure but does not move, not with respiration nor with cardiac beats. In PNX, lung sliding and lung pulse are absent. Absence of lung sliding and lung pulse may be objectified using M-mode which yields that characteristic pattern known as the '*stratosphere sign*' (Fig. 7.5). Furthermore, B-lines cannot be detected in case of PNX since such a

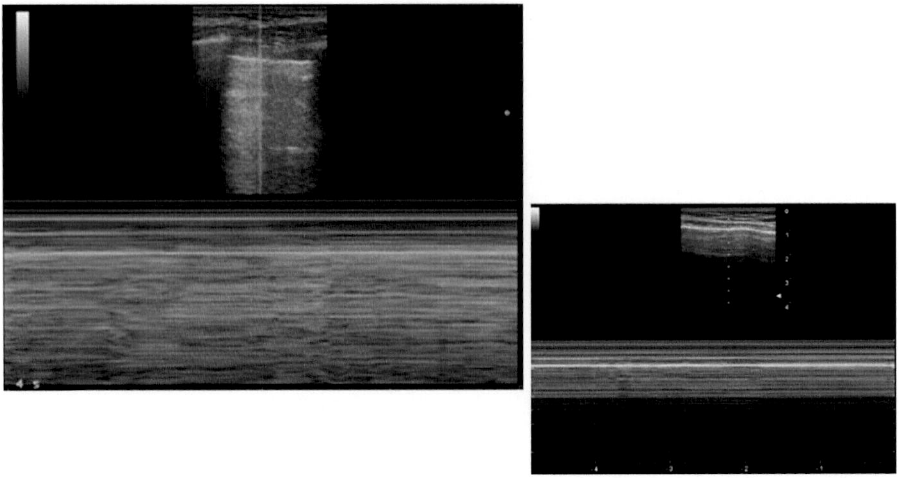

Fig. 7.5 Typical PNX M-mode pattern: the so-called 'stratosphere sign' (see text)

artifact originates from the interlobular septa covered by the visceral pleura which does not slide onto the parietal one in this specific pathological condition. When PNX is present, there are also points where the visceral pleura adheres again to the parietal pleura depicting the physical lateral limit of the intrapleural air layer. This transition point between PNX and normal lung can be detected with PLUS and it is known as '*lung point*'. The lung point is a highly specific sign which represents a point on the chest wall where the typical sonographic pattern of PNX (absence of lung sliding and B-lines) into the normal pattern of lung sliding (Fig. 7.6A).

In case of PNX, air in the pleural space tends to accumulate in the non-dependent areas of the chest. When the patient lies in the supine position, the areas of interest correspond to the anterior and inferior part of the chest at the third and fourth intercostal spaces between the parasternal and the mid-clavicular lines. The exam must start placing the probe in this area as discussed above (Figs. 7.3 and 7.4). Then, moving the probe laterally and inferiorly, further intercostal spaces need to be examined in order to evaluate the extension of PNX or to confirm the diagnosis looking for the lung point (Fig. 7.6B).

The sonographic diagnosis of PNX includes the following sings:

- Absence of lung sliding;
- Absence of B-lines;
- Absence of lung pulse;
- Presence of lung point(s).

However, the absence of lung sliding alone does not allow to confirm PNX diagnosis, since several other conditions, like massive consolidations, pulmonary contusions, ARDS, and pleural adhesions, may cause a motionless pleural line. These conditions are frequent in critically ill patients and in emergency conditions. For

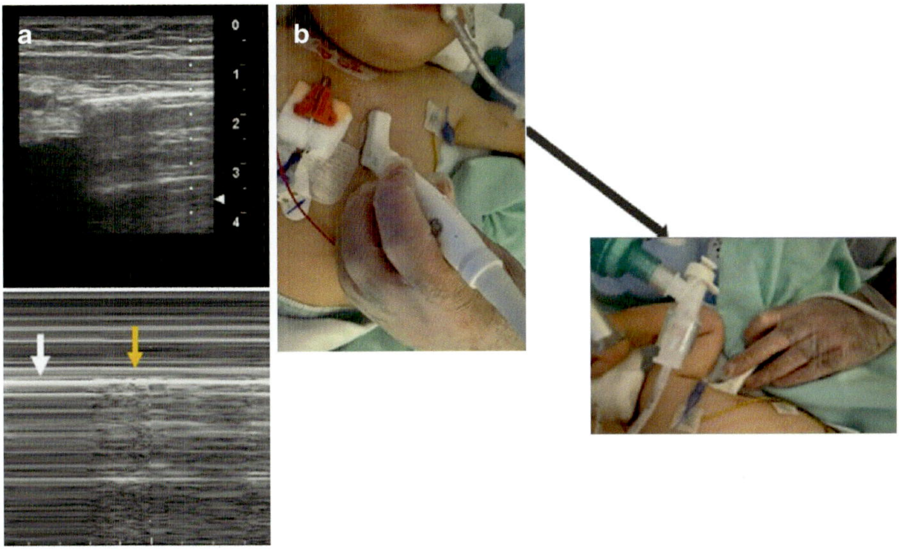

Fig. 7.6 **A.** Lung Point(s): highly specific sign which represents the transition point between the typical sonographic pattern of PNX (absence of lung sliding and of B-lines) (white arrow) into the normal pattern of lung sliding (yellow arrow) **B.** Searching for lung point(s)—moving the probe laterally on the chest wall—allows PNX extension evaluation. In fact, lung point(s) depict the physical limit of PNX and can be employed to detect the extension of PNX, but not its volume

these reasons, when PLUS is applied in these specific situations, the specificity of the absent lung sliding in predicting PNX has been proved to be lower. Recently, some authors have also hypothesized that the contraction of the recruited intercostal muscles in a dyspneic patient due to PNX may generates artifacts mimicking lung sliding even it should be absent. In 2014, Cavaliere and coworkers have published a case series of 8 spontaneously breathing patients who had undergone pneumonectomy and presenting a sign mimicking the lung sliding on the same side of the pneumonectomy. This sign was not present during controlled mechanical ventilation when patients were sedated and paralyzed but it was recognizable after weaning when they were spontaneously breathing. Therefore, for all these reasons, a safe diagnosis or rule-out of PNX by PLUS must necessarily rely also on the other sonographic signs particularly the B-lines and the lung points.

In case of PNX, the visualization of even one isolated B-line in the non-dependent areas proves the adherence of the visceral pleura to the parietal pleura. Visualization of B-lines allows to rule-out PNX with a true negative rate of 100%. Obviously, the only absence of B-lines is not an indicator of PNX. Looking at this sign, there is a condition in which the sonographer could be misled: in case of subcutaneous emphysema comet-tail artifacts mimicking B-lines can be seen. These artifacts are known as ‘E-lines’ (*E* for emphysema). Compared with B-lines, E-lines originates from the subcutaneous tissues and not from the pleural line which cannot be seen due to the air above the pleura and outside the thorax. So, E-lines have not to be confused with B-lines. To avoid misdiagnosis, the sonographer must be sure to visualize the bat sign, the pleural line between two ribs and deeper, then the same depth of the pleural line on both sides of the chest should be observed.

PNX is characterized by the absence of both lung sliding and lung pulse due to the presence of air between the two pleural layers. Thus, visualization of lung pulse allows to rule out PNX. This sign is very useful to differentiate PNX from other conditions characterized by the absence of lung sliding. In a study on patients with cardiac activity but absent lung sliding due to massive atelectasis and main-stem intubation, lung pulse was a common finding which allowed diagnosis with 93% sensitivity.

As already written above, the lung point is 100% specific for PNX diagnosis. Unfortunately, the sensitivity of this sign is low because in the case of massive PNX with complete lung collapse where no lung points can be visualized. On the contrary, in the stable patient and especially in the case of small radio-occult PNX (*i.e.* after central vein puncture attempts), sensitivity of the lung point is higher and when the lung point is detected PNX can be diagnosed. In case PNX confirmation, the lung point is useful to assess PNX extension.

However, in emergency conditions, absence of any movement of the pleural line, either lung sliding or lung pulse, coupled with absence of B-lines allows prompt diagnosis of PNX without the need for searching the lung point.

PLUS has been proved to be more accurate than CXR in ruling out PNX especially for those small radio-occult PNXs.

The international Liaison Committee on Lung Ultrasound for the International Consensus Conference on Lung Ultrasound (ICC-LUS)—in the international evidence-based recommendations for point-of-care lung ultrasound published in 2012 on Intensive Care Medicine—proposes the use of a flow chart suggesting the correct sequence and how to combine the four sonographic signs to rule out or rule in PNX.

7.5 How to Diagnose or Rule-out Hemothorax

Hemothorax is a pathological condition characterized by the presence of blood between the two pleural layers. The presence of fluid between the two pleural layers can be easily detected using PLUS as a fluid mass (Fig. 7.7).

In the evaluation of hemothorax, the micro-convex transducer is preferable. If not available, a phased array transducer can be used. In neonates, small infants, and preterm newborns also the same linear probe with which the puncture has been performed can be used.

The optimal site to detect a pleural effusion in a supine patient is at the posterior axillary line just above the diaphragm.

PLUS is more accurate in distinguishing pleural effusion from atelectasis than CXR presenting 100% sensitivity and 90% specificity.

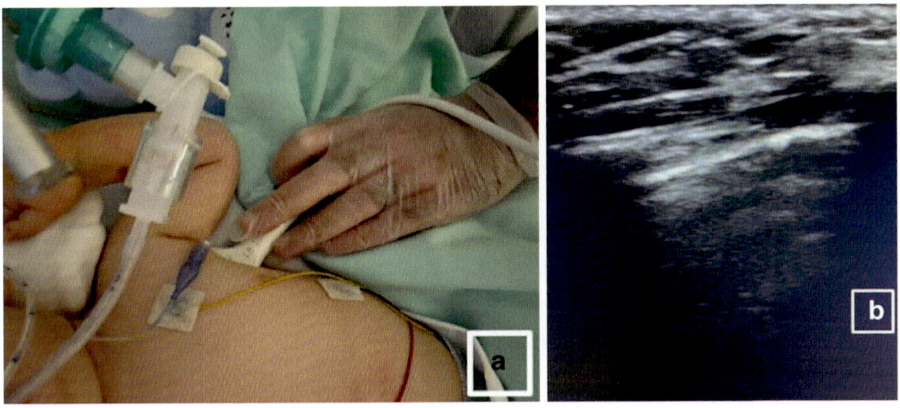

Fig. 7.7 **A.** To detect pleural effusion the transducer is placed longitudinally on the lateral and posterior regions of the chest wall, just above the diaphragm; **B.** *Curtain Sign* allowing to rule-out pleural effusion

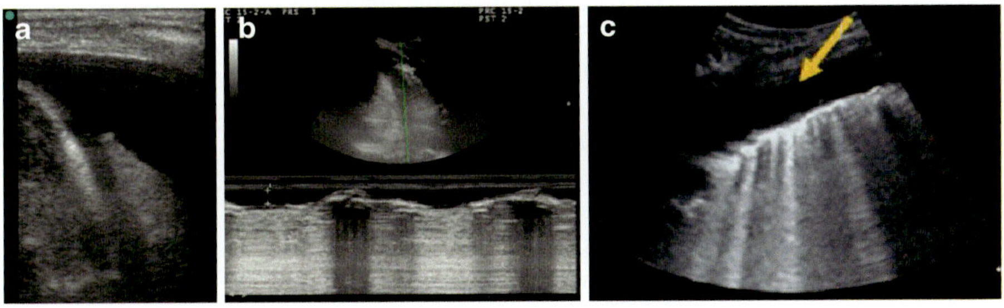

Fig. 7.8 **A.** Fluid mass between the two pleural layers (pleural effusion) and **B.** the M- mode documenting the *Sinusoid Sign* (respiratory movements of the lung within the effusion); **C.** loculated and corpuscular fluid mass with internal echoes between the two pleural layers (yellow arrow)

In case of hemothorax or other kind of pleural effusions both the following signs are present:

- a fluid mass between the parietal and visceral pleura;
- respiratory movements of the lung within the effusion, the so called '*sinusoid sign*'.

The sinusoid sign is a dynamic sign showing the variation of the distance between the two pleural layers during the respiratory cycle. This sign may be easily objectified using M-mode as a sinusoid movement of the visceral pleura (Fig. 7.6B).

PLUS has the potential also for diagnosing the nature of the effusion. Effusion may be a free fluid mass, in this case, using PLUS, it appears as an anechoic mass between the visceral and parietal pleura. Visualization of internal echoes, either of mobile particles in corpuscular effusions or septa in loculated effusion, is highly suggestive of exudate or hemothorax (Fig. 7.8). However, while most transudates are anechoic, some exudates are also anechoic. In the latter case, thoracentesis may be needed for further characterization.

Finally, in case of hemothorax PLUS plays a major role in guiding chest drainage procedure if needed.

7.6 Evidence Supporting the Role of Pleural and Lung Ultrasound as a Part of the 'Global Use' of Ultrasound Applied to the Procedure of Central Venous Access and its Clinical Usefulness

Even if performed by ultrasound guidance, neonatal and pediatric central venous cannulation remains a delicate and potentially dangerous procedure especially when puncturing the subclavian vein in the supraclavicular area or the transition tract between the subclavian vein and the brachiocephalic vein and when accessing the axillary vein at the thorax. The risk of pleuro-pulmonary mechanical complications is high especially in neonates or in low weight premature newborns. Therefore, today it is strongly recommended to have the ultrasound equipment available soon after the procedure for early ultrasound detection of respiratory life-threatening complications especially in case of difficult puncture of the subclavian or axillary vein, and particularly if the patient suffers from shortness of breath or complains of discomfort or pain worsening after catheter placement.

Several observational prospective studies and some meta-analyses have been published on the accuracy of ultrasound to detect respiratory complications after central veins puncture both in adults and pediatric patients. In these studies, sensitivity, and specificity of PLUS for identification of post-procedural PNX were nearly 100%. There were 13 PNXs in 13 observational prospective studies, all were identified by PLUS, whereas only 10 were identified by the CXR. Obviously, this already well-known superiority of PLUS when compared with CXR for PNX detection is consistent with the above-mentioned literature and has been confirmed also when performed soon after the procedure of central veins puncture to rule-out a post-procedural so-called radio-occult PNX. In fact, in most cases, the damage of pleura during the procedure of central veins puncture substantially results in a small radio-occult PNX which is usually missed by the conventional CXR by definition. PLUS has been shown to be more sensitive than supine CXR and similar to CT scan in the detection of post-procedural iatrogenic PNX. Even if a radio-occult small PNX in a stable patient is not usually drained, follow-up, observation and sonographic monitoring is mandatory as in some patients it may quickly progress to cause hemodynamic instability. As mentioned above, the location of the lung point(s) in the supine patient allows to predict the PNX extension which can be monitored over time looking at the changes of lung point(s) location on the chest wall. For detection and monitoring of effusions and hemothorax, PLUS is proved to be more accurate than supine CXR and is as accurate as CT scan both in adults and pediatrics. Particularly when anterior–posterior view in the supine patient is considered, CXR has low sensitivity. Moreover, often pleural effusion might be erroneously interpreted as atelectasis on CXR and vice versa.

Bedside PLUS, performed by adequately trained physicians, allows faster diagnosis of pleuro-pulmonary complications compared with CXR. In fact, in published studies, the average mean time required for bedside sonographic diagnosis of PNX after central venipuncture was about 5 minutes as compared to an average mean time to CXR completion of more than 1 hour and an average mean time to CXR interpretation of more than 2 hours.

PLUS is a non-ionizing, highly accurate and rapid diagnostic technique whose spread and systematic use among clinicians should be encouraged since it has been proved to significantly reduce the exposure of neonates and children to several unnecessary ionizing radiation with obvious benefits.

However, to gain its maximum effectiveness, PLUS should be clinically integrated and performed by adequately trained healthcare providers. Although already existing training programs are heterogeneous in setup, learning and assessment methods, it has been proved that even a brief training and a few supervised exams may allow safe and reproducible recognition of the signs for PNX diagnosis on video clips. Krishnan and coworkers showed that high accuracy in excluding PNX was achieved after a simple training with a 5-minute online training video, and that this knowledge was retained for at least 6 months. See et al. have found that 10 supervised PLUS exams are sufficient to attain a high level of accuracy, greater than 95%, among ultrasound-naïve respiratory therapists. Published evidence prove that PLUS is relatively easy to teach and easy to learn. All standardized training programs focused on central vascular access devices placement should include formal and practical education on pleural and lung ultrasound aimed at training operators to recognize the pleural line to avoid its damage during the procedure and to rule-out potential pleuro-pulmonary complications after a difficult puncture, especially when accessing subclavian or axillary veins.

PLUS guidance is also useful to assist chest tube placement in case of confirmed pneumothorax or hemothorax to be drained. There are no studies in neonates and small infants about these procedures, but it is probable that PLUS may provide similar advantages. Furthermore, some authors have successfully performed a PLUS-guided drainage of a tension pneumomediastinum.

Published studies confirm that PLUS is an excellent and powerful tool for detection of PNX, also in neonates, and hemothorax. When performed by appropriately trained healthcare providers in a clinically integrated manner its cost-effectiveness attains its maximum.

7.7 Take Home Messages and Practical Considerations

- The pleura and the lung must be visualized before every puncture of a central vein during pre-procedural evaluation of all possible venous options. In fact, proximity and contiguity with the pleural line should be considered when choosing the safest vein to be punctured and proper approach.
- The pleura must be visualized during the procedure when performing an approach to central venipuncture at risk for potential pleural damage.
- Soon after the procedure, PLUS must be performed in order to rule-out or diagnose potential pleuro-pulmonary complications, mainly PNX and hemothorax, in any difficult puncture of the subclavian or axillary vein, and particularly if the patient complains of shortness of breath, discomfort or pain worsening after catheter placement.
- The micro-convex probe or the same linear probe with which central venipuncture has been performed can be used for pleural line evaluation. The linear probe is effective in neonates, preterm newborns, and small infants also for diagnosis of hemothorax. In older children, the linear probe allows exclusion or diagnosis of PNX, whilst in order to confirm hemothorax, the micro-convex probe is preferred.
- In the supine patient, the probe must be positioned in the parasternal area to exclude or confirm PNX. The probe must be placed perpendicular to two or more consecutive ribs and it can be moved laterally and inferiorly to evaluate PNX extension.
- The probe must be placed in the dependent areas of the lung, between posterior and middle axillary lines and just above the diaphragm, in order to exclude or diagnose pleural effusions like hemothorax after central venipuncture.
- If PNX is confirmed, its progression can be monitored over time using PLUS.
- If PNX or hemothorax needs to be drained, PLUS can be used to guide the procedure of chest drainage placement.

Bibliography

1. Ablordeppey EA, Drewry AM, Beyer AB, Theodoro DL, Fowler SA, Fuller BM, Carpenter CR. Diagnostic accuracy of central venous catheter confirmation by bedside ultrasound versus chest radiography in critically ill patients: a systematic review and meta-analysis. Crit Care Med. 2017;45(4):715–24. https://doi.org/10.1097/CCM.0000000000002188.
2. Alrajhi K, Woo MY, Vaillancourt C. Test characteristics of ultrasonography for the detection of pneumothorax: a systematic review and meta-analysis. Chest. 2012;141:703–8.
3. Ambroggio L, Sucharew H, Rattan MS, et al. Lung ultrasonography: a viable alternative to chest radiog- raphy in children with suspected pneumonia? J Pediatr. 2016;176(93–98):e7. https://doi.org/10.1016/j.jpeds.2016.05.033.
4. Ball CG, Kirkpatrick AW, Feliciano DV. The occult pneumothorax: what have we learned? Can J Surg. 2009;52:E173–9.

5. Ball CG, Kirkpatrick AW, Laupland KB, et al. Factors related to the failure of radiographic recognition of occult post-traumatic pneumothoraces. Am J Surg. 2005;189:541–6.
6. Biasucci DG, La Greca A, Scoppettuolo G, Pittiruti M. What's really new in the field of vascular access? Towards a global use of ultrasound. Intensive Care Med. 2015;41(4):731–3. https://doi.org/10.1007/s00134-015-3728-y.
7. Biasucci DG, Ricci Z, Conti G, Cogo P. Sonographic dynamic assessment of lung injury in a child with hypoplastic left heart syndrome undergoing extracorporeal membrane oxygenation. Pediatr Pulmonol. 2014;49(12):E147–50. https://doi.org/10.1002/ppul.23059.
8. Brooks A, Davies B, Smethhurst M, Connolly J. Emergency ultrasound in the acute assessment of haemothorax. Emerg Med J. 2004;21:44–6.
9. Cavaliere F, Zamparelli R, Soave MP, Gargaruti R, Scapigliati A, De Paulis S. Ultrasound artifacts mimicking pleural sliding after pneumonectomy. J Clin Anesth. 2014;26(2):131–5.
10. Coley BD. Pediatric chest ultrasound. Radiol Clin N Am. 2005;43:405–18.
11. Crocoli A, Tornesello A, Pittiruti M, et al. Central venous access devices in pediatric malignancies: a position paper of Italian Association of Pediatric Hematology and Oncology. J Vasc Access. 2015;16(2):130–6. https://doi.org/10.5301/jva.5000314.
12. Detaille T, Pirotte T, Veyckemans F. Vascular access in the neonate. Best Pract Res Clin Anaesthesiol. 2010;24:403–18.
13. Dominguez A, Gaspar HA, Preto M, Ejzenberg FE. Point-of-care lung ultrasound in paediatric critical and emergency care. J Paediatr Child Health. 2018;54(9):945–52. https://doi.org/10.1111/jpc.14067.
14. Escourrou G, De Luca D. Lung ultrasound decreased radiation exposure in preterm infants in a neonatal intensive care unit. Acta Paedi- atr. 2016;105(5):e237–9. https://doi.org/10.1111/apa.13369.
15. Hill SL, Edmisten T, Holtzman G, Wright A. The occult pneumothorax: an increasing diagnostic entity in trauma. Am Surg. 1999;65:254–8.
16. International Liaison Committee on Lung Ultrasound (ILC-LUS) for the International Consensus Conference on Lung Ultrasound (ICC-LUS), Volpicelli G, Elbarbary M, Blaivas M, et al. International evidence-based recommendations for point-of-care lung ultrasound. Intensive Care Med. 2012;38(4):577–91. https://doi.org/10.1007/s00134-012-2513-4.
17. Krishnan S, Kuhl T, Ahmed W, Togashi K, Ueda K. Efficacy of an online education program for ultrasound diagnosis of pneumothorax. Anesthesiology. 2013;118:715–21.
18. Lamperti M, Bodenham AR, Pittiruti M, et al. International evidence-based recommendations on ultrasound-guided vascular access. Intensive Care Med. 2012;38(7):1105–17. https://doi.org/10.1007/s00134-012-2597-x.
19. Lamperti M, Biasucci DG, Disma N, Pittiruti M, Breschan C, Vailati D, Subert M, Traškaitė V, Macas A, Estebe JP, Fuzier R, Boselli E, Hopkins P. European Society of Anaesthesiology guidelines on peri-operative use of ultrasound-guided for vascular access (PERSEUS vascular access). Eur J Anaesthesiol. 2020;37(5):344–76. https://doi.org/10.1097/EJA.0000000000001180. Erratum in: Eur J Anaesthesiol. 2020 Jul;37(7):623
20. Lanza C, Russo M, Fabrizzi G. Central venous cannulation: are routine chest radiographs necessary after B-mode and colour Doppler sonography check? Pediatr Radiol. 2006;36(12):1252–6.
21. Lichtenstein D, Goldstein I, Mourgeon E, Cluzel P, Grenier P, Rouby JJ. Comparative diagnostic performances of auscultation, chest radiography, and lung ultrasonography in acute respiratory distress syndrome. Anesthesiology. 2004;100:9–15.
22. Lichtenstein D, Hulot JS, Rabiller A, Tostivint I, Meziere G. Feasibility and safety of ultrasound-aided thoracentesis in mechanically ventilated patients. Intensive Care Med. 1999;25:955–8.
23. Lichtenstein D, Meziere G, Biderman P, Gepner A. The comet-tail artifact, an ultrasound sign ruling out pneumothorax. Intensive Care Med. 1999;25:383–8.
24. Lichtenstein DA, Lascols N, Prin S, Mezière G. The lung pulse: an early ultrasound sign of complete atelectasis. Intensive Care Med. 2003;29:2187–92.

25. Lichtenstein DA, Menu Y. A bedside ultrasound sign ruling-out pneumothorax in the critically ill. Lung sliding Chest. 1995;108:1345–8.
26. Lichtenstein DA, Meziere GA. Relevance of lung ultrasound in the diagnosis of acute respiratory failure: the BLUE protocol. Chest. 2008;134:117–25.
27. Lichtenstein DA, Mezière G, Biderman P, Gepner A. The lung point: an ultrasound sign specific to pneumothorax. Intensive Care Med. 2000;26:1434–40.
28. Lichtenstein DA, Mezière G, Lascols N, et al. Ultrasound diagnosis of occult pneumothorax. Crit Care Med. 2005;33:1231–8.
29. Lichtenstein DA. Ultrasound in the management of thoracic disease. Crit Care Med. 2007;35:S250–61.
30. Lichtenstein DA. Whole body ultrasonography in the critically ill. Berlin-Heidelberg: Springer; 2010.
31. Monti JD, Younggren B, Blankenship R. Ultrasound detection of pneumothorax with minimally trained sonographers: a preliminary study. J Spec Oper Med. 2009;9:43–6.
32. Noble VE, Lamhaut L, Capp R, Bosson N, Liteplo A, Marx JS, Carli P. Evaluation of a thoracic ultrasound training module for the detection of pneumothorax and pulmonary edema by prehospital physician care providers. BMC Med Educ. 2009;9:3.
33. Pietersen PI, Madsen KR, Graumann O, Konge L, Nielsen BU, Laursen CB. Lung ultrasound training: a systematic review of published literature in clinical lung ultrasound training. Crit Ultrasound J. 2018;10(1):23. https://doi.org/10.1186/s13089-018-0103-6.
34. Pittiruti M, LaGreca A. How to choose the most appropriate ultrasound-guided approach for central line insertion: introducing the rapid central venous assessment protocol. In: Lumb P, Karakitsos D, editors. Critical care ultrasound. Philadelphia, PA: Saunders; 2014. p. 76–9.
35. Raimondi F, Rodriguez Fanjul J, Aversa S, et al. Lung ultrasound for diagnosing pneumothorax in the critically ill neonate. J Pediatr. 2016;175:74–8. https://doi.org/10.1016/j.jpeds.2016.04.018.
36. Raimondi F, Yousef N, Migliaro F, Capasso L, De Luca D. Point-of-care lung ultrasound in neonatology: classification into descriptive and functional applications. Pediatr Res. 2018; https://doi.org/10.1038/s41390-018-0114-9.
37. Reissig A, Kroegel C. Accuracy of transthoracic sonography in excluding post-interventional pneumothorax and hydropneumothorax. Comparison to chest radiography. Eur J Radiol. 2005;53:463–70.
38. Rocco M, Carbone I, Morelli A, et al. Diagnostic accuracy of bedside ultrasonography in the ICU: feasibility of detecting pulmonary effusion and lung contusion in patients on respiratory support after severe blunt thoracic trauma. Acta Anaesthesiol Scand. 2008;52:776–84.
39. Sajadieh H, Afzali F, Sajadieh V, Sajadieh A. Ultrasound as an alternative to aspiration for determining the nature of pleural effusion, especially in older people. Ann N Y Acad Sci. 2004;1019:585–92.
40. Sartori S, Tombesi P, Trevisani L, Nielsen I, Tassinari D, Abbasciano V. Accuracy of transthoracic sonography in detection of pneumothorax after sonographically guided lung biopsy: prospective comparison with chest radiography. AJR Am J Roentgenol. 2007;188:37–41.
41. See KC, Ong V, Wong SH, et al. Lung ultrasound training: curriculum implementation and learning trajectory among respiratory therapists. Intensive Care Med. 2016;42:63–71.
42. Soldati G, Testa A, Pignataro G, Portale G, Biasucci DG, Leone A, Gentiloni Silveri N. The ultrasonographic deep sulcus sign in traumatic pneumothorax. Ultrasound Med Biol. 2006;32:1157–63.
43. Sperandeo M, Maggi M, Catalano D, Trovato G. No sliding, no pneumothorax: thoracic ultrasound is not an all-purpose tool. J Clin Anesth. 2014;26(5):425–6. https://doi.org/10.1016/j.jclinane.2014.04.005.
44. Singh Y, Tissot C, Fraga MV, Yousef N, Cortes RG, Lopez J, Sanchez-de-Toledo J, Brierley J, Colunga JM, Raffaj D, Da Cruz E, Durand P, Kenderessy P, Lang HJ, Nishisaki A, Kneyber MC, Tissieres P, Conlon TW, De Luca D. International evidence-based guidelines on point of care ultrasound (POCUS) for critically ill neonates and children issued by the POCUS

working Group of the European Society of paediatric and neonatal intensive care (ESPNIC). Crit Care. 2020;24(1):65. https://doi.org/10.1186/s13054-020-2787-9. PMID: 32093763; PMCID: PMC7041196
45. Volpicelli G, Caramello V, Cardinale L, Mussa A, Bar F, Frascisco MF. Detection of sonographic B-lines in patients with normal lung or radiographic alveolar consolidation. Med Sci Monit. 2008;14:CR122–8.
46. Weinberger SE, Drazen JM. Diagnostic procedures in respiratory diseases. In: Kasper DL, Braunwald E, Hauser S, Longo D, Jameson JL, Fauci AS, et al., editors. Harrison's principles of internal medicine. 6th ed. New York: McGraw-Hill; 2005. p. 1505–8.
47. Yang PC, Luh KT, Chang DB, Wu HD, Yu CJ, Kuo SH. Value of sonography in determining the nature of pleural effusion: analysis of 320 cases. AJR Am J Roentgenol. 1992;159:29–33.
48. Yousefifard M, Baikpour M, Ghelichkhani P, et al. Screening performance characteristic of ultrasonography and radiography in detection of pleural effusion; a meta-analysis. Emerg (Tehran). 2016;4(1):1–10.

Chapter 8
Technique and Devices for Securement of the Catheter and Protection of the Exit Site

Mauro Pittiruti

After completing the maneuver of insertion, the securement of the catheter and protection of the exit site are of paramount importance for the optimal performance of the venous access device (VAD) and for the minimization of complications such as infection, catheter dislodgment and venous thrombosis.

The exit site of the catheter is a relevant route of bacterial contamination (so called 'extra-luminal' route), and the prevention of infection is based on the proper choice of the exit site and its appropriate protection. Both for peripheral and central VADs, an exit site placed in a skin area of relevant bacterial contamination will increase the risk of infection. Skin contamination by bacteria and fungi is particularly high in skin areas that are humid, hairy, or close to natural or artificial connections with the digestive tract (mouth, anus, gastrostomy, enterostomy, etc.) or with the respiratory tract (nose, mouth, tracheostomy, etc.) or with any other skin breech (surgical drains, thoracostomy, nephrostomy, etc.). Examples of central VADs at high risk for infection are CICCs with the exit site at the neck or close to a tracheostomy, or FICCs inserted in the common femoral vein and coming out of the inguinal groove, or PICCs with the exit site to close to the axilla. Also, regardless of its location, the exit site should be appropriately protected by using one or more of the following strategies: tunneling, glue, proper securement devices, and semipermeable transparent membranes.

For both peripheral and central VADs, the choice of the exit site is very important also for the prevention of dislodgment. An exit site placed in a very unstable area such as the neck or the groin will be associated with a high risk of catheter dislodgment. Though, the choice of a skin area with minimal movements and maximal stability (for example: the infraclavicular region, mid-arm, mid-thigh, etc.) will not be enough for preventing dislodgment. Additional strategies should be added, such

M. Pittiruti (✉)
Department of Surgery, Catholic University Hospital, Rome, Italy

D. G. Biasucci et al. (eds.), *Vascular Access in Neonates and Children*,
https://doi.org/10.1007/978-3-030-94709-5_8

as proper securement device (skin-adhesive sutureless device or subcutaneous anchorage), cyanoacrylate glue, and semipermeable transparent membranes.

Finally, proper securement of the catheter has also a major role in preventing venous thrombosis. Catheter-related thrombosis is a phenomenon caused by the catheter insertion itself (damage of the vein wall integrity), by the permanence of the catheter inside the vein (obstacle to the blood flow), and by the possible endothelial irritation due to the infused solutions. Though, another major cause of catheter-related thrombosis is the friction of the catheter on the vein wall caused by the instability of the device. This occurs frequently both as 'mechanical thrombophlebitis' for peripheral short cannulas and as major venous thrombosis for central VADs, particularly for catheters with the exit site in the groin area or at the neck. Many clinical studies have shown that an optimal securement of the catheter is associated with a reduction of the risk of venous thrombosis.

In this chapter we will discuss different techniques and devices that may directly or indirectly enhance catheter securement and/or protection of the exit site, with a resulting favorable impact on the risk of infection, dislodgment, and thrombosis.

8.1 Protocols for Choosing the Exit Site

Different protocols have been described for the proper choice of the exit site of a VAD. These protocols take into considerations the different aspects discussed above: the contamination of the skin, its humidity, the stability of the region, and so on.

The first protocol of this kind was described by Dawson in 2013, as a guide for the proper choice of the exit site of a PICC (i.e., an ultrasound guided central VAD inserted in the deep veins of the arm): the so-called 'ZIM' (Zone Insertion Method). The ZIM has become rapidly popular for all PICC insertions, both in children and in adults. The basic concept of Dawson's ZIM is that the ideal area for the exit site at the arm is the middle third of the arm ('green' zone): catheters coming out of the skin in the distal third ('red' zone), close to the antecubital fossa, will be too unstable, while an exit site in the proximal third ('yellow' zone), close to the axilla, will be easily contaminated by the local bacterial flora. In short, when the only reasonable puncture site is located in the yellow zone (for instance, because of the caliber of the veins), any effort should be done for obtaining an exit site in the green zone, tunneling the catheter. Interestingly, the ZIM method is useful in clinical practice both for defining when tunneling is needed (i.e., when the ideal puncture site is in the yellow zone and not in the green zone) and for estimating how long the tunnel must be (i.e., long enough to obtain the exit site in the green area).

In recent papers, similar Zone Insertion Methods have been described also for CICCs and FICCS.

The so-called Central ZIM divides the neck/chest area in three zones: the red zone corresponds to the neck, the yellow zone to the supraclavicular region, and the green zone to the infraclavicular region. The red zone is an area of high skin contamination (due to the bacteria coming from the mouth and the nose) and high instability; non-tunneled CICC inserted in this area are prone to infection, dislodgment, and venous thrombosis. The yellow zone is the area where central venipuncture is often performed: ultrasound-guided access to the internal jugular vein (IJV), brachio-cephalic vein (BCV), subclavian vein (SBV) and external jugular vein (EJV) is commonly performed with the puncture site in this area. The yellow zone may be also acceptable as exit site in many patients, for example in older children without tracheostomy. On the other hand, in neonates and in infants (and in any patient with tracheostomy), an exit site in the yellow zone is not appropriate, and the catheter should be tunneled so to obtain an exit site in the green zone. Finally, the green zone is an ideal area both as puncture site and as exit site.

The so-called Femoral ZIM divides the groin/thigh area in three zones. The red zone corresponds to the area close to the knee, quite unstable and not recommended as exit site (this is also an area where venipuncture is quite difficult, as the superficial femoral vein is too deep). The yellow zone is the groin area and the upper third of the thigh; while venipuncture is almost always quite easy in this area, since the common femoral vein is quite large and easy to access (with the possible exceptions of very small premature neonates and very obese children), the exit site is not ideal since it is an unstable and highly contaminated area (inguinal groove, close to the urinary tract and to the perineum). FICCs with exit site at the groin are acceptable for limited period; if a FICC is planned to stay in place for more than 48 h and the only option is the venipuncture in the yellow zone, the catheter should be tunneled to the green zone (mid-thigh). Direct access to the superficial femoral vein at mid-thigh would represent probably the ideal solution, as the exit site is in a clean and stable area, with no tunneling required, but this venous access is feasible only in older children, as in neonates and infants the superficial femoral vein is too small.

Very recently, the 'ZIM' has been proposed also for the insertion of peripheral VADs in the upper limb. Different versions have been proposed, usually considering 'green' zones that corresponds to an ideal exit site (the forearm; the area above the antecubital fossa), 'yellow' zones where the exit site is not ideal but acceptable for cannulas inserted in emergency and expected to stay in place for less than 24 h (the dorsal side of the hand and of the wrist; the antecubital fossa), and 'red' zones where the insertion of a short peripheral cannula is consistently discouraged (the ventral side of the wrist).

8.2 Tunneling

Tunneling is a powerful technical tool for obtaining the 'ideal' exit site independently from the choice of the puncture site. The most typical example is the insertion of ultrasound guided CICCs in neonates, where the brachio-cephalic vein (BCV) represents the safest and easiest access to the central veins; though, the puncture site of ultrasound-guided access to the BCV is located in the supraclavicular area, which is a rather unstable area for the exit site; therefore, in this situation it is mandatory to tunnel the catheter so to move the exit site far from the puncture site, to a stable and clean skin area (typically, to the infraclavicular region) (Fig. 8.1).

Catheter tunneling is a simple and safe maneuver that can be applied to any central VAD (CICC, PICC or FICC), as long as the catheter is inserted using the modified Seldinger technique (needle venipuncture—guidewire through needle—introducer over guidewire—catheter through introducer). Though theoretically possible, the tunneling maneuver has never been described for ECC.

A recently published protocol, so-called RAVESTO (Rapid Assessment of Venous Exit Site and Tunneling Options) lists and describes all the possible options for tunneling PICCs, CICCs, and FICCs.

PICC tunneling (Figs. 8.2 and 8.3) is indicated whenever the best puncture site appears to be in the yellow zone. Tunneling has dramatically increased the

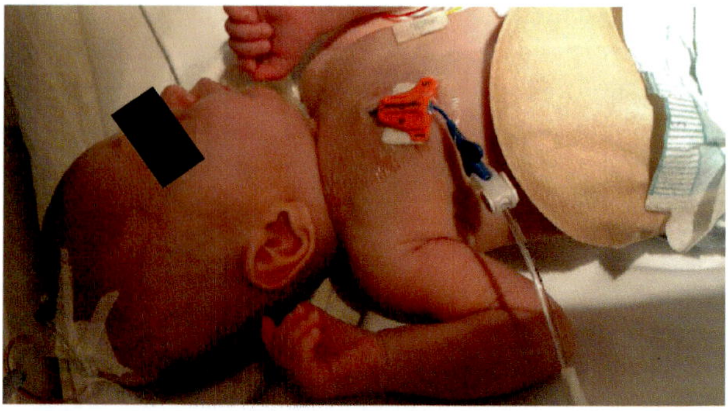

Fig. 8.1 Tunneled CICC in neonate (puncture of the brachio-cephalic vein and tunneling to the infra-clavicular area)

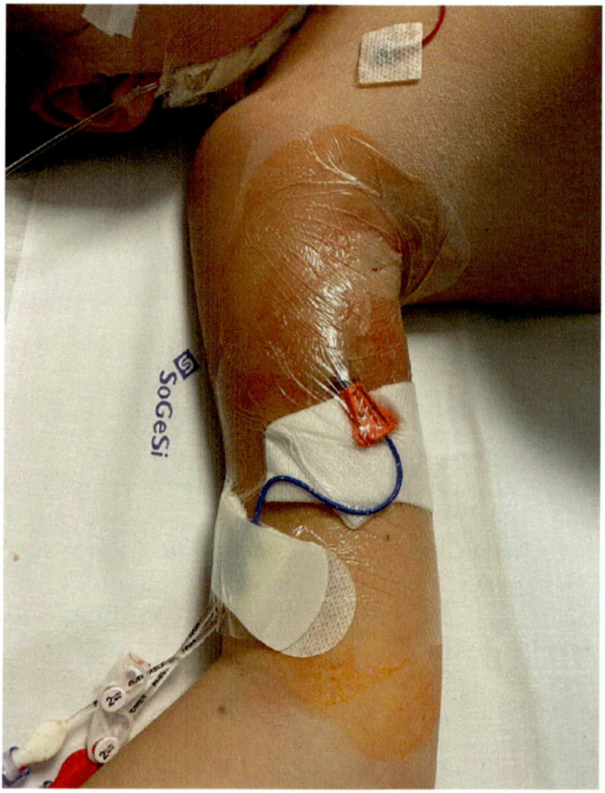

Fig. 8.2 Tunneled PICCs in children: puncture site in Dawson's yellow zone and exit site in the green zone

Fig. 8.3

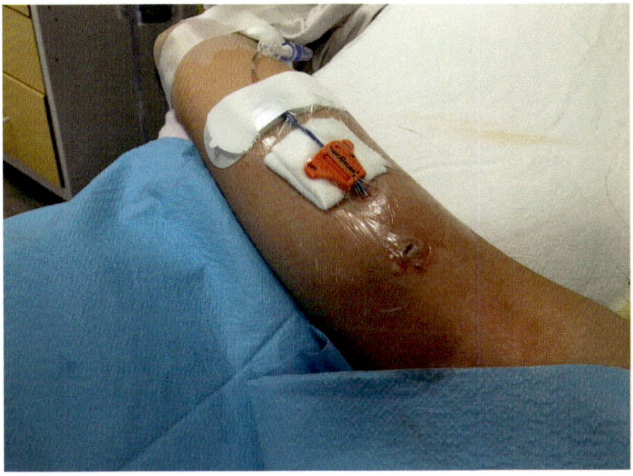

feasibility of PICC insertion in children, considering that the availability of a vein of proper caliber is the main limitation to PICCs in this age group. Current PICCs (i.e., peripherally inserted central catheters inserted in the deep veins of the arm adopting ultrasound guidance and modified Seldinger technique) should be in polyurethane and power injectable; as such, they are available of no less than 3Fr of caliber (i.e., 1 mm). Considering that the inner diameter of the vein should be at least three times the external diameter of the catheter, the smallest acceptable vein for PICC insertion must have a diameter of 3 mm. Veins of this caliber are rare in the green zone of the arm of small children, but they may be present in the yellow zone; in these cases, the vein is punctured in the yellow zone but the catheter is subsequently tunneled so to obtain an exit site in the green zone. The technique of PICC tunnelling is described in Figs. 8.4, 8.5, and 8.6.

Several options of CICC tunneling are described in the RAVESTO protocol: (a) CICC with puncture site in the supraclavicular area but tunneled downward, so to obtain an exit site in the infraclavicular area (typically in neonates and infants after access to the BCV, but also in critically ill children with tracheostomy) (Figs. 8.7, 8.8, and 8.9); (b) CICC with puncture site in the infraclavicular area but tunneled downward so to obtain an exit site in the lower chest area (this may be used in children, after access to the axillary vein, if a cuffed catheter is indicated: see below) (Fig. 8.10); (c) CICC with puncture site in the supra/infraclavicular area but tunneled to the arm (so-called 'chest-to-arm' tunneling) so to have an exit site similar to a PICC (this strategy is adopted when an exit site at the arm is preferred but the insertion of a PICC is unfeasible); (d) CICC with puncture site in the supra/infraclavicular area but tunneled to the back, so to obtain an exit site in the scapular region

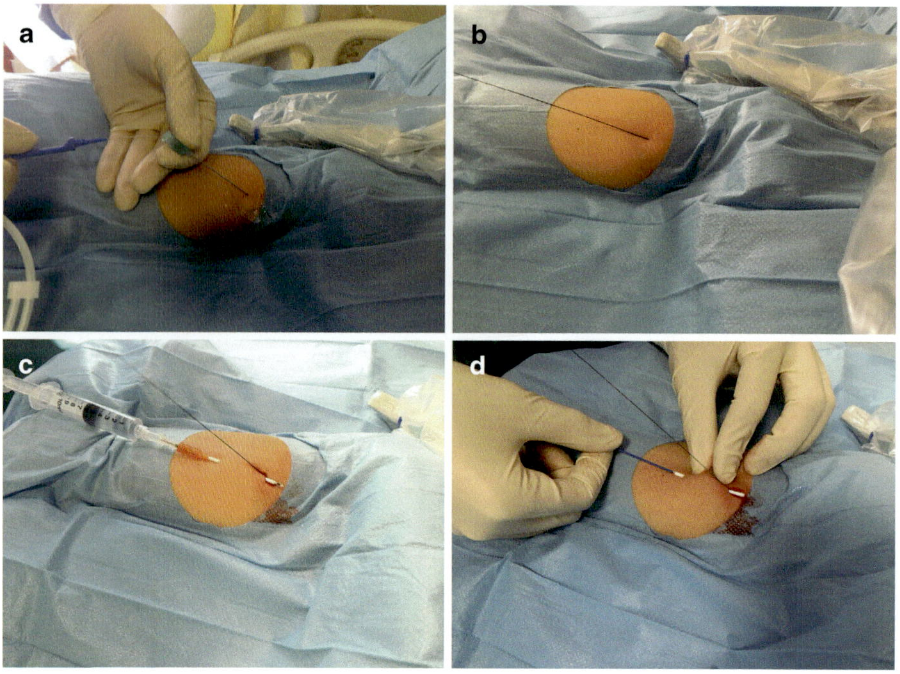

Fig. 8.4 Technique of insertion of a tunneled PICC. (**a**) venipuncture; (**b**) insertion of the guidewire; (**c**), preparation of the tunnel using a 14G short cannula; (**d**) removal of the needle from the cannula and insertion of the catheter

(this 'back tunneling' has been used in non-collaborative children at high risk for pulling out the catheter, since the catheter exit site is out of reach, but also in critically neonates and children who must stay pronated most of the day) (Fig. 8.11). The technique of CICC tunnelling is described in Figs. 8.12, 8.13, and 8.14.

The typical indication for tunneling a FICC is when the puncture site is at the groin (access to the common femoral vein) and the planned exit site is at mid-thigh. In short, an exit site at mid-thigh can be achieved either by direct puncture of the superficial femoral vein at mid-thigh or by puncture of the common femoral vein at the groin, with subsequent tunneling to the mid-thigh area. In both cases, the catheter will be relatively protected by the risk of complications (infection, dislodgment, thrombosis). The technique of FICC tunnelling is described in Figs. 8.15 and 8.16.

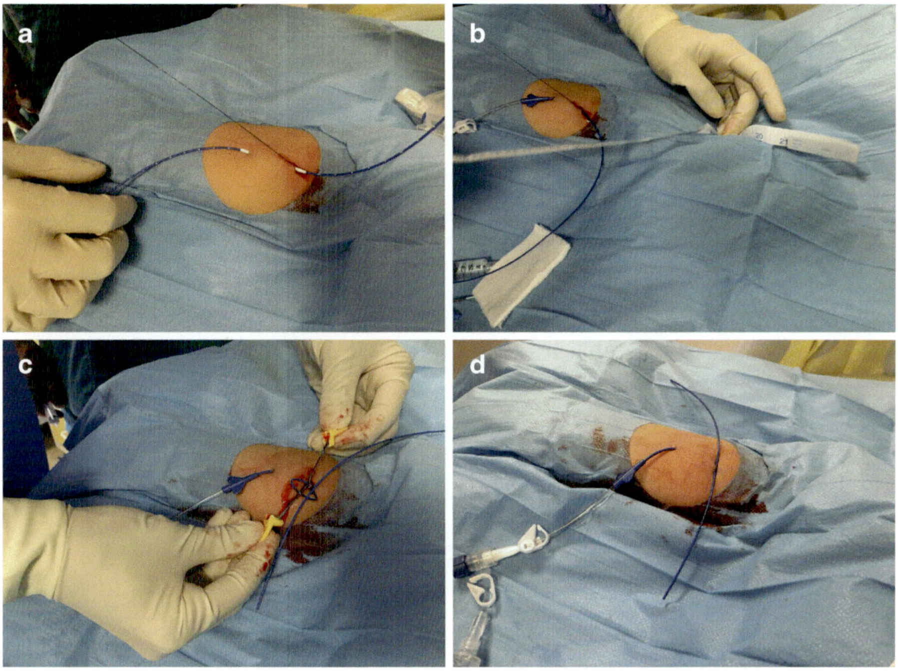

Fig. 8.5 Technique of insertion of a tunneled PICC. (**a**) passage of the catheter through the cannula; (**b**) length estimation based on surface landmarks; (**c**) insertion of the micro-introducer over the guidewire and insertion of the guidewire; (**d**) completed insertion of the catheter

Different techniques of tunnelling are available. In most cases, it is recommended to use metallic tunnelers. The tip of the catheter is connected to one end of the tunneler and the tunnel is made passing the device into the subcutaneous tissue.

A short tunneling can be achieved using a short peripheral cannula (Fig. 8.17). The needle-cannula is passed in the subcutaneous tissue from the puncture site to the planned exit site; the needle is removed, and the catheter is passed inside the cannula. A 4-5Fr catheter can be threaded through a 14G cannula, while a 3Fr catheter can adapt to a 16G cannula. The main disadvantages of this technique are (a) that the needle is sharp (and not blunt as most metallic tunnelers) so that it may cause subcutaneous bleeding, and (b) that the tunnel cannot be longer than 3–4 cm.

'Pseudo-tunneling' refers to the technique of extended subcutaneous route, i.e., a long trajectory of the needle in the subcutaneous tissue from the skin to the vein; this is not a real tunnel, since the puncture site and the exit site coincide.

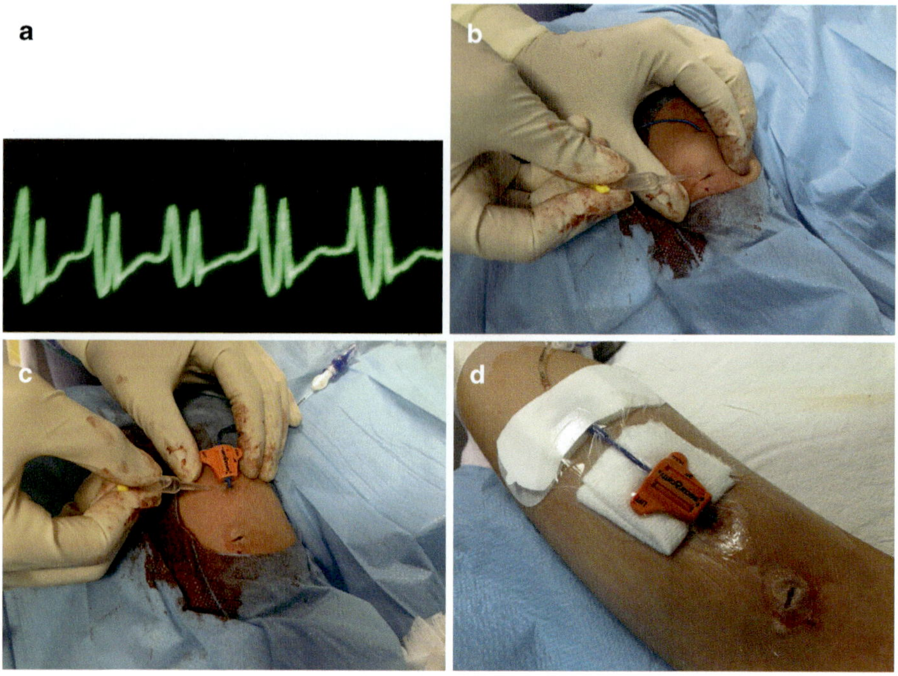

Fig. 8.6 Technique of insertion of a tunneled PICC. (**a**), tip location by intra-cavitary ECG; (**b**) closure of the puncture site by cyanoacrylate glue; (**c**) sealing of the exit site by cyanoacrylate glue; (**d**) final dressing

Fig. 8.7 Tunnelled CICCs in neonates and infants: tunneling to the infra-clavicular area

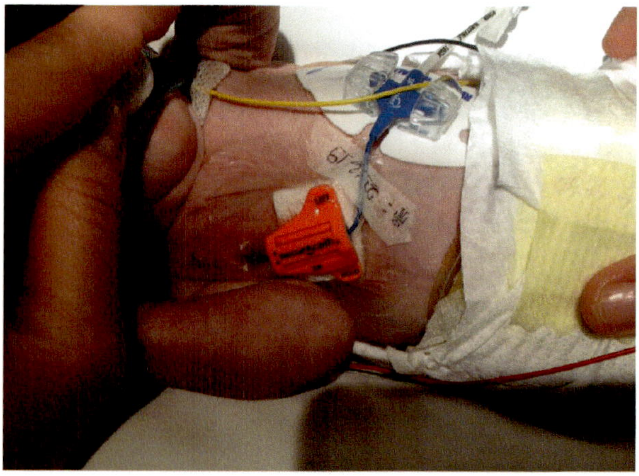

Fig. 8.8

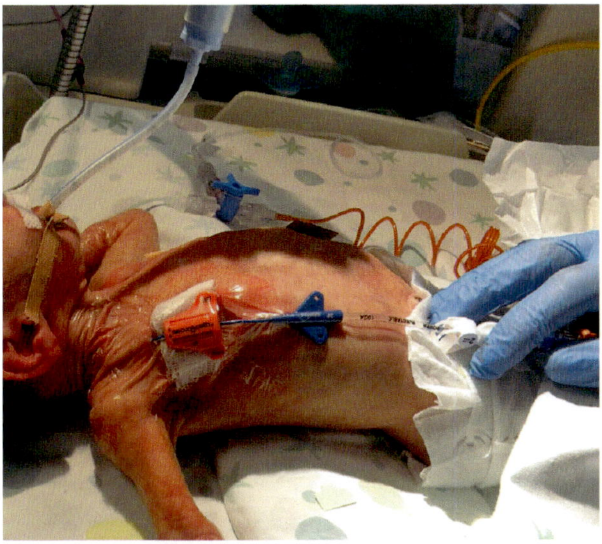

Fig. 8.9

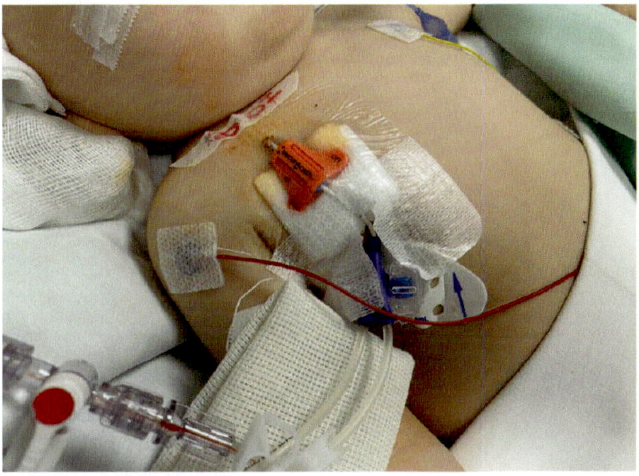

Fig. 8.10 Tunnelled CICC: tunneling to the lateral chest

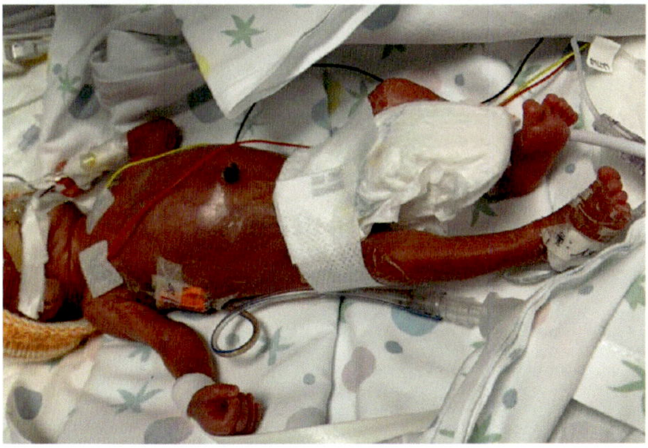

Fig. 8.11 CICC tunneled to the back

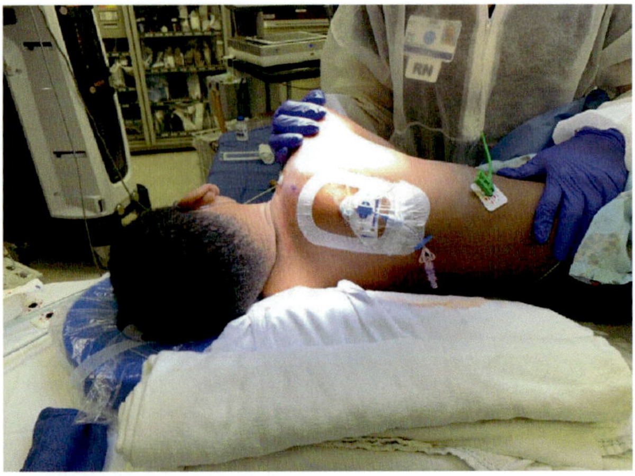

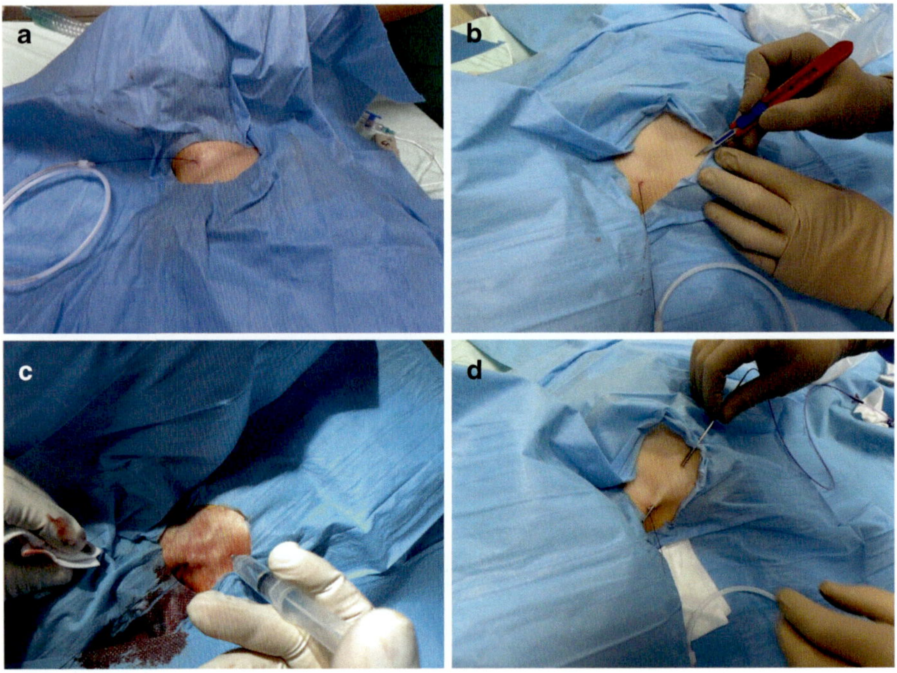

Fig. 8.12 Technique of insertion of a tunneled CICC. (**a**) puncture of the BCV and insertion of the guidewire; (**b**) small incision of the exit site; (**c**) preparation of the tunnel by hydro-dissection; (**d**) passage of the metallic tunneler

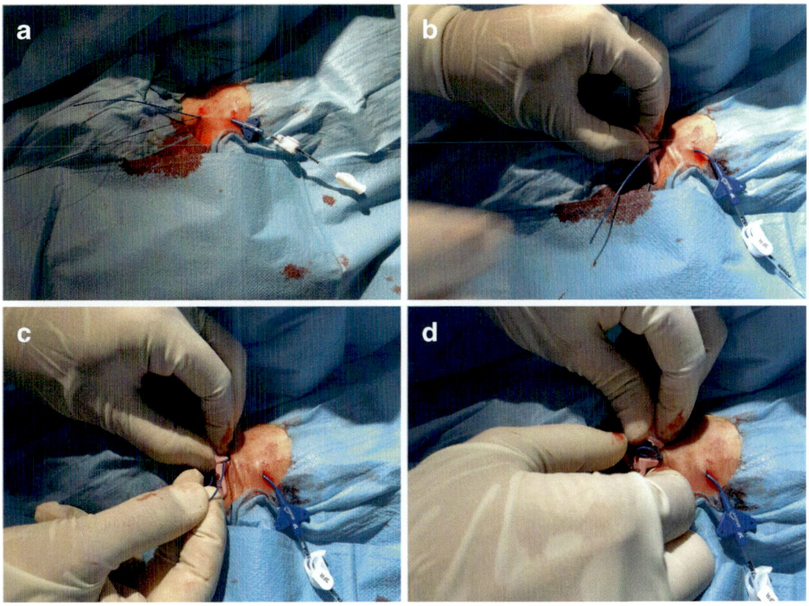

Fig. 8.13 Technique of insertion of a tunneled CICC. (**a**) passage of the catheter through the tunnel; (**b**) insertion of the micro-introducer-dilator over the guidewire; (**c**) removal of the dilator and of the guidewire; (**d**) insertion of the catheter through the micro-introducer

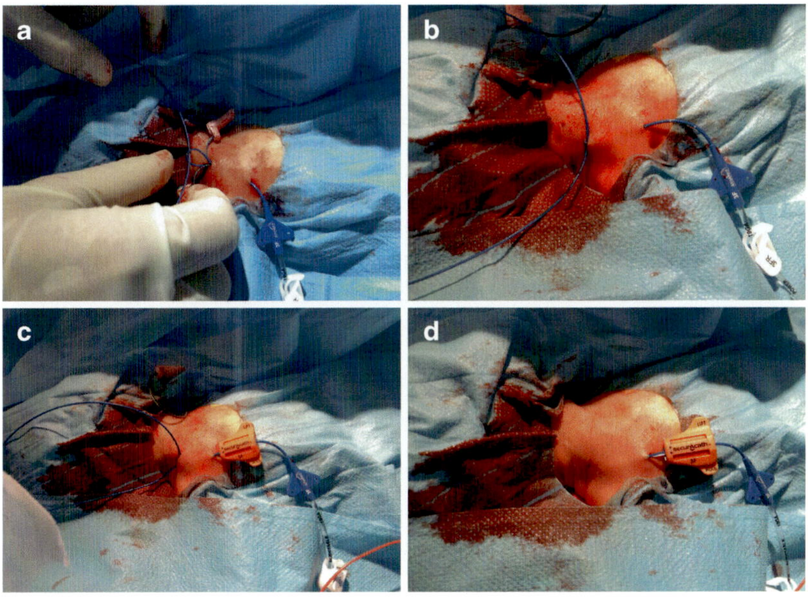

Fig. 8.14 Technique of insertion of a tunneled CICC. (**a**) peel away of the micro-introducer during the insertion of the catheter; (**b**) complete insertion of the catheter; (**c**) after tip location, securement with subcutaneous anchorage; (**d**) glue over the puncture site and over the exit site

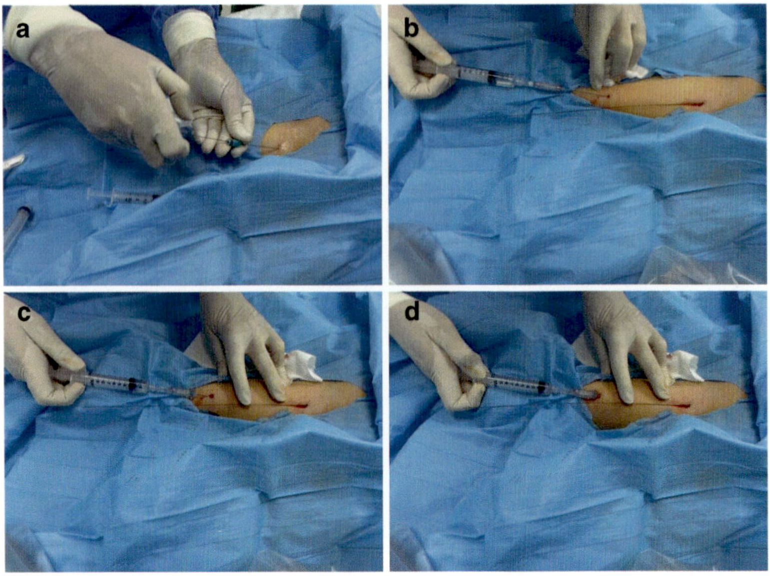

Fig. 8.15 Technique of insertion of a tunneled FICC. (a) venipuncture and insertion of guidewire; (b) local anesthesia on the planned exit site; (c and d) preparation of tunnel by hydro-dissection

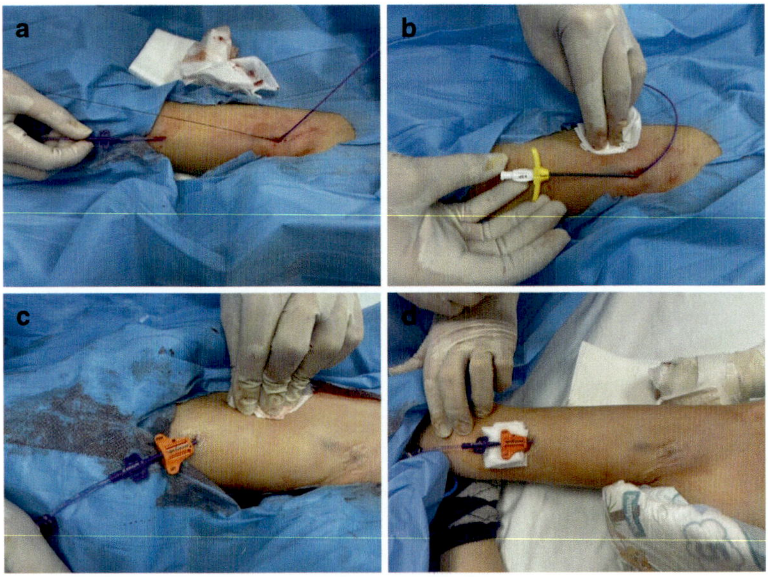

Fig. 8.16 Technique of insertion of a tunneled FICC. (a) passage of the catheter through the tunnel; (b) insertion of the micro-introducer-dilator; (c) insertion of the catheter through the introducer; (d) securement by subcutaneous anchorage and protection by cyanoacrylate glue

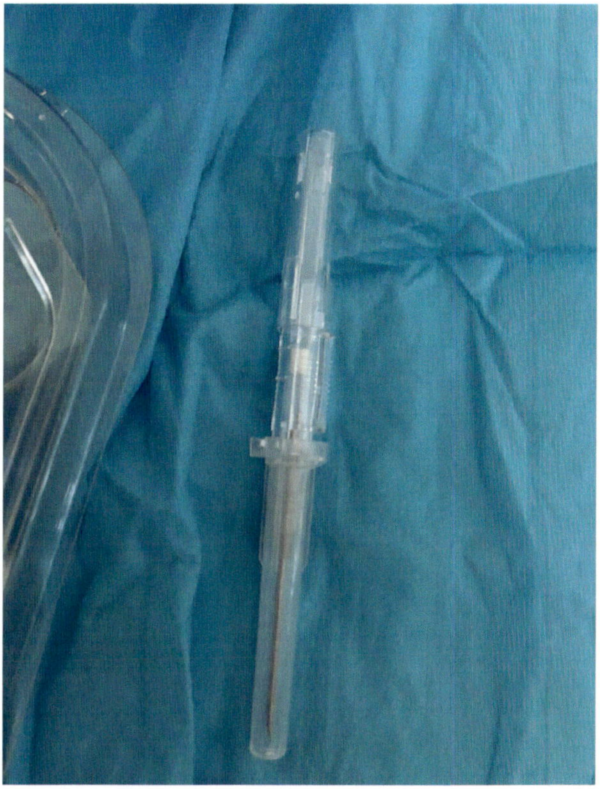

Fig. 8.17 16G short needle cannula, used for tunnelling

8.3 Catheter securement

Since a decade, sutures have been recognized as an inappropriate and dangerous method for securing external catheters. The stitches that secure the wing to the skin are inevitably associated with multiple chronic infective granulomas, with overgrowth of germs in the proximity of the exit site, increasing the risk of bacterial contamination by the extra-luminal route. All current guidelines recommend avoiding stitches as method of securement and adopt sutureless methods such as (a) skin-adhesive sutureless devices that keep the wing attached to the skin; (b) semipermeable transparent dressing with integrated securement; (c) subcutaneous anchorage systems (SAS).

Skin-adhesive sutureless systems (Figs. 8.18 and 8.19) and transparent dressing with integrated securement have the advantage of being relatively inexpensive and easy to apply, but the disadvantage of requiring a weekly replacement. Also, during the replacement maneuver, there is some risk of accidental catheter dislodgment.

Subcutaneously anchorage (SAS) (Figs. 8.20 and 8.21) is probably the most effective strategy currently available for catheter securement. SAS must be applied at the time of insertion and stays in place as long as the catheter is in place, as no

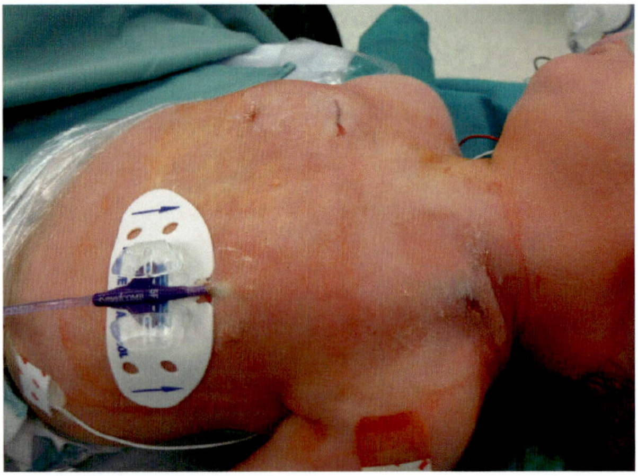

Fig. 8.18 Tunneled CICC secured by skin adhesive sutureless device (StatLock)

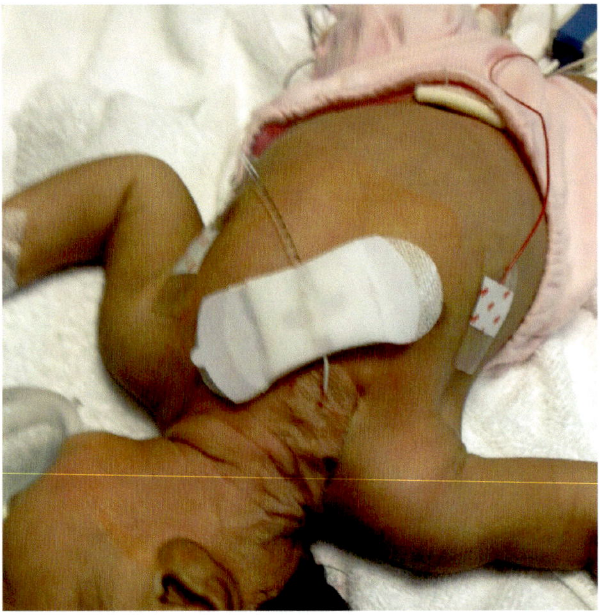

Fig. 8.19 Tunneled CICC secured by skin adhesive sutureless device (GripLok)

routine replacement is required. Though SAS are more expensive than the other securement devices, they are surely cost-effective (a) when the VAD is expected to stay in place for more than 5 weeks, and (b) when the risk of accidental dislodgment is estimated to be high. Recent clinical studies have demonstrated the high effectiveness of SAS in preventing dislodgment in neonates and children, as well as their safety. The main limitation of SAS is that they are not available for catheter smaller than 3Fr or bigger than 12Fr: this implies that they cannot be used for ECC in neonates or for peripheral VADs, except for midline catheters. In all other central VADs

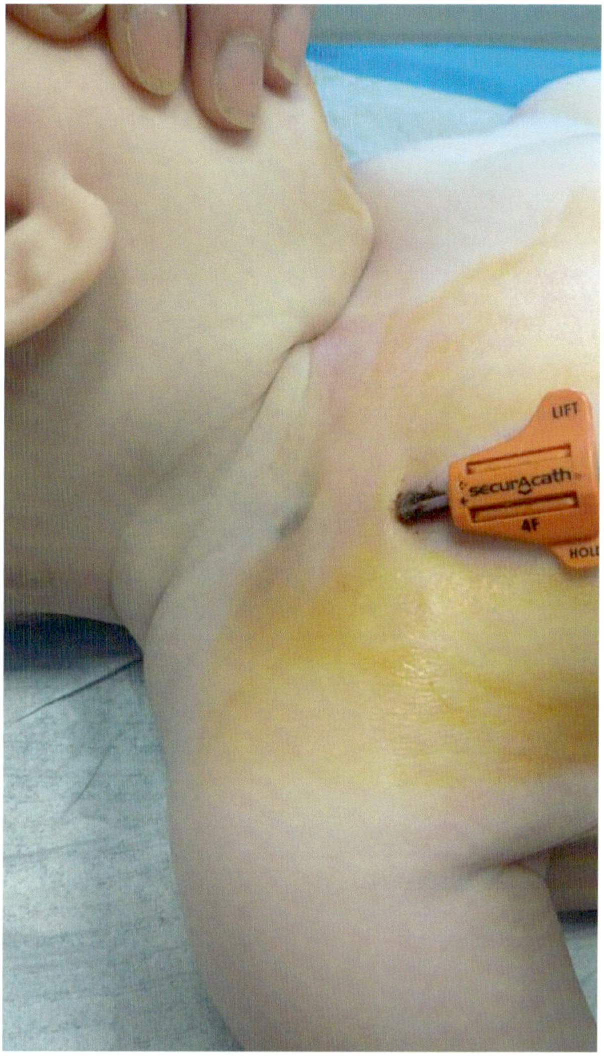

Fig. 8.20 Tunneled CICC secured by subcutaneous anchorage (Securacath)

(PICCs, CICCs, FICCs) in infants and children, the adoption of SAS is certainly beneficial and cost-effective and should be recommended. Figure 8.22 shows the technique of SAS placement. Though not specifically recommended by the manufacturers, many centers place a sterile gauze under the SAS, so to avoid pressure damage to the skin (Fig. 8.23).

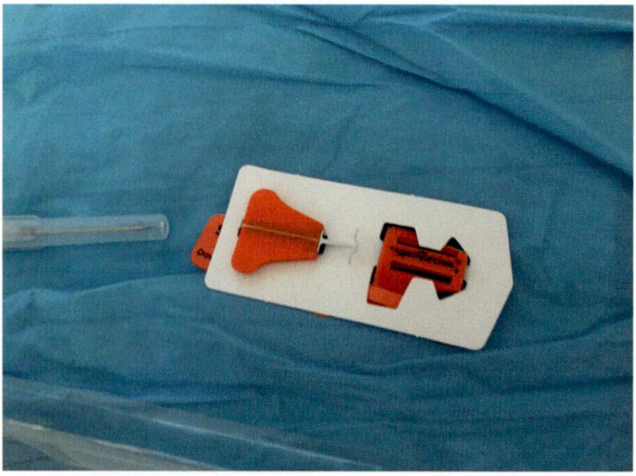

Fig. 8.21 Subcutaneously anchored securement device (Securacath)

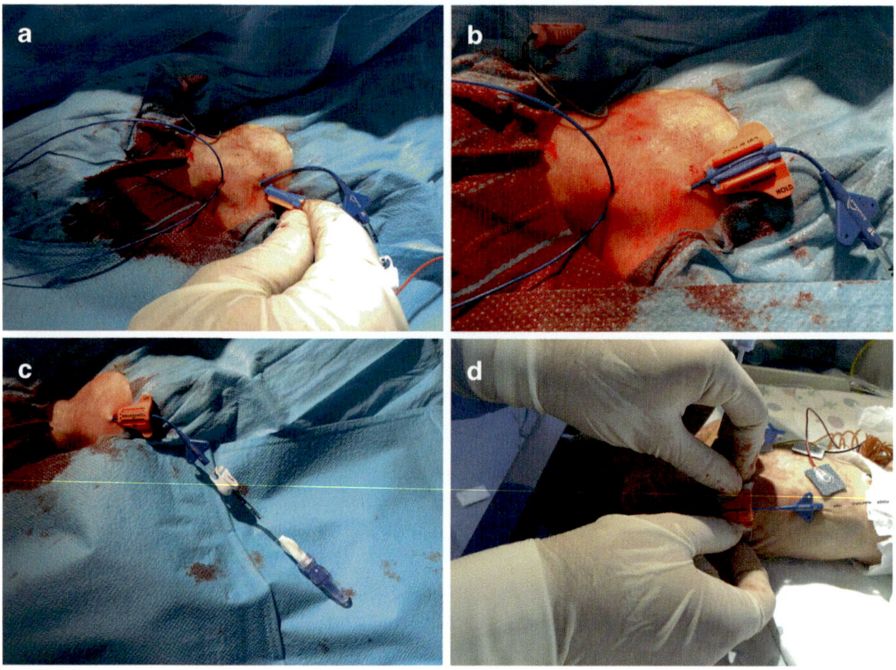

Fig. 8.22 Placement of subcutaneous anchorage. (**a**) insertion of the lower part of the device; (**b**) placement of the catheter over the groove; (**c**), closure of the device placing the upper part over the lower part, so to block the catheter; (**d**) a gauze is placed under the device

8.4 Cuffed catheters

The only other strategy that allows a definitive securement of an external central VAD as effective as the SAS is the use of tunneled-cuffed catheters. As opposed to uncuffed catheters, which can be either tunneled or non-tunneled (depending on the

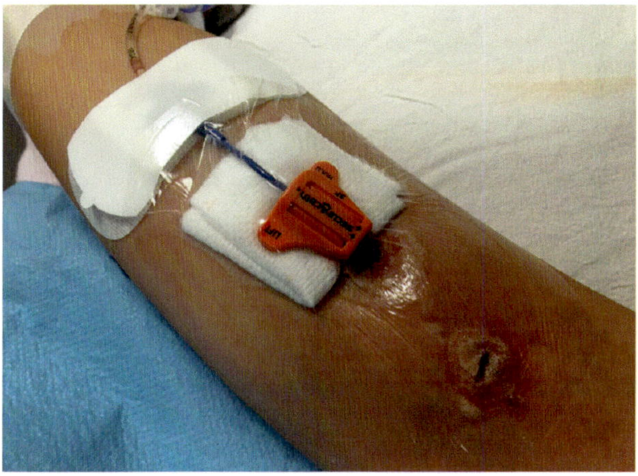

Fig. 8.23 Tunneled PICC secured by subcutaneous anchorage: a gauze is visible just under the Securacath

clinical situation), cuffed catheters are supposed to be always tunneled: the cuffed tract of the catheter is placed inside the tunnel, so that the cuff can progressively anchor the catheter to the subcutaneous tissue, by the slowly development of a sterile chronic inflammatory reaction. Recent studies have discussed the benefits of cuffed-tunneled catheters compared to uncuffed tunneled catheters secured with SAS. In both cases, tunneling has a proven role in reducing the risk of bacterial contamination by the extraluminal route, but - as regards securement - SAS may have some advantage over cuffs: (a) it is immediately effective as securement (while the cuff requires a few weeks before the chronic inflammation secures the catheter); (b) the cost of a cuffed catheter is superior to the cost of an uncuffed catheter + SAS; (c) the incidence of cuff-related complications (infection, dislodgment, etc.) seems to be higher than the incidence of SAS-related complications; (d) cuff-related complications always imply the removal of the VAD, while SAS-related complications do not; (e) removal of a cuffed catheter often requires sedation or local anesthesia, while removal of a catheter secured with SAS is rapid and painless. It is quite likely than in the next future cuffed-tunneled catheters will be replaced by uncuffed tunneled catheters secured with SAS.

8.5 Cyanoacrylate glue

Cyanoacrylate glue is one of the most effective and versatile technologies introduced in the world of venous access in the last decade. Glue for venous access is used in minimal amounts (0.15–0.35 ml) (Fig. 8.24) and should preferably be either butyl-cyanoacrylate or octyl-butyl-cyanoacrylate, since octyl-cyanoacrylate dries too slowly.

When inserting VADs, glue is potentially useful for many different goals: (a) it is highly effective in stopping any bleeding or oozing from the exit site soon after

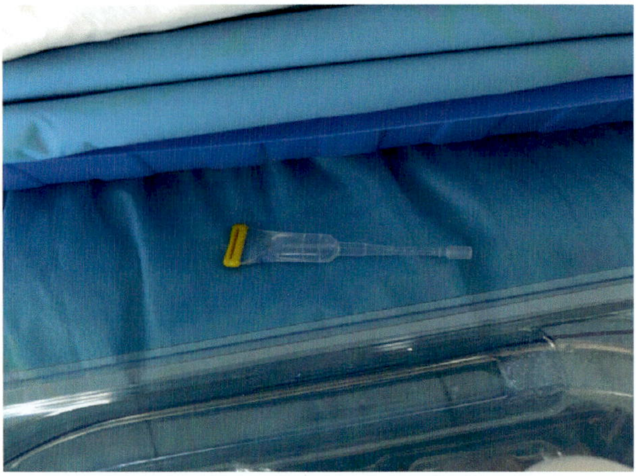

Fig. 8.24 Vial of 0.5 ml cyanoacrylate glue

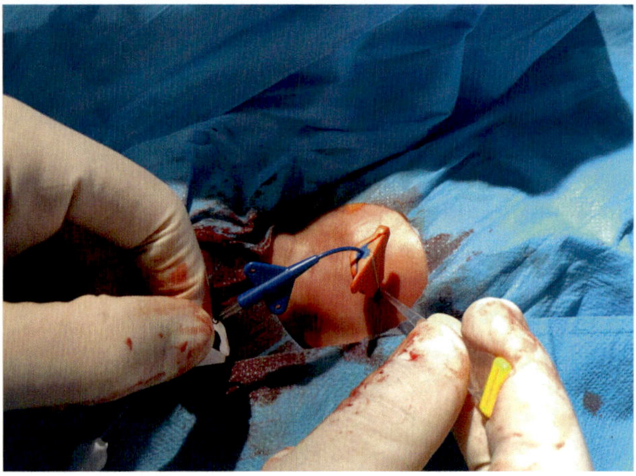

Fig. 8.25 Cyanoacrylate glue for sealing the exit site

insertion (and such action is also quite cost-effective, as it avoids the risk for an unscheduled dressing change, as it may occur when bleeding is excessive); (b) closing the breach of the exit site, glue effectively reduces the extraluminal contamination by bacteria; (c) it contributes to proper securement of the catheter, preventing dislodgment; (d) last, it is precious for closing skin incisions without the need of stitches.

Glue has been shown to be effective and safe as additional securement of short peripheral cannulas and ECC, used together with semipermeable transparent dressing. It has been shown to be safe, effective, and cost-effective in any CICC, PICC or FICC, where it significantly reduces the risk of local bleeding and infection by sealing the exit site (Fig. 8.25). Also, it is the first option for skin closure (Fig. 8.26) after placement of ports or tunneled catheters.

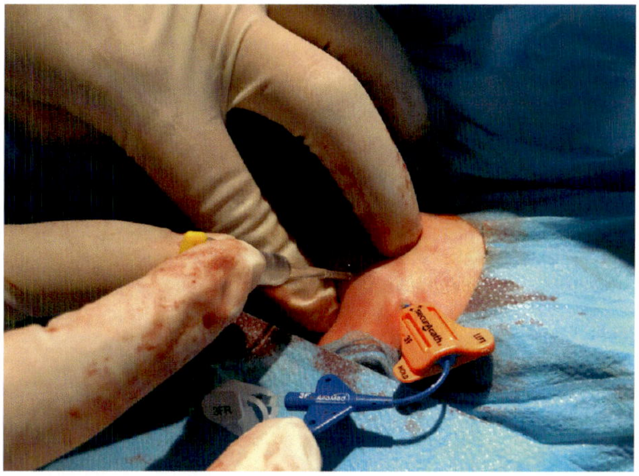

Fig. 8.26 Cyanoacrylate glue for closing the puncture site

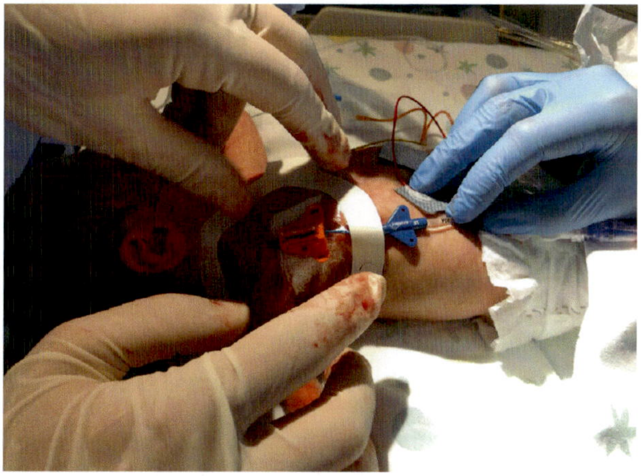

Fig. 8.27 Semipermeable transparent membrane over the exit site

Clinical studies have shown glue to be safe even on the skin of premature newborns. In vitro studies have demonstrated that the long-term use of glue does not alter the chemical and physical properties of polyurethane catheters.

Obviously, even if glue represents an important strategy for the protection of the exit site, it must be always used in association with semipermeable transparent membranes.

8.6 Semipermeable Transparent Membranes

Sterile semipermeable transparent dressings in polyurethane are the best protection of the exit site and of the area surrounding the emergency of the catheter from the skin, also contributing to catheter securement (Fig. 8.27). Gauze dressings should not be used routinely for covering the exit site of venous access devices, as they offer no protection at all from bacterial contamination, and they do not contribute to catheter securement. In short, current guidelines recommend that all exit sites of peripheral and central VADs should be protected by transparent membranes: they must be applied properly and replaced weekly.

Commercially available transparent dressings may have different clinical performance, since they have different degrees of transparency, of skin adhesiveness, of permeability, etc.; some transparent dressings are bordered (a feature that decreases the risk of unscheduled dressing change), while some have integrated securement devices. One important feature is permeability, which becomes critical in premature newborns, characterized by a very high trans-epidermal water loss (TEWL). In all neonates, infants, and children, we recommend using transparent membranes with high MVTR (Moisture Vapor Transfer Rate). A transparent membrane with poor permeability (MVTR <1500)—if used in a child with high perspiration—will be associated with accumulation of humidity below the dressing and possible maceration of the skin. For the same reason, the adoption of transparent dressings with chlorhexidine-releasing gel pad should be always avoided in pediatric patients, since the transpiration of the skin area covered by the gel pad will be completely abolished; furthermore, the chlorhexidine released by the gel, acting on the macerated skin, may increase the local damage to the epidermidis.

8.7 Conclusions

In short, proper catheter securement and proper protection of the exit site require a multimodal strategy that should include: (a) wise choice of the exit site and the adoption—when needed—of tunneling techniques; (b) sutureless securement devices (preferably: subcutaneous anchorage for central VADs with caliber 3Fr or bigger); (c) cyanoacrylate glue (to be used for all VADs); (d) semipermeable transparent dressings (to be used for all VADs).

Catheter securement and protection of the exit site is still an unsolved issue for UVC (see chapter below), though in the future cyanoacrylate glue may play a role in this regard.

The association of cyanoacrylate glue and semipermeable transparent dressing is currently the best securement/protection strategy for ECC and short peripheral cannulas.

Long peripheral cannulas, midline catheters and all external central VADs should be secured and protected by a triple strategy: cyanoacrylate glue, sutureless device, and transparent dressing. In most central VADs, the most effective and cost-effective sutureless device is the SAS (subcutaneous anchored securement).

Bibliography

1. Barone G, Pittiruti M, Ancora G, Vento G, Tota F, D'Andrea V. Centrally inserted central catheters in preterm neonates with weight below 1500 g by ultrasound-guided access to the brachio-cephalic vein. J Vasc Access. 2021 May;22(3):344–52. https://doi.org/10.1177/1129729820940174.
2. Biasucci DG, Pittiruti M, Taddei A, Picconi E, Pizza A, Celentano D, Piastra M, Scoppettuolo G, Conti G. Targeting zero catheter-related bloodstream infections in pediatric intensive care unit: a retrospective matched case-control study. J Vasc Access. 2018 Mar;19(2):119–24. https://doi.org/10.5301/jva.5000797.
3. Cellini M, Bergadano A, Crocoli A, Badino C, Carraro F, Sidro L, Botta D, Pancaldi A, Rossetti F, Pitta F, Cesaro S. Guidelines of the Italian Association of Pediatric Hematology and Oncology for the management of the central venous access devices in pediatric patients with onco-hematological disease. J Vasc Access. 2020;10:1129729820969309. https://doi.org/10.1177/1129729820969309.
4. Crocoli A, Martucci C, Sidro L, Delle Donne D, Menna G, Pittiruti M, De Pasquale MD, Strocchio L, Natali GL, Inserra A. Safety and effectiveness of subcutaneously anchored securement for tunneled central catheters in oncological pediatric patients: A retrospective study. J Vasc Access. 2021;4:11297298211009364. https://doi.org/10.1177/11297298211009364.
5. D'Andrea V, Barone G, Pezza L, Prontera G, Vento G, Pittiruti M. Securement of central venous catheters by subcutaneously anchored suturless devices in neonates. J Matern Fetal Neonatal Med. 2021;9:1–4. https://doi.org/10.1080/14767058.2021.1922377.
6. D'Andrea V, Pezza L, Barone G, Prontera G, Pittiruti M, Vento G. Use of cyanoacrylate glue for the sutureless securement of epicutaneo-caval catheters in neonates. J Vasc Access. 2021;8:11297298211008103. https://doi.org/10.1177/11297298211008103.
7. Dawson R. PICC Zone Insertion Method™ (ZIM™): A Systematic Approach to Determine the Ideal Insertion Site for PICCs in the Upper Arm. Journal of the Association for Vascular Access. 2011;16(3):156–65.
8. Giustivi D, Gidaro A, Baroni M, Paglia S. Tunneling technique of PICCs and Midline catheters. J Vasc Access. 2021;16:11297298211002579.
9. Gorski L, Hadaway L, Hagle M, et al. Infusion therapy standards of practice. J Infus Nurs. 2021;44(1S Suppl 1):S1–S224.
10. Ostroff MD, Pittiruti M, Ostroff MD, Pittiruti M. Alternative exit sites for central venous access: Back tunneling to the scapular region and distal tunneling to the patellar region. J Vasc Access. 2020 Jul;9:1129729820940178.
11. Pinelli F, Pittiruti M, Van Boxtel T, Barone G, Biffi R, Capozzoli G, Crocoli A, Elli S, Elisei D, Fabiani A, Garrino C, Graziano U, Montagnani L, Prato AP, Scoppettuolo G, Zadra N, Zanaboni C, Zerla P, Konstantinou E, Jones M, Rosay H, Simcock L, Stas M, Pepe G. GAVeCeLT-WoCoVA Consensus on subcutaneously anchored securement devices for the securement of venous catheters: Current evidence and recommendations for future research. J Vasc Access. 2020;2:1129729820924568. https://doi.org/10.1177/1129729820924568.
12. Pittiruti M, Scoppettuolo G, Dolcetti L, Celentano D, Emoli A, Marche B, Musarò A. Clinical experience of a subcutaneously anchored sutureless system for securing central venous catheters. Br J Nurs. 2019;28(2):S4–S14. https://doi.org/10.12968/bjon.2019.28.2.S4.

Part II
Venous Access in Neonates

Chapter 9
Peripheral Venous Access in Neonates

Giovanni Barone, Vito D'Andrea, and Mauro Pittiruti

The appropriate type of vascular access device, peripheral or central, is chosen in order to accommodate the needs of the neonate (parenteral nutrition, intravenous medication, etc.). The choice of vascular access is also related to many other factors such as gestational age, birth weight, comorbidities, previous history of infusion therapy, and ability/resources available for inserting and maintaining the device.

As general rule, the vascular access device should be of the smallest outer diameter with the fewest number of lumens and should be the least invasive as possible, still considering the prescribed intravenous therapy.

Peripheral venous access (PVA) is certainly the less invasive venous access device; though, venous cannulation may be a challenging procedure especially in small preterm neonates, even under perfect conditions (i.e., in ventilated and sedated).

9.1 Indication

The key question is: is a venous access really needed? In fact, even in neonates, a large variety of clinical situations can be managed without establishing venous access. If the newborn really needs a venous access, we should consider three issues:

G. Barone
Neonatal Intensive Care Unit, Ospedale 'Infermi', Rimini, Italy

V. D'Andrea
Neonatal Intensive Care Unit, University Hospital Fondazione Policlinico Gemelli IRCCS, Rome, Italy
e-mail: vito.dandrea@policlinicogemelli.it

M. Pittiruti (✉)
Department of Surgery, Catholic University Hospital, Rome, Italy

D. G. Biasucci et al. (eds.), *Vascular Access in Neonates and Children*,
https://doi.org/10.1007/978-3-030-94709-5_9

1. Anticipated duration of intravenous therapy. When the anticipated duration of infusion therapy is less than 6 days, PVA should be preferred as first option unless a central access is needed for other reason.
2. Infusate characteristics. Do not use peripheral catheters for continuous vesicant therapy, parenteral nutrition, or infusates with an osmolarity greater than 900 mOsm/L.
3. Need of vein preservation for long term access. Every human being is born with a limited number of veins suitable for venous access. Neonates, especially preterm ones, might need repeated venous cannulations, therefore it is crucial to consider the opportunity of preserving the vasculature for future venous accesses.

9.2 Device

We should use peripheral venous catheter of the smallest gauge possible, while still compatible with the prescribed therapy. Peripheral venous cannulas of small caliber (22G–26G) are appropriate for most infusion therapies. Peripheral catheters larger than 20G are likely to cause phlebitis; on the contrary, small gauge catheters minimize the insertion-related trauma, and this aspect is particularly relevant in preterm infants. For this reason, 24G–26G catheters are appropriate for extremely low birth weight infant (< 1000 grams) and 22G–24G for the other neonates. Larger catheters (20G) may be considered when rapid fluid replacement is required.

Steel winged venous access devices should be used only for single-dose administrations and should not be left in place.

9.3 Procedure

Care should be taken when performing invasive procedures in neonates: aseptic precautions and awareness of best practice to avoid nosocomial infection are crucial. Furthermore, the skin of preterm babies is particularly fragile in the first week of life and the bones of chronically ill preterm babies may develop rickets and are vulnerable to fractures.

Equipment needed:

- Gloves
- 22G, 24G or 26G short cannula with safety mechanism, based on infant characteristics; 26G cannulas are preferred for very small neonates.
- Vein visualization device (such as NIR: see Chap. 5), if needed
- 2 ml syringe, pre-filled with normal saline.
- Short extension connected to a needle-free device with neutral displacement (ideally, with straight fluid path design and minimal dead space).
- 2% chlorhexidine in 70% IPA.

- Cyanoacrylate glue.
- Semipermeable transparent dressing with high permeability (i.e., high moisture vapor transmission rate).

Technique:

1. Before starting, choose a suitable vein. Avoid using site such as the antecubital fossa and long saphenous veins, potentially useful for insertion of epicutaneo-cava catheters. If a scalp vein is chosen (Fig. 9.1), hair removal might be necessary. Assess the condition of the skin and evaluate previous site of intravenous access, in order to identify previous venipuncture-related or infusion-related complications (e.g., phlebitis, infiltration), so to avoid these areas. When veins are difficult to visualize, cannulation success may be improved by visible light devices or by NIR technology. If using visible light devices, adopt only cold light sources so to avoid thermal burns. For near-infrared light devices follow the manufacturer's instructions and try to identify bifurcating veins and tortuosity which might make the puncture unsuccessful. Always avoid blind venipuncture: veins should be properly identified either by direct eye visualization or by device-assisted visualization.

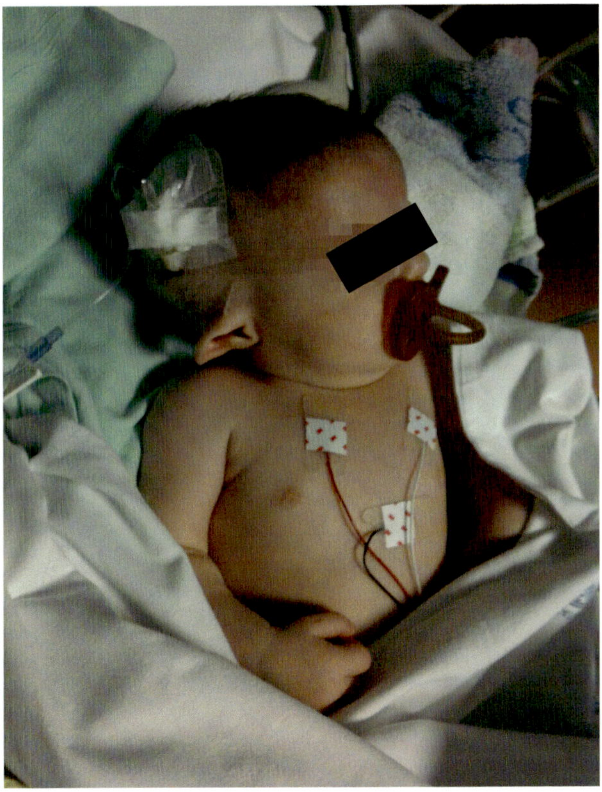

Fig. 9.1 Peripheral venous cannula on the scalp

2. Adjust the height of the incubator and ensure you have adequate lighting.
3. Consider sucrose analgesia and swaddling, when appropriate.
4. Hygiene of the hands (alcohol-based gel rub)
5. Wear non-sterile gloves.
6. Clean site with alcoholic 2% chlorhexidine wipes and let it dry for 30 seconds.
7. Flush the short extension set with normal saline to remove air.
8. Firmly grip the limb using your fingers as a tourniquet whilst stretching the skin, to stabilize the vein. It may be helpful if an assistant holds the limb.
9. With the cannula bevel facing upwards, puncture the skin and vein together at an angle of approximately 35°. Carefully advance the cannula until blood appears in the hub.
10. Withdraw the needle holding it with your thumb and middle finger, while simultaneously advancing the cannula into the vein with your forefinger.
11. Attach the short extension set and the needle-free device.
12. Flush the cannula with normal saline to check patency.
13. Secure the cannula using cyanoacrylate glue. Sterile strips may be used, but they are potentially harmful to the delicate skin of the newborn and far less effective than glue.
14. Cover with semipermeable transparent membrane (Fig. 9.2). Avoid dressings and strapping that obscure the entry site of the line as this can make detection of extravasation difficult. Ensure dressing is not circumferential to the limb.
15. Place a splint only exceptionally, if needed. Cannula in antecubital fossa often require immobilization, but this may cause stress and discomfort to the neonate.
16. Document site, date, time of insertion, number of attempts made, gauge of device and initials of inserter.

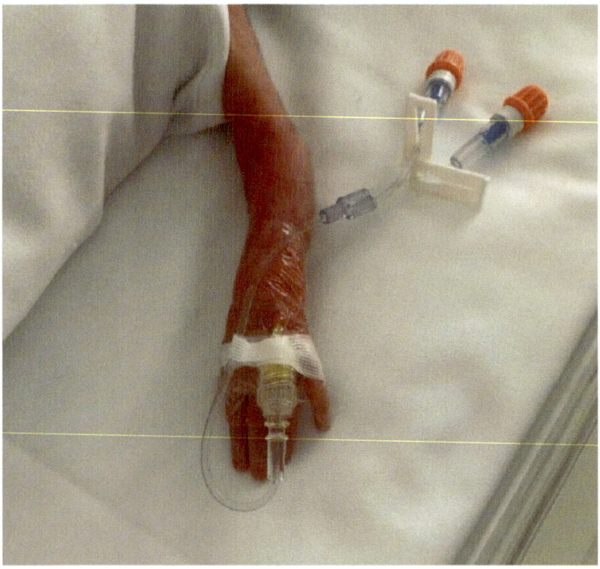

Fig. 9.2 24G cannula placed on the hand and secured with cyanoacrylate glue and semipermeable transparent dressing

It's common sense to avoid multiple punctures in newborns. In most neonatal intensive care units, there is an unspoken rule regarding vein cannulation: "three strikes and you're out". Though, we recommend to ask for help even after your second unsuccessful attempt.

9.4 Complications

Complications related to PVA and infusions include:

1. Infections. Premature neonates are at high risk of infection due to the immaturity of immune system. Local infection of the exit site is common and may be secondary to inappropriate skin antisepsis at time of insertion or to detachment and contamination of the dressing. When exit site infection is suspected at visual inspection, the cannula must be removed. PVA-related blood stream infections are rare.
2. Phlebitis. It can be bacterial (due to contamination of the exit site), mechanical (typically secondary to inappropriate stabilization of the cannula or to excessive caliber of the cannula compared to the vein), or chemical (due to infusion of irritant/vesicant solutions that are not compatible with the peripheral route). Figure 9.3 shows the effect of an extravasation (potassium) after placement of a peripheral cannula on the hand. The risk of phlebitis is related to vesicant or irritant drugs, parenteral nutrition, or infusates with an osmolarity greater than 900 mOsm/L. For this reason, PVA should be used for parenteral nutrition only for short periods (few days).
3. Infiltration/extravasation. Non-irritant solutions cause 'infiltration', which is not harmful but inevitably associated with loss of the venous access. Leakage of irritant/vesicant solutions in the surrounding tissues is named 'extravasation' and may be associated not only with loss of the venous access but also with severe local damage. For example, leakage of parenteral nutrition in the subcutaneous tissue might cause skin ulceration, secondary infection, and scar. Sometimes skin necrosis could happen if the extravasation is not properly managed, and the infusion contained high irritant solutions like calcium.
4. Occlusion of the lumen is frequent for small caliber cannulas and should be prevented by periodic flushing with saline.

9.5 The RaSuVA Protocol (Rapid Superficial Vein Assessment)

As stated earlier, every human being is born with a limited number of veins suitable for venous access. Sometimes neonates—especially preterm ones—need repeated venous cannulations. The puncture and cannulation of these veins is commonly

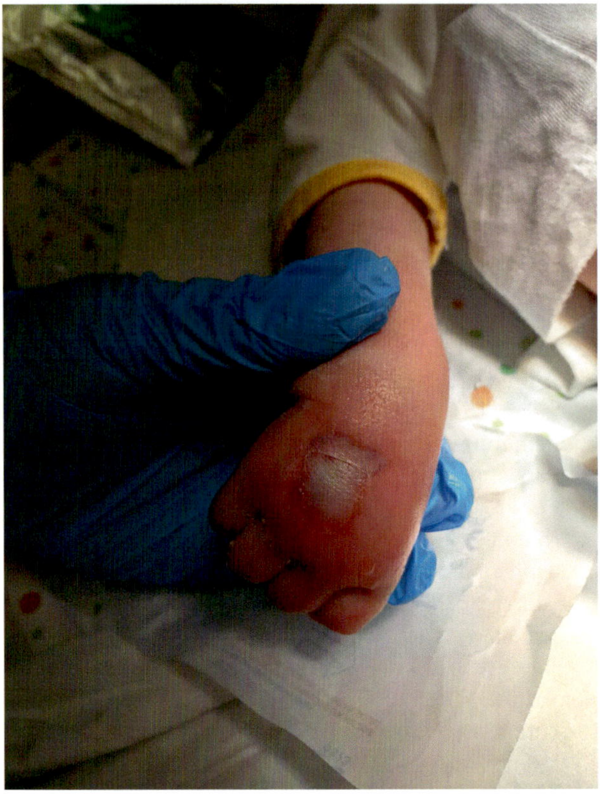

Fig. 9.3 Extravasation (peripheral cannula inappropriately used for potassium-enriched solutions)

performed by direct visualization, though new technologies such as 'Near-Infra-Red' (NIR) technique are very promising.

However, the choice of the vein most suitable for the insertion may be difficult and mainly relies upon an empiric decision, depending usually on the operator's preference and experience, often after a non-systematic assessment of the main superficial veins.

We suggest an easy and repeatable protocol for a rational and systematic evaluation of the superficial veins in neonates, as a potential guide for choosing the most appropriate approach in each situation.

The Rapid Superficial Vein Assessment—RaSuVA—is a sequential assessment of seven sites, systematically explored 'from foot to head', first on the right and then on the left side. The assessment may be performed by direct eye evaluation or also using a device with NIR technology. Each area of the upper and lower limbs is explored with and without tourniquet. The seven sites include (1) medial malleolus, (2) lateral malleolus, (3) popliteal fossa, (4) back of the hand and wrist, (5) antecubital fossa, (6) anterior scalp veins, (7) posterior scalp veins. After RaSuVA, the clinician can build a map of all the suitable veins for venous access. We advise to keep this map in the medical notes of the patient, recording time by time and attempt by attempt which veins have been used. This easy protocol can help to preserve veins in newborns which might need multiple cannulations and would also help to choose the best intravenous device.

This protocol is also useful to define a list of preferred options in each patient depending on the type of the vascular access device to insert (peripheral or central). Using RaSuVA, each unit can build its own policy. For example, the insertion of PVA may preferably be performed in the lower limbs (excluding the saphenous vein) as a first option or on the back of the hand and at the wrist as a second option. On the other hand, the insertion of a central line may be performed at the antecubital fossa (first option) or at the saphenous vein at the medial malleolus (second option). Even at a teaching institution, it must be accepted that there are patients in whom it is imperative that the most skilled practitioner available must be in charge for the very first attempt of venous cannulation; sometimes in such patients, there is no room for training, and RaSuVA could help to identify such patients.

RaSuVA is a simple and rapid assessment tool designed to optimize and rationalize the use of veins in newborn babies.

Bibliography

1. Atay S, Sen S, Cukurlu D. Incidence of infiltration/extravasation in newborns using peripheral venous catheter and affecting factors. Rev Esc Enferm USP. 2018;52:e03360.
2. Bell L. Infusion nursing: an evidence-based approach: third edition. Crit Care Nurse [Internet]. 2011;31(3):1–92. Available from: http://ccn.aacnjournals.org/cgi/doi/10.4037/ccn2011161
3. Chopra V, Flanders SA, Saint S, Woller SC, O'Grady NP, Safdar N, et al. The Michigan appropriateness guide for intravenous catheters (MAGIC): results from a multispecialty panel using the RAND/UCLA appropriateness method. Ann Intern Med. 2015;163(6):S1–39.
4. Danski MTR, Mingorance P, Johann DA, et al. Incidence of local complications and risk factors associated with peripheral intravenous catheter in neonates. Rev Esc Enferm USP. 2016;50(1):22–8.
5. Gorski L, Hadaway L, Hagle M, et al. Infusion therapy standards of practice. J Infus Nurs. 2021;44(1S Suppl 1):S1–S224.
6. Gorski LA, Hagle ME, Bierman S. Intermittently delivered IV medication and pH: Reevaluating the evidence. J Infus Nurs. 2015;38:27–46.
7. Incekar MC, Yildiz S, Selalmaz M, et al. Turkish validation of the infiltration scale in infants. J Pediatr Nurs. 2019;44:e13–9.
8. Infusion Nursing Society. Policies and Procedures for infusion therapy: Neonate to adolescent [Internet]. 2nd ed. 2016. Available from: http://www.bumc.bu.edu/irb/irbguidance/
9. Legemaat M, Carr P, van Rens RM, et al. Peripheral intravenous cannulation: complication rates in the neonatal population: a multicenter observational study. J Vasc Access. 2016;17(4):360–5.
10. O'Grady NP, Alexander M, Burns LA, et al; Healthcare infection control practices advisory committee. Guidelines for the prevention of intravascular catheter-related infections. Am J Infect Control. 2011;39(4, suppl 1):S1-S34.
11. Ullman AJ, Bernstein SJ, Brown E, Aiyagari R, Doellman D, Faustino EVS, Gore B, Jacobs JP, Jaffray J, Kleidon T, Mahajan PV, McBride CA, Morton K, Pitts S, Prentice E, Rivard DC, Shaughnessy E, Stranz M, Wolf J, Cooper DS, Cooke M, Rickard CM, Chopra V. The Michigan

appropriateness guide for intravenous catheters in Pediatrics: miniMAGIC. Pediatrics 2020 Jun;145(Suppl 3):S269-S284. https://doi.org/10.1542/peds.2019-3474I. PMID: 32482739.
12. Wallis MC, McGrail M, Webster J, Marsh N, Gowardman J, Playford EG, et al. Risk factors for peripheral intravenous catheter failure: a multivariate analysis of data from a randomized controlled trial. Infect Control Hosp Epidemiol [Internet]. 2014;35(1):63–8. Available from: http://www.ncbi.nlm.nih.gov/pubmed/24334800
13. Wynsma LA. Negative outcomes of intravascular therapy in infants and children. AACN Clin Issues. 1998;9(1):49–63.

Chapter 10
Umbilical Venous Catheters

Roberta Centorrino, Valentina Dell'Orto, and Daniele De Luca

10.1 Indications

The umbilical venous catheter (UVC) is an extremely common vascular access device in neonates of any gestational age, given the immediate accessibility of the umbilical vein and the relative simplicity of its placement. UVC presents peculiar characteristics that one must keep in mind to optimize its use. First, the tip of the UVC must be placed at the entrance of right atrium, at the junction between atrium and inferior vena cava. This position is considered to be safe and associated with minimal incidence of complications. In some emergency situations a sub-hepatic position has also been regarded as clinically acceptable (so-called 'umbilical venous sub-hepatic catheter', UVSHC). Noteworthily, the UVC is a central venous access device, since the tip is located in the right atrium or in the inferior vena cava, while UVSHC should be regarded as a peripheral venous access. Also, the 'sub-hepatic' position is associated with severe thrombotic and infective complications and should be adopted only as an emergency: UVSHC should be replaced as soon as possible. The different indications of UVC and UVSHC are described in Table 10.1.

The umbilical vein is only accessible early after birth (first 48 h), although cases of UVC placement have been reported even in 2-week-old neonates. This strictly depends on the umbilical vein conditions (ability to identify the vein, patency of the lumen, and wall tissue elasticity). Maintaining the moisture of the umbilical cord

R. Centorrino · V. Dell'Orto · D. De Luca (✉)
Division of Pediatrics and Neonatal Critical Care, Medical Centre "A.Béclère", South Paris University Hospital, APHP and South Paris-Saclay University, Paris, France
e-mail: Valentina.dellorto@aphp.fr

D. G. Biasucci et al. (eds.), *Vascular Access in Neonates and Children*,
https://doi.org/10.1007/978-3-030-94709-5_10

Table 10.1 Type of umbilical catheter and clinical indication

Clinical indication	Type of catheter
Critically ill neonates <1000–1250 g	UVC
Critically ill SGA neonates	UVC
Critically ill neonates >1000–1250 g and AGA	UVC
Infusion of solutions non-compatible with the peripheral route	UVC
Measurement of central venous pressure or $ScvO_2$	UVC
Rashkind procedure	UVC (dedicated device)
Neonatal resuscitation	UVSHC
Exchange-transfusion[a]	UVSHC or UVC
Other extra-corporeal therapies[b]	UVSHC or UVC

Abbreviations: AGA: appropriate for gestational age; $ScvO_2$: Oxygen saturation of central venous blood; SGA: small for gestational age; UVC: Umbilical vein catheter (central venous access device); UVSHC: Umbilical vein sub-hepatic catheter (peripheral venous access device)

[a]Exchange-transfusion may be performed through UVSHC, UVC or also other vascular accesses including peripheral lines: an UVC is not strictly needed

[b]These may include different techniques such as continuous veno-venous hemo(dia)filtration, single-pass albumin dialysis, and plasma exchange. These techniques may be possible with UVC of high diameter

may theoretically increase the chance of a late UVC insertion. A delayed separation of the umbilical cord may be associated with congenital immunodeficiency or local infection; thus, placing an UVC in this setting might be less safe. Delayed UVC placement (after one week of postnatal age) should be performed only in case of emergency (such as resuscitation, severe hypoglycemia, or exchange-transfusion), if rapid placement of a venous access is unavailable. Since the umbilical vein is not supposed to remain patent after birth, its use in these conditions may theoretically increase the risk of complications.

UVC is officially considered the ideal emergency vascular access for neonatal delivery room resuscitation, according to current guidelines. UVCs are typically used for intravenous administration of parenteral nutrition and drugs, for blood sampling, and for blood transfusions. At the time of insertion, it is often not easy to predict the clinical course of the newborn, so there is a risk of overuse UVCs, especially in preterm infants.

In a quality improvement document aiming to reduce unnecessary placement of UVCs, Shahid et al. developed consensus guidelines providing indications for UVC placement on the basis of gestational age, severity of illness, and ease of establishing a peripheral intravenous vascular access. They recommend the use of UVC in all preterm infants ≤28 weeks, and in newborns ≥29 weeks mechanically ventilated or with $FiO_2 > 40\%$ on continuous positive airway pressure and/or hemodynamically unstable and/or needing inotropes or fluids bolus, or with difficulty on establishing a peripheral intra-venous (PIV) access.

10.2 Insertion Technique

UVCs are placed by direct insertion, as the umbilical vein lumen is visible and accessible after having cut the umbilical cord. The catheter is threaded through the umbilical vein, which has a length of 1–3 cm and a diameter of 3–6 mm. The umbilical vein reaches the left branch of the portal vein, close to the common trunk of the portal vein. The Arantius venous duct (AVD) connects the left branch of the portal vein with the inferior vena cava (IVC). The connection between AVD and the portal vein is close to the end of the umbilical vein. Thus, an umbilical catheter may find its way into AVD and IVC or may be blocked in the portal circulation. Figure 10.1 depicts the anatomical structures with the different UVC routes and the placement of both a UVC and a UVSHC.

Insertion procedure:

- *Cleaning the cord and surrounding skin.* This is meant to remove blood, amniotic fluid, *vernix caseosa*, meconium and debris.
- *Disinfection and preparation of a sterile area.* Skin antisepsis must be performed with 2% chlorhexidine in iso-propyl-alcohol (IPA), since iodine compounds must be avoided as they may induce hypothyroidism in both term and preterm patients. Though, an excessive amount of alcoholic chlorhexidine (or an excessive exposure time) may cause chemical skin burns in extremely preterm neonates. Therefore, the minimal amount of antiseptic should be used (see Chap. 21), and after 30 seconds the skin should be washed with normal saline so to reduce contact time with the immature skin.
- *Placement of a sterile umbilical tape at the base of the cord.* This is useful to reduce blood loss (especially from umbilical arteries and especially if UVC is placed early after birth).
- *Cutting the umbilical cord.* This must be done within the Wharton jelly and 0.5–1 cm above the umbilical tape. It is advised to leave at least 1 cm if an umbilical arterial catheter (UAC) is to be inserted, as this maneuver may be difficult in a short cord.
- *Umbilical vein identification.* The umbilical vein is usually patent; if not, it may be slightly dilated by a small forceps or a stylet. In some cases, a 4-vessel cord may be found because of the presence of a fully patent second umbilical vein or an umbilical vein with varicosity/aneurism. These anomalies are usually associated with complex congenital malformations but may also occur in normal neonates. Care should be applied to cannulate the true umbilical vein, avoiding a varix.

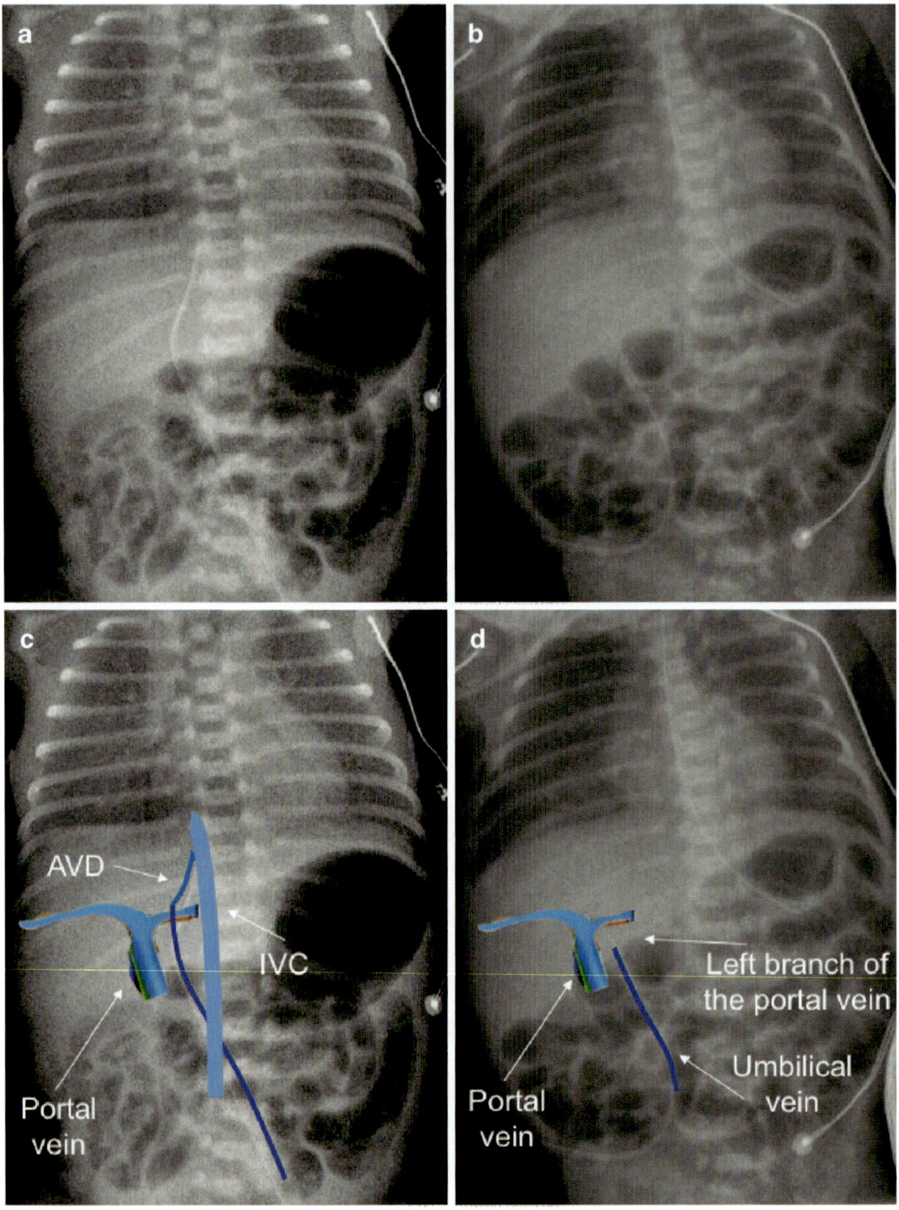

Fig. 10.1 Typical radiological imaging of the trajectory of a UVC ("babygram"). Panel A and B show an UVC and UVSHC, respectively. Panel C and D illustrate the anatomical structures. Abbreviations: AVD: Arantius venous duct; IVC: Inferior vena cava

- *Removal of clots visible at the vein surface.* This can be done by using gauzes and normal saline irrigation.
- *Choice of the catheter.* The catheter diameter must be chosen according to the vein size. Since the umbilical vein has no flow once the cord is disconnected from the placenta, the catheter can be as large as possible. A catheter completely filling the venous lumen may reduce the risk of displacement or reflux around the catheter in case of high flow infusion. The functional closure of the AVD occurs minutes or hours after birth; the anatomical closure occurs during the first week of life (even later in preterm babies). Functional closure can be overcome by an appropriately sized and stiff catheter or by various maneuvers (see below). On the contrary, anatomical closure of the AVD makes the UVC placement impossible.
- *Catheter priming and insertion.* The catheter should be filled with normal saline, 5–10% glucose solution, or a mix of both, or other appropriate solutions, depending on the clinical needs. The catheter must be inserted gently, with a cephalad direction, towards the head or the left shoulder. In case of double lumen UVC, both lumens must be filled. There are several formulae to calculate the ideal length of insertion to place an UVC (see below), though they currently have little role, since the whole maneuver should be performed under ultrasound control. Once placed at the desired depth, blood should be slowly aspirated to assess the patency, and the position of the tip must be verified by real time ultrasound. The insertion usually requires a single operator, but a second operator might be important for facilitating the maneuvers of tip location.
- *Catheter malpositions and maneuvers to aid placement of UVC.* Sometimes the catheter does not advance towards the IVC but is blocked inside the portal circulation. If resistance is felt approximately 1–2.5 cm below the estimated insertion depth for UVCC placement, the catheter tip is likely to be stuck at the bifurcation of right and left portal veins. This is a frequent occurrence when the catheter is threaded in a 'blind' fashion inside the vasculature. The best prevention of this difficulty is to adopt an ultrasound-based tip navigation, according to the Neo-ECHOTIP protocol (see Chap. 6). We recommend that the progression of the UVC should be always performed under direct ultrasound visualization, placing the probe in the epigastric area, between the umbilical cord and the xyphoid. Using a small sectorial probe 7–8 MHz, it is possible to follow step by step the progression of the catheter inside the liver, until it reaches the junction between IVC and right atrium. A small pression with the probe may be helpful to direct the catheter to the target, avoiding misdirection inside the liver. When the maneuver is 'blind' (without ultrasound), several techniques may be used for facilitating the passage of the catheter into the IVC (for example, the so called 'pressure technique': a gentle pressure on the right upper abdomen is applied with two fingers, while advancing the catheter; or, the so called 'hand liver mobilization',

for the purpose of obtain better alignment between the umbilical vein, AVD and IVC). Many other maneuvers have been described (‘two catheters technique’, ‘right lateral decubitus insertion’, etc.): though easy and harmless, most of them are of uncertain effectiveness and should be replaced by ultrasound-based tip navigation.

- *Tip location.* UVC position has been traditionally verified by X-ray, but ultrasound is gaining popularity as it is quicker, more accurate, safer, easy repeatable at bedside, less expensive and rapidly available at bedside (since it is already used in neonatal critical care for many other purposes). Ultrasound is favored over chest-x ray because it can reveal the tip position, catheter migration, and anatomical anomalies during the procedure; also, it avoids radiation exposure. Radiological confirmation can be flawed by abnormal anatomy, such as in congenital diaphragmatic hernias. As suggested by many authors, ultrasound should be regarded today as the gold standard for catheter position confirmation. Considering that ultrasound is also precious as a tip navigation technique, facilitating the catheter progression through the IVC up to the junction with the right atrium, it is reasonable to adopt the Neo-ECHOTIP protocol for both ultrasound-based tip navigation and tip location of UVC. Figure 10.2 depicts the correct position of a UVC at the junction between IVC and right atrium. Less common methods for verifying the central position of the UVC tip are (a) fluoroscopy (which can be justified only in very rare clinical situations, as in the case of neonates with congenital heart defects who undergo hemodynamic procedures), (b) intracavitary ECG (which is considered the gold standard for centrally inserted central venous catheters, but it may be logistically difficult for UVC), and (c) monitoring venous pressure while advancing the catheter (Fig. 10.3). The different methods of tip location are shown in Table 10.2.

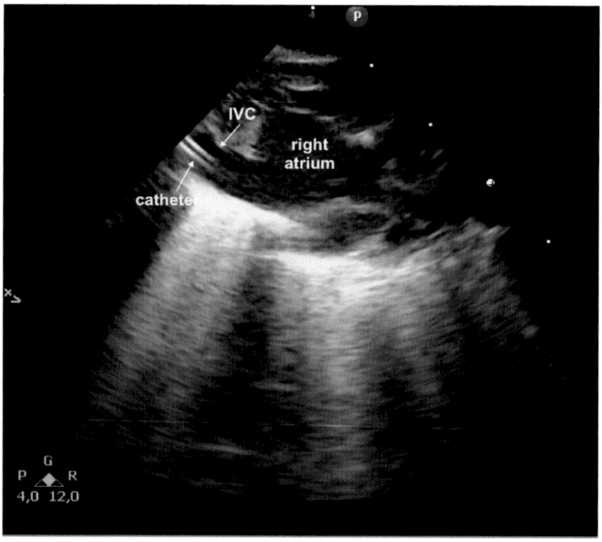

Fig. 10.2 Ultrasound-based tip location. An UVC is visualized as a “double track” image in the proximity of the junction between the IVC and the right atrium. Abbreviations: IVC: Inferior vena cava

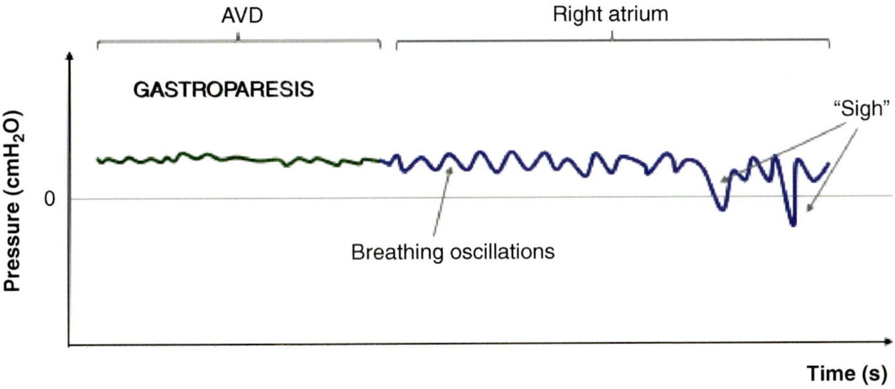

Fig. 10.3 Pressure tracing obtained while advancing the UVC. CVP (blue curve) is easily recognizable as an undulating line around a normal mean value of 5–8 cmH_2O with negative inflections during inspiration. Deep inflections are evident during "sighs". AVD pressure (green curve) have similar values but is more constant and freer from any respiratory change. Abbreviations: AVD: Arantius venous duct; CVP: central venous pressure; UVC: umbilical venous catheter

Table 10.2 Different methods of tip location for UVCs

Name	Technique	Pro's	Con's
Ultrasound based tip location	Direct visualization of the catheter (if needed, enhanced by 'bubble test': See Chap. 6)	Intraprocedural method. Useful also for tip navigation. Very accurate. Safe, inexpensive, easily repeatable.	Requires minimal ultrasound training
X-ray	Radiological landmark: Tip position between T9 and T10		Post-procedural method. Not useful for tip navigation. Inaccurate. Expensive, time-consuming, unsafe (x-ray exposure)
Intracavitary ECG method	The highest peak of the P-wave corresponds to the junction between superior vena cava and right atrium	Intraprocedural method. Very accurate and rapid (does not require calculations or measurements)	Needs special cable (ECG adapter). Not useful for tip navigation
Pressure method	Appearance of a CVP curve while advancing the UVC	Intraprocedural method. Rapid and relatively accurate.	Needs pressure line and sensor. Not useful for tip navigation

- *Securement and stabilization.* Once the tip position is checked, the catheter needs to be secured and stabilized. Different methods may be used to secure the UVC. Various combinations of sutures, tape, gels, and dedicated dressings can be used, but none of these methods have been shown to be superior, as they have not been investigated in rigorous studies. However, attention should be provided to the skin of preterm neonates as this may easily be injured both by surgical sutures and by some skin adhesive securement systems. Clinical studies are also investigating the possible role of cyanoacrylate glue in securing the UVC to the cord.

10.3 Materials

UVCs should be preferably in polyurethane. Several diameters, lengths, and number of lumens are available. Table 10.3 summarized the types of UVC commonly available within the EU market. Clinicians should be aware that the marks on the catheters used to estimate the insertion depth may be often inaccurate and vary between the tools. As regards the caliber of the UVC, 3.5Fr catheters are usually recommended for infants weighing more than 3.5 kg and 5Fr catheters for infants weighing more than 3.5 kg. Double and triple-lumen catheters are available if simultaneous administration of incompatible solutions is anticipated.

UVC maintenance may require additional devices such as high-pressure valves, single or multiple stopcocks with needle free connectors and port protectors, or protective bags filled with antiseptic agents.

10.4 Contraindications

Contraindications to UVC placement are mainly secondary to anatomical variations and thrombotic complications. UVC may be also unsuitable in abdominal wall malformations such as laparoschisis and omphalocele. In some cases of laparoschisis, UVC placement may be feasible, although other venous accesses should be preferred.

Vascular anomalies such as tortuous umbilical veins, persistence of the right umbilical vein (which should disappear around 7 weeks' gestation), anomalies of the umbilical/portal junction or aneurysms of the umbilical or portal veins can make UVC placement difficult or impossible. These anomalies may be associated with chromosomopathies, genetic syndromes, or major congenital malformations.

UVCs are also contraindicated in case of IVC thrombosis, a rare neonatal condition associated with acquired and inherited thrombophilia (66–72). Since UVC passes through the portal vein, it is debated if its presence may significantly affect gut hemodynamics. Properly placed UVCs are safe, but a UVC misplaced into the AVD or inside the portal circulation increases the risk of necrotizing enterocolitis (NEC). Thus, when NEC is suspected or diagnosed (albeit this condition is rare

Table 10.3 Characteristics of some polyurethane UVCs commonly available on the EU market

Manufacturer (model)	Diameter (Fr)	Available lumens	Length (cm)	Max flow (mL/min) [Prox./dist.]	Dead volume (mL) [Prox./dist.]
Vygon	2.5	1	30	3	0.21
	3.5	1	40	1.5	0.34
	4	1	40	18	0.36
	4	2	20	2 × 11	0.26 × 2
	4	2	40	12/11	0.26 × 2
	4	2	40	7/6	0.28 × 2
	5	1	40	24	0.46
	5	2	40	9/7	0.30 × 2
	5	3	38	–	0.32/0.19/0.19
	8	1	40	79	0.84
	8	3	38	–	0.77/0.33/0.33
Plastimed	3.5	1	30	–	–
	3.5	1	40	–	–
	4	2	15	10/9	0.15/0.13
	4	2	20	9/8	0.20/0.15
	4	2	30	7/6	0.25/0.20
	5	1	30	–	–
	5	2	30	13/12	0.30/0.25
	7	1	30	–	–
Covidien-Medtronic	2.5	1	25	–	–
	3.5	1	25	–	–
	3.5	2	38	–	–
	5	1	25	–	–
	5	3	38	–	–
	8	3	38	–	–

The table should not be considered comprehensive, as variations may happen according to market or industrial policy changes. Technical details have been collected from manufacturer where they were immediately available on their illustrative sheet or website. Different UVC and different characteristics may exist in other markets. These data are not meant to be used for clinical decisions, as readers are required to check these details with the manufacturer or its representatives

during the first week of life) the UVC should be removed or its tip location reconsidered. In some cases of thoraco-abdominal surgery, UVCs may be relatively contraindicated if the presence of the catheter impedes surgery.

10.5 Complications

UVCs are generally considered to be safe. Though, they may be associated with several complications. UVCs are probably safer than epicutaneo-caval catheters (ECCs) and their risk of thrombosis and vascular occlusion is lower than femoral catheters. Nonetheless, UVCs have a very high rate of dislodgment or dysfunction (28.6 per 1000 catheter/days).

One relevant non-infective complication is migration of UVC after insertion, which may occur in 50%, 63% or even in 90% of cases. It is commonly attributed to the drying of Wharton jelly and the secondary shortening of the umbilical cord. A prospective cohort study quantified the direction and the magnitude of catheter tip migration. The authors described an inward migration pattern during the first 48 h after UVC placement, followed later by an outward migration. The inward migration was explained by cord stump contraction over time together with an increase in lung volume (favored by ventilation, surfactant administration), the outward migration instead was likely to result from gradual distension of the abdomen as the bowel fills with gas. A significant variation of the abdominal girth should be considered as a possible cause of UVC migration and about half the infants included in studies experienced migration, mainly inward within 24 and 48 h from the catheter insertion. The risk of tip migration is a strong reason for adopting ultrasound-based tip location, which can be repeated at any time after insertion, even daily, with minimal cost and minimal invasiveness.

UVCs are also potentially associated with other severe non-infective complications.

UVC with the tip in the atrium may be associated with cardiac arrhythmias (mainly atrial flutter and paroxysmal supraventricular tachycardia). Cardiac tamponade caused by UVC is rare (0.5–2% incidence) but life-threatening, and it can occur even when the catheter is properly positioned.

UVSHC are particularly dangerous, being associated with liver abscess or necrosis, portal thrombosis, air in the portal system and other hepatic complications. Catheter-related portal vein thrombosis has been described as a rare event but is increasingly recognized thanks to the spreading of frequent ultrasound evaluations when the UVC is in place and after its removal. Reported incidence varies from 2.2% to 43% due to differences in study design and methodology. Umbilical catheters have also been associated with the development of intracardiac thrombosis, pulmonary embolism and renal vein thrombosis. In a recent prospective cohort study position of the tip of the catheter in the portal system or in the DV and was significantly associated with an increased incidence of NEC in preterm infants was found.[59]

Table 10.4 reports non-infective complications of UVC, as described in the literature.

Care is required for prevention of infective complications, the requirement for sterility being the same as in other central vascular access. UVCs are placed in neonates who, by definition, are immunocompromised compared to older children. Moreover, UVCs are often placed in preterm neonates who are even at higher risk for sepsis. UVCs have been associated with colonization in 22%–59% of cases and with bloodstream infection in 3%–8% of cases. In patients requiring long-term central venous access, bloodstream infection is reduced by nearly half after the adoption of a dedicated vascular access team in NICU. Also, other authors showed that line bundles and dedicated line care teams decrease the risk of infection.

Table 10.4 Non-infective complications of umbilical catheters

	UVC	UVSHC
Meckel's diverticulum perforation	X	X
Atrial flutter	X	
Atrial fibrillation	X	
Paroxystic supra-ventricular tachycardia	X	
Other arrhythmias	X	
Pleural effusion	X	
Pericardial effusion/ tamponade	X	
Rupture and/or migration	X	X
Liver abscess[a]		X
Peritoneal perforation	X	
Wharton's jelly embolism	X	X
Portal hypertension		X
Myocardial infarction	X	X
Veno-biliary fistula		X
Portal air		X
Liver rupture		X
Thrombosis	X	X
Infusate reflux[b]	X	X
Cardiogenic shock	X	X
Unexplained cardiac arrest	X	X

The list should not be considered exhaustive, and conditions are listed just on the basis of their literature description. Some of these complications may be associated and some may be related to pre-existing underlying conditions. A direct cause-effect relationship cannot be proven in some cases. Overall, UVSHC are associated with increased risk of complications if compared to UVC

[a]Liver abscess can be infectious or sterile. In this latter case they usually resolve spontaneously

[b]Reflux around the catheter lumen is especially frequent with UVSHC, narrow catheters and high flow infusions

On the other hand, the best strategy of infection prevention is the prompt removal of the UVC. UVC-associated bloodstream infection rates increase with time up to 42 per 1000 UVC-days by day 10 from insertion. The most significant increase appears after day 4 from insertion: therefore, UVCs should not be kept longer than 4 days. Though CDC guidelines suggest that UVC may remain in situ for up to two weeks (based on low quality evidence), we recommend prompt removal within few days, followed by placement of a different central venous access, if required, or by a peripheral venous access. An ECC may be the best choice to replace the UVC if there is no need for hemodynamic monitoring, frequent blood sampling or transfusions. ECCs have a lower infectious risk than UVC and may stay longer. If there is no need for parenteral nutrition or high osmolarity infusion, a peripheral venous access would be acceptable; though, it must be reminded that leaving an UVC in place will reduce costs and the number of venipunctures. On the contrary, in critically ill or unstable neonates, an ultrasound guided central venous access (via the brachio-cephalic vein or the femoral vein) will be more useful than an ECC and associated with longer dwelling time and less rate of infective complications.

10.6 Clinical Management

There are several important issues to be addressed about the optimal clinical management of patients with a UVC. Some of them have received extensive research with data from meta-analyses. Each NICU should have a written protocol including a comprehensive bundle for the decision to insert a UVC and its management. Having this tool has proven to reduce the use of UVCs, save resources and potentially decrease complications.

10.6.1 How to Calculate the Depth of Insertion to Place an UVC?

There are several methods to estimate or measure the depth of insertion of a UVC. None of the methods is really accurate. All of them have drawbacks and there is no clear data to prefer one method over another. However, length estimation is currently less important than in the past, since the introduction of ultrasound for tip navigation and tip location. The safest and most accurate method for advancing the catheter is under ultrasound control (tip navigation). Once gently advanced up to the estimated depth, aspiration should always be attempted, and blood return should be prompt. Care should be applied when drawing blood from a UVC in preterm neonates as this may significantly decrease cerebral oxygenation and should be performed slowly. Once the catheter is in position, intraprocedural confirmation of the tip with ultrasound must be performed (tip location). Table 10.5 reports the main methods available to calculate the depth of insertion, their advantages, and pitfalls.

10.6.2 When Should we Use Multiple Lumen UVCs?

A Cochrane meta-analysis of three randomized controlled trials found a decrease in the number of additional venous access accesses when using a multiple lumen-UVC, but only during in the first week of life. However, there was also a significant

Table 10.5 Different methods to estimate or the insertion depth for UVC

Name	Technique/Formula	Pro's	Con's
Shukla-Ferrara formula	(BW × 3 + 9)/3	Easy and similar to UAC formula	May be wrong in SGA patients
Modified Shukla-Ferrara formula	(BW × 3 + 9)/2	Easy and similar to UAC formula	May be wrong in SGA patients
Dunn's nomogram	Determined by shoulder-umbilical length on The Dunn nomogram	Accurate	Cumbersome (require unusual measurements)
Minimal weight calculation	(BW × 1.5) + 5.5	Easy	May be wrong in SGA patients
Surface anatomy method	Umbilicus to nipple distance—1 cm	Very accurate	Cumbersome (require unusual measurements)
Lateral look method	Umbilicus to the mid-xiphoid-to-bed distance	Rapid	Measurement prone to errors especially in most preterm babies and in incubators

Birth weight and length are to be considered in kilograms and centimeters, respectively
Abbreviations: BW: birth weight; CVP: Central venous pressure; SGA: small for gestational age; UAC: Umbilical artery catheters; UVC: Umbilical venous catheter

increase in catheter malfunction [risk ratio 3.69 (95% CI 0.99, 13.81); $p = 0.05$; risk difference 0.15 (95% CI 0.03, 0.27); $p = 0.01$). The data should be balanced with the higher cost of multiple lumen catheters. Double and triple-lumen catheters should be used selectively, only when simultaneous administration of incompatible solutions is anticipated.

10.6.3 Should Antimicrobial-Impregnated Central Venous Catheters be Used?

Polyurethane UVCs that release antimicrobial silver ions have recently become available. Such catheters are theoretically associated with reduced risk of infection since they decrease both endoluminal and extraluminal colonization. A randomized controlled study has demonstrated that these silver-impregnated UVCs are effective in decreasing the risk of catheter-related bloodstream infections in preterm infant. The use of such UVCs for prevention of CRBSI in preterm infants has been recommended by SHEA guidelines in 2014.

10.6.4 Should Prophylactic Antibiotics be Used before or after UVC Placement?

There is only one study on this subject and thus there is insufficient evidence to answer this question. However, it is highly recommended to avoid the use prophylactic antibiotics before or after UVC placement, in line with other data aiming to reduce antibiotic pressure and bacterial selection in NICUs.

10.6.5 Should Heparin be Used for Prevention of UVC Occlusion/Malfunction?

As for all other central venous access devices, there is no evidence that heparin lock or continuous heparin infusing may be beneficial in reducing lumen occlusion or catheter malfunction.

10.6.6 Should Heparin be Used for Prevention of UVC-Related Thrombosis?

The question is important especially in situations where the risk of thrombosis is high such as, critically ill neonates, polycythemia, etc.; however, data from a randomized clinical trial showed no effect of adding a continuous heparin infusion on UVC-related thrombosis.

10.7 Particular Considerations during Newborn Transportation

Critically ill neonates may be transferred by a mobile NICU which are fully equipped with all monitoring. The placement of a UVC line is almost invariably the quickest way to provide central or secured vascular access to give life-saving drugs. During transportation, particular care should be applied when securing the catheter; additional sutures or glue may be used in order to avoid displacement due to vibration, changes in relative speed or altitude. The tip position should be checked during transportation using portable ultrasound devices.

Bibliography

1. Abdellatif M, Ahmed A, Alsenaidi K. Cardiac tamponade due to umbilical venous catheter in the newborn. BMJ Case Rep. 2012 Jul;13:2012.
2. Ades A, Sable C, Cummings S, Cross R, Markle B, Martin G. Echocardiographic evaluation of umbilical venous catheter placement. J Perinatol. 2003;23:24–8.
3. Adesanya O, Naqvi M. Term neonate with liver laceration, obstructive uropathy, and ascites-secondary to extravasation of Total parenteral nutrition: a complication of Malpositioned umbilical venous catheter. Glob Pediatr Health. 2016 Oct 12;3:2333794X16670494.
4. Adiego-Calvo I, Saviron-Cornudella R, Martinez-Payo C, Rubio-Aranda E, Sancho-Sauco J, Cisneros-Gimeno AI, Perez-Perez P, Lerma-Puertas D, Whyte-Orozco J. Are congenital malformations more frequent in fetuses with intrahepatic persistent right umbilical vein? A comparative study. Taiwan J Obstet Gynecol. 2016;55:782–5.
5. Aitken J, Williams FL. A systematic review of thyroid dysfunction in preterm neonates exposed to topical iodine. Arch Dis Child Fetal Neonatal Ed. 2014;99:F21–8.
6. Aiyagari R, Song JY, Donohue JE, Yu S, Gaies MG. Central venous catheter-associated complications in infants with single ventricle: comparison of umbilical and femoral venous access routes. Pediatr Crit Care Med. 2012;13:549–53.
7. Akar M, Dilli D, Sandal G, Öncel MY, Erdeve Ö, Dilmen U. Prenatally diagnosed umbilical vein aneurysm with good prognosis. J Clin Ultrasound. 2012;40:368–9.
8. Amer A, Broadbent RS, Edmonds L, Wheeler BJ. Central venous catheter-related tachycardia in the Newborn. Case Report and Literature Review Case Rep Med. 2016;6206358.
9. Anderson J, Leonard D, Braner DA, Lai S, Tegtmeyer K. Videos in clinical medicine. Umbilical vascular catheterization. N Engl J Med. 2008 Oct 9;359(15): e18.
10. Arnts IJ, Bullens LM, Groenewoud JM, Liem KD. Comparison of complication rates between umbilical and peripherally inserted central venous catheters in newborns. J Obstet Gynecol Neonatal Nurs. 2014;43:205–15.
11. Aydin B, Dilli D, Uzunaliç N, Zenciroğlu A, Okumuş N, Cinar HG, Aydin M, Ipek MS. Calcified thrombosis of the inferior vena cava extending to renal veins in a newborn with homozygous MTHFR a1298c mutation. Genet Couns. 2012;23:523–7.
12. Balain M, Oddie SJ, McGuire W. Antimicrobial-impregnated central venous catheters for prevention of catheter-related bloodstream infection in newborn infants. Cochrane Database Syst Rev. 2015;9:CD011078.
13. Barone G, Pittiruti M, Biasucci DG, Elisei D, Iacobone E, La Greca A, Zito Marinosci G, D'Andrea V. Neo-ECHOTIP: a structured protocol for ultrasound-based tip navigation and tip location during placement of central venous access devices in neonates. J Vasc Access. 2021 Apr;5:11297298211007703.
14. Bertini G, Elia S, Ceciarini F, Dani C. Reduction of catheter-related bloodstream infections in preterm infants by the use of catheters with the AgION antimicrobial system. Early Hum Dev. 2013;89:21–5.
15. Butler-O'Hara M, Buzzard CJ, Reubens L, McDermott MP, DiGrazio W, D'Angio CT. A randomized trial comparing long-term and short-term use of umbilical venous catheters in premature infants with birth weights of less than 1251 grams. Pediatrics. 2006;118:e25–35.
16. Butler-O'Hara M, D'Angio CT, Hoey H, Stevens TP. An evidence-based catheter bundle alters central venous catheter strategy in newborn infants. J Pediatr. 2012;160:972–7.
17. Chang PT, Taylor GA. Umbilical venous catheter malposition and errors in interpretation in newborns with Bochdalek hernia. Pediatr Radiol. 2015;45:982–8.

18. Chen HJ, Chao HC, Chiang MC, Chu SM. Hepatic extravasation complicated by umbilical venous catheterization in neonates: a 5-year, single-center experience. Pediatr Neonatol. 2020 Feb;61(1):16–24.
19. Chen HN, Lee ML, Tsao LY. Exchange transfusion using peripheral vessels is safe and effective in newborn infants. Pediatrics. 2008;122:e905–10.
20. Costa S, De Carolis MP, Savarese I, Manzoni C, Lacerenza S, Romagnoli C. An unusual complication of umbilical catheterisation. Eur J Pediatr. 2008;167:1467–9.
21. Curry S, Honeycutt M, Goins G, Gilliam C. Catheter-associated bloodstream infections in the NICU: getting to zero. Neonatal Netw. 2009 May-Jun;28(3):151–5.
22. De Luca D, Romain O, Yousef N, Andriamanamirija D, Shankar-Aguilera S, Walls E, Sgaggero B, Aube N, Tissières P. Biomonitoring in neonatal critical care. J Ped Puericulture 2015; 28, 276-300. [article in French].
23. Demirel N, Aydin M, Zenciroglu A, Bas AY, Yarali N, Okumus N, Cinar G, Ipek MS. Neonatal thrombo-embolism: risk factors, clinical features and outcome. Ann Trop Paediatr. 2009;29:271–9.
24. Derinkuyu BE, Boyunaga OL, Damar C, Unal S, Ergenekon E, Alimli AG, Oztunali C, Turkyilmaz C. Hepatic complications of umbilical venous catheters in the neonatal period: the ultrasound Spectrum. J Ultrasound Med. 2018 Jun;37(6):1335–44.
25. DeWitt AG, Zampi JD, Donohue JE, Yu S, Lloyd TR. Fluoroscopy-guided umbilical venous catheter placement in infants with congenital heart disease. Congenit Heart Dis. 2015;10:317–25.
26. Dhua AK, Singh B, Kumar D, Awasthy N. Broken umbilical vein catheter as an embolus in a neonate – an unusual preventable complication. J Neonatal Surg. 2013;2:45.
27. Dongara BA, Patel DV, Nimbalkar SM, Potana N, Nimbalkar AS. Umbilical Venous Catheter Versus Peripherally Inserted Central Catheter in Neonates: A Randomized Controlled Trial. J Trop Pediatr. 2017 Jan 10;pii:fmw099.
28. Dubbink-Verheij GH, Visser R, Roest AA, et al. Thrombosis after umbilical venous catheterisation: prospective study with serial ultrasound. Arch Dis Child Fetal Neonatal Ed. 2020 May;105(3):299–303.
29. Dubbink-Verheij GH, Visser R, Tan RNGB, Roest AAW, Lopriore E, Te Pas AB. Inadvertent migration of umbilical venous catheters often leads to malposition. Neonatology. 2019;115(3):205–10.
30. Elser HE. Options for securing umbilical catheters. Adv Neonatal Care. 2013;13(6):426–9.
31. Escourrou G, De Luca D. Lung ultrasound decreased radiation exposure in preterm infants in a neonatal intensive care unit. Acta Paediatr. 2016;105:e237–9.
32. Fleming SE, Kim JH. Ultrasound-guided umbilical catheter insertion in neonates. J Perinatol. 2011;31:344–9.
33. Franta J, Harabor A, Soraisham AS. Ultrasound assessment of umbilical venous catheter migration in preterm infants: a prospective study. Arch Dis Child Fetal Neonatal Ed. 2017 May;102(3):F251–5.
34. Garland JS, Alex CP, Sevallius JM, Murphy DM, Good MJ, Volberding AM, Hofer LL, Gordon BJ, Maki DG. Cohort study of the pathogenesis and molecular epidemiology of catheter-related bloodstream infection in neonates with peripherally inserted central venous catheters. Infect Control Hosp Epidemiol. 2008 Mar;29(3):243–9.
35. Gazula S. Umbilical venous catheter insertion in gastroschisis. Indian J Pediatr. 2014;81:1261–2.
36. Gorski L, Hadaway L, Hagle ME, McGoldrick M, Orr M, Doellman D. Umbilical cathethers. In: Gorski L, Hadaway L, Hagle ME, McGoldrick M, Orr M, Doellman D, editors. Infusion therapy standards of practise; 2021. p. S90–3.
37. Grizelj R, Vukovic J, Bojanic K, et al. Severe liver injury while using umbilical venous catheter: case series and literature review. Am J Peri – natol. 2014;31:965–74.
38. Gupta AO, Peesay MR, Ramasethu J. Simple measurements to place umbilical catheters using surface anatomy. J Perinatol. 2015 Jul;35(7):476–80.

39. Gupta R, Drendel AL, Hoffmann RG, Quijano CV, Uhing MR. Migration of central venous catheters in neonates: a radiographic assessment. Am J Perinatol. 2016 May;33(6):600–4.
40. Hagerott HE, Kulkarni S, Restrepo R, et al. Clinico-radiologic features and treatment of hepatic lesions caused by inadvertent infusion of parentera l nutrition in liver parenchyma due to malposition of umbilical vein catheters. Pediatr Radiol. 2014;44:810–5.
41. Hargitai B, Toldi G, Marton T, Ramalingam V, Ewer AK, Bedford Russell AR. Pathophysiological mechanism of extravasation via umbilical venous catheters. Pediatr Dev Pathol. 2019 Jul–Aug;22(4):340–3.
42. Hoellering A, Tshamala D, Davies MW. Study of movement of umbilical venous catheters over time. J Paediatr Child Health. 2018 Dec;54(12):1329–35.
43. Hoellering AB, Koorts PJ, Cartwright DW, Davies MW. Determination of umbilical venous catheter tip position with radiograph. Pediatr Crit Care Med. 2014 Jan;15(1):56–61.
44. Hüning BM, Horsch S, Roll C. Blood sampling via umbilical vein catheters decreases cerebral oxygenation and blood volume in preterm infants. Acta Paediatr. 2007;96:1617–21.
45. Inglis GD, Davies MW. Prophylactic antibiotics to reduce morbidity and mortality in neonates with umbilical venous catheters. Cochrane Database Syst Rev. 2005;4:CD005251.
46. J Pediatr. 2006;148:546–8.
47. Kaae R, Kyng KJ, Frederiksen CA, et al. Learning curves for training in ultrasonography-based examination of umbilical catheter placement: a piglet study. Neonatology. 2020;117(2):144–50.
48. Kabra NS, Kumar M, Shah SS. Multiple versus single lumen umbilical venous catheters for newborn infants. Cochrane Database Syst Rev. 2005;3:CD004498.
49. Karatza A, Tsamandas A, Varvarigou A, Davlouros P, Pavlou V, Mantagos S. Supernumerary umbilical vein in a hydropic neonate with hypertrophic cardiomyopathy. Fetal Pediatr Pathol. 2011;30:173–6.
50. Karber BC, Nielsen JC, Balsam D, Messina C, Davidson D. Optimal radiologic position of an umbilical venous catheter tip as determined by echocardiography in very low birth weight newborns. J Neonatal Perinatal Med. 2017;10(1):55–61.
51. Katheria AC, Fleming SE, Kim JH. A randomized controlled trial of ultrasound-guided peripherally inserted central catheters compared with standard radiograph in neonates. J Perinatol. 2013;33(10):791–4.
52. Kdous M, Khlifi O, Brahem M, Khrouf M, Amari S, Ferchiou M, Zhioua F. Extensive Thrombosis of the Inferior Vena Cava and Left Renal Vein in a Neonate. Case Rep Obstet Gynecol. 2015;2015:569797.
53. Keir A, Giesinger R, Dunn M. How long should umbilical venous catheters remain in place in neonates who require long-term (≥5-7 days) central venous access? J Paediatr Child Health. 2014 Aug;50(8):649–52.
54. Kieran EA, Laffan EE, O'Donnell CP. Estimating umbilical catheter insertion depth in newborns using weight or body measurement: a randomised trial. Arch Dis Child Fetal Neonatal Ed. 2016;101:F10–5.
55. Kieran EA, Laffan EE, O'Donnell CP. Positioning newborns on their back or right side for umbilical venous catheter insertion. Acta Paediatr. 2016;105:e443–7.
56. Kieran EA, O'Donnel CPF. Accuracy of length measurements on neonatal umbilical catheters. Arch Dis Fetal Neonatal Ed. 2014;99:F520–1.
57. Kishigami M, Shimokaze T, Enomoto M, Shibasaki J, Toyoshima K. Ultrasound-guided umbilical venous catheter insertion with alignment of the umbilical vein and ductus venosus. J Ultrasound Med. 2020 Feb;39(2):379–83.
58. Kumar N, Murki S. Bilateral pleural effusion complicating umbilical venous catheterization. Indian Pediatr. 2013;50:1157–8.
59. Kumar N, Uhing MR, Powell M. Congenital absence of ductus venosus: an umbilical catheter with an abnormal path. J Perinatol. 2009;29:646–8.

60. Kumar SV, Chandra V, Balakrishnan B, Batra M, Kuriakose R, Kannoly G. A retrospective single centre review of the incidence and prognostic significance of persistent foetal right umbilical vein. J Obstet Gynaecol. 2016;36:1050–5.
61. Lee HN, Kwon SH, Oh JH. Successful transumbilical retrieval of a broken umbilical venous catheter in a 1-day-old new born baby. Cardiovasc Intervent Radiol. 2015;38:484–7.
62. Lei T, Xie HN, Feng JL. Prenatal diagnosis of four-vessel umbilical cord with supernumerary vein varix: A case report and literature review. J Obstet Gynaecol Res. 2017;43:1200–4.
63. Li J, Kong JY, James TE, Chandran S. Umbilical lines in a sick, extremely low birth weight infant: clinical quandary of X-ray images. BMJ Case Rep. 2016 Jun;22:2016.
64. Lide B, Lindsley W, Foster MJ, Hale R, Haeri S. Intrahepatic Persistent Right Umbilical Vein and Associated Outcomes: A Systematic Review of the Literature. J Ultrasound Med. 2016;35:1–5.
65. Lim-Dunham JE, Vade A, Capitano HN, Muraskas J. Characteristic sonographic findings of hepatic erosion by umbilical vein catheters. J Ultrasound Med. 2007 May;26(5):661–6.
66. Longhini F, Jourdain G, Ammar F, Mokthari M, Boithias C, Romain O, Letamendia E, Tissieres P, Chabernaud JL, De Luca D. Outcomes of Preterm Neonates Transferred Between Tertiary Perinatal Centers. Pediatr Crit Care Med. 2015;16:733–8.
67. Mahajan V, Rahman A, Tarawneh A, Sant'anna GM. Liver fluid collection in neonates and its association with the use of a specific umbilical vein catheter: report of five cases. Paediatr Child Health. 2011;16:13–5.
68. Manzoni P, De Luca D, Stronati M, Jacqz-Aigrain E, Ruffinazzi G, Luparia M, Tavella E, Boano E, Castagnola E, Mostert M, Farina D. Prevention of nosocomial infections in neonatal intensive care units. Am J Perinatol. 2013;30:81–8.
69. Marschall J, Mermel LA, Fakih M, et al. Society for Healthcare Epidemiology of America. Strategies to prevent central line-associated bloodstream infections in acute care hospitals: 2014 update. Infect Control Hosp Epidemiol. 2014 Jul;35(7):753–71.
70. Meinen RD, Bauer AS, Devous K, Cowan E. Point-of-care ultrasound use in umbilical line placement: a review. J Perinatol. 2020 Apr;40(4):560–6.
71. Mele R, Panesar LE, Heyden M, Sridhar S, Brandon D. Neonatal nurse practitioner use of ultrasonography to Verify umbilical venous catheter placement in the neonatal intensive care unit. Adv Neonatal Care. 2020 Aug;20(4):294–300.
72. Michel F, Brevaut-Malaty V, Pasquali R, et al. Comparison of ultrasound and X-ray in determining the position of umbilical venous catheters. Resuscitation. 2012;83:705–9.
73. Montaruli E, Pfister RE, Wildhaber BE. Sterile hepatic abscess secondary to administration of parenteral fluids via an umbilical venous catheter in a premature baby. J Pediatr Gastroenterol Nutr. 2011;53:575–6.
74. Morag I, Shah PS, Epelman M, et al. Childhood outcomes of neonates diagnosed with portal vein thrombosis. J Paediatr Child Health. 2011;47:356–60.
75. Mutlu M, Parıltan BK, Aslan Y, Eyüpoğlu İ, Kader Ş, Aktürk FA. Comparison of methods and formulas used in umbilical venous catheter placement. Turk Pediatri Ars. 2017 Mar 1;52(1):35–42.
76. Narang S, Roy J, Stevens TP, Butler-O'Hara M, Mullen CA, D'Angio CT. Risk factors for umbilical venous catheter-associated thrombosis in very low birth weight infants. Pediatr Blood Cancer. 2009;52:75–9.
77. O'Grady NP, Alexander M, Burns LA, et al. Healthcare infection control practices advisory committee (HICPAC). Guidelines for the prevention of intravascular catheter-related infections. Clin Infect Dis. 2011 May;52(9):e162–93.
78. Oestreich AE. Umbilical vein catheterization—appropriate and inappropriate placement. Pediatr Radiol. 2010;40:1941–9.
79. Parra Buitrago A, Valencia Zuluaga NA, Uribe Murillo AF. Inferior vena cava thrombosis and endocarditis in a premature patient: case report. Rev Chil Pediatr. 2014;85:708–13. [Article in Spanish]

80. Pennaforte T, Klosowski S, Alexandre C, Ghesquière J, Rakza T, Storme L. Intérêt du refoulement hépatique pour repositionner un cathéter veineux ombilical "sous-hépatique" dans la veine cave inférieure [Increased success rate in umbilical venous catheter positioning by posterior liver mobilization]. Arch Pediatr. 2010 Oct;17(10):1440-1444. French.
81. Plooij-Lusthusz AM, van Vreeswijk N, van Stuijvenberg M, Bos AF, Kooi EMW. Migration of umbilical venous catheters. Am J Perinatol. 2019 Nov;36(13):1377–81.
82. Pulickal AS, Charlagorla PK, Tume SC, Chhabra M, Narula P, Nadroo AM. Superiority of targeted neonatal echocardiography for umbilical venous catheter tip localization: accuracy of a clinician performance model. J Perinatol. 2013;33(12):950–3.
83. Quaak MS, Draaisma JM. A four-vessel umbilical cord. Arch Dis Child Fetal Neonatal Ed. 2017;102:F115.
84. Rahal H, Radouani MA, Knouni H, Barkat A. Deep vein thrombosis due to protein C deficiency in a neonate. Arch Pediatr. 2015;22:1035–8. [Article in French]
85. Ramasethu J. Complications of vascular catheters in the neonatal intensive care unit. Clin Perinatol. 2008;35:199–222.
86. Reynolds PR, Banerjee S, Meek JH. Alcohol burns in extremely low birthweight infants: still occurring. Arch Dis Child Fetal Neonatal Ed. 2005;90:F10.
87. Rosenblatt J, Loberstajn A, Coulomb A, Stos B, Garel C, Abarah B, Bénifla JL, Jouannic JM. Intra-abdominal umbilical vein varix associated with fetal cardiac failure: a pitfall to the prenatal diagnosis of α-zero-thalassemia. Fetal Diagn Ther. 2013;34:59–62.
88. Rubortone SA, Costa S, Perri A, D'Andrea V, Vento G, Barone G. Real-time ultrasound for tip location of umbilical venous catheter in neonates: a pre/post intervention study. Ital J Pediatr. 2021 Mar 18;47(1):68.
89. Sanderson E, Yeo KT, Wang AY, Callander I, Bajuk B, Bolisetty S, Lui K. NICUS network. Dwell time and risk of central-line-associated bloodstream infection in neonates. J Hosp Infect. 2017 Jun 23;pii:S0195-6701(17)30345-6.
90. Saul D, Ajayi S, Schutzman DL, Horrow MM. Sonography for complete evaluation of neonatal intensive care unit central support devices: a pilot study. J Ultrasound Med. 2016;35:1465–73.
91. Scalabre A, Gorincour G, Hery G, Gamerre M, Guys JM, de Lagausie P. Evolution of congenital malformations of the umbilical-portal-hepatic venous system. J Pediatr Surg. 2012;47:1490–5.
92. Schlesinger AE, Braverman RM, DiPietro MA, Pictorial essay. Neonates and umbilical venous catheters: normal appearance, anomalous positions, complications, and potential aid to diagnosis. AJR Am J Roentgenol. 2003;180:1147–53.
93. Scott MV, Fujii AM, Behrman RH, Dillon JE. Diagnostic ionizing radiation exposure in premature patients. J Perinatol. 2014 May;34(5):392–5.
94. Selvam S, Humphrey T, Woodley H, English S, Kraft JK. Sonographic features of umbilical catheter-related complications. Pediatr Radiol. 2018 Dec;48(13):1964–70.
95. Shabeer MP, Abiramalatha T, Gibikote S, Rebekah G, Thomas N. Bedside sonography performed by neonatology residents to confirm central vascular catheter position in neonates – a prospective diagnostic evaluation study. J Neonatal Perinatal Med. 2021;14(1):101–7.
96. Shah PS, Shah VS. Continuous heparin infusion to prevent thrombosis and catheter occlusion in neonates with peripherally placed percutaneous central venous catheters. Cochrane Database Syst Rev. 2008;2:CD002772.
97. Shahid S, Dutta S, Symington A, Shivananda S; McMaster University NICU. Standardizing umbilical catheter usage in preterm infants. Pediatrics 2014 Jun;133(6): e1742–e1752. https://doi.org/10.1542/peds.2013-1373. Epub 2014 May 19.
98. Sheta A, Al-Awad EH, Soraisham AS. Supraventricular tachycardia associated with umbilical venous catheterization in neonates. J Clin Neonatol. 2018;7:166–9.
99. Shibata M, Kanehiro H, Shinkawa T, Fujita Y, Yada K, Kamamoto T, Arai I, Nishikubo T, Sakata M, Kobayashi H, Takeda M, Nonomura A, Takahashi Y. A neonate with umbilical

arteriovenous malformation showing hemorrhagic shock from massive umbilical hemorrhage. Am J Perinatol. 2009;26:583–6.
100. Simanovsky N, Ofek-Shlomai N, Rozovsky K, Ergaz-Shaltiel Z, Hiller N, Bar-Oz B. Umbilical venous catheter position: evaluation by ultrasound. Eur Radiol. 2011;21:1882–6.
101. Sinha A, Fernandes CJ, Kim JJ, Fenrich AL Jr, Enciso J. Atrial flutter following placement of an umbilical venous catheter. Am J Perinatol. 2005;22:275–7.
102. Smorgick N, Herman A, Wiener Y, Halperin R, Sherman D. Prenatal thrombosis of the inferior vena cava and the renal veins. Prenat Diagn. 2007;27:603–7.
103. Stevens TP, Schulman J. Evidence-based approach to preventing central line-associated bloodstream infection in the NICU. Acta Paediatr Suppl. 2012;101:11–6.
104. Stoll BJ, Hansen NI, Adams-Chapman I, Fanaroff AA, Hintz SR, Vohr B, Higgins RD. National Institute of Child Health and Human Development neonatal research network. Neurodevelopmental and growth impairment among extremely low-birth-weight infants with neonatal infection. JAMA. 2004 Nov 17;292(19):2357–65.
105. Stroud MH, Trautman MS, Meyer K, et al. Pediatric and neonatal interfacility transport: results from a national consensus conference. Pediatrics. 2013;132:359–66.
106. Sulemanji M, Vakili K, Zurakowski D, Tworetzky W, Fishman SJ, Kim HB. Umbilical Venous Catheter Malposition Is Associated with Necrotizing Enterocolitis in Premature Infants. Neonatology. 2017;111:337–43.
107. Takada H, Yoshikawa H, Imaizumi M, Kitamura T, Takeyama J, Kumaki S, Nomura A, Hara T. Delayed separation of the umbilical cord in two siblings with Interleukin-1 receptor-associated kinase 4 deficiency: rapid screening by flow cytometer.
108. Tal L, Angelo JR, Akcan-Arikan A. Neonatal extracorporeal renal replacement therapy – a routine renal support modality? Pediatr Nephrol. 2016;31:2013–5.
109. Taylor T, Massaro A, Williams L, et al. Effect of a dedicated percutaneously inserted central catheter team on neonatal catheter-related bloodstream infection. Adv Neonatal Care. 2011;11:122–8.
110. Thaker VV, Leung AM, Braverman LE, Brown RS, Levine B. Iodine-induced hypothyroidism in full-term infants with congenital heart disease: more common than currently appreciated? J Clin Endocrinol Metab. 2014;99:3521–6.
111. Tissot C, Buchholz H, Mitchell MB, et al. First pediatric transatlantic air ambulance transportation on a Berlin heart EXCOR left ventricular assist device as a bridge to transplantation. Pediatr Crit Care Med. 2010;11:e24–5.
112. Traen M, Schepens E, Laroche S, van Overmeire B. Cardiac tamponade and pericardial effusion due to venous umbilical catheterization. Acta Paediatr. 2005 May;94(5):626–8.
113. Tsui BC, Richards GJ, Van Aerde J. Umbilical vein catheterization under electrocardiogram guidance. Paediatr Anaesth. 2005;15:297–300.
114. Türk E, Soylar R, Akca T, Serter S, Karaca İ. Venobiliary fistula related to umbilical venous catheter in a newborn. Pediatr Int. 2015;57:478–80.
115. Ullman AJ, Bernstein SJ, Brown E et al. The Michigan appropriateness guide for intravenous catheters in Pediatrics: miniMAGIC. Pediatrics 2020 Jun;145(Suppl 3): S269S284. https://doi.org/10.1542/peds.2019-3474I. PMID: 32482739.
116. Unal S, Ekici F, Cetin İİ, Bilgin L. Heparin infusion to prevent umbilical venous catheter related thrombosis in neonates. Thromb Res. 2012;130:725–8.
117. Vali P, Fleming SE, Kim JH. Determination of umbilical catheter placement using anatomic landmarks. Neonatology. 2010;98(4):381–6.
118. Verheij G, Smits-Wintjens V, Rozendaal L, Blom N, Walther F, Lopriore E. Cardiac arrhythmias associated with umbilical venous catheterisation in neonates. BMJ Case Rep. 2009;pii:bcr04.2009.1778.
119. Verheij GH, te Pas AB, Smits-Wintjens VE, Šràmek A, Walther FJ, Lopriore E. Revised formula to determine the insertion length of umbilical vein catheters. Eur J Pediatr. 2013 Aug;172(8):1011–5.

120. Verheij GH, Te Pas AB, Witlox RS, Smits-Wintjens VE, Walther FJ, Lopriore E. Poor accuracy of methods currently used to determine umbilical catheter insertion length. Int J Pediatr. 2010.
121. Weng YH, Chiu YW. Comparison of efficacy and safety of exchange transfusion through different catheterizations: femoral vein versus umbilical vein versus umbilical artery/vein. Pediatr Crit Care Med. 2011;12:61–4.
122. Williams S, Chan AK. Neonatal portal vein thrombosis: diagnosis and management. Semin Fetal Neonatal Med. 2011 Dec;16(6):329–39.
123. Wyckoff MH, Aziz K, Escobedo MB, Kapadia VS, Kattwinkel J, Perlman JM, Simon WM, Weiner GM, Zaichkin JG. Part 13: neonatal resuscitation: 2015 American Heart Association guidelines update for cardiopulmonary resuscitation and emergency cardiovascular care (reprint). Pediatrics. 2015;136(Suppl 2):S196–218.
124. Yigiter M, Arda IS. Hiçsönmez a hepatic laceration because of malpositioning of the umbilical vein catheter: case report and literature review. J Pediatr Surg. 2008;43:E39–41.
125. Yumani DF, van den Dungen FA, van Weissenbruch MM. Incidence and risk factors for catheter-associated bloodstream infections in neonatal intensive care. Acta Paediatr. 2013;102:e293–8.

Chapter 11
Epicutaneo-Cava Catheters

Vito D'Andrea, Giorgia Prontera, Serena Rubortone, and Mauro Pittiruti

11.1 Introduction

Central venous access devices are often required in neonates, particularly in preterm babies or in newborns who are candidate to intensive care procedures, surgery, or parenteral nutrition. A venous access device is 'central' when its tip is located in the superior vena cava (SVC) or in the right atrium (RA) or in the inferior vena cava (IVC). According to the terminology adopted by the WoCoVA Foundation (WoCoVA = World Congress on Vascular Access), central venous access devices in neonates should be classified as follows:

- Umbilical venous catheter (UVC)—inserted in the umbilical vein, tip at the junction between RA and IVC.
- Epicutaneo-cava catheters (ECC)—inserted in superficial veins of the limb or the scalp, tip in the SVC or at the junction between RA and SVC
- Centrally Inserted Central Catheters (CICC)—inserted by ultrasound guidance in deep veins of the supra/infraclavicular area, tip at the junction between RA and SVC
- Femorally Inserted Central Catheters (FICC)—inserted by ultrasound guidance in deep veins of the groin and the thigh, tip in the IVC or at the junction between RA and SVC.

V. D'Andrea · G. Prontera · S. Rubortone
Neonatal Intensive Care Unit, University Hospital Fondazione Policlinico Gemelli IRCCS, Rome, Italy
e-mail: vito.dandrea@policlinicogemelli.it; serenaantonia.rubortone@policlinicogemelli.it

M. Pittiruti (✉)
Department of Surgery, Catholic University Hospital, Rome, Italy

D. G. Biasucci et al. (eds.), *Vascular Access in Neonates and Children*,
https://doi.org/10.1007/978-3-030-94709-5_11

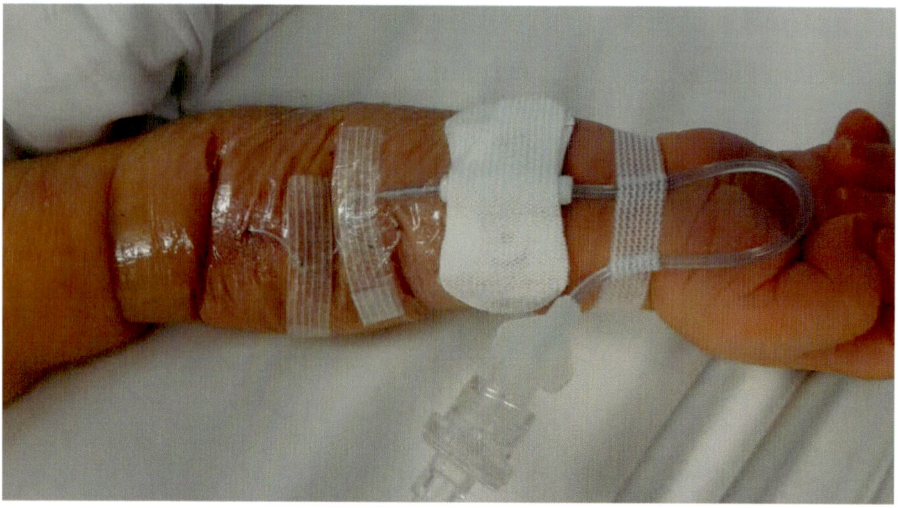

Fig. 11.1 Epicutaneo-cava catheter inserted in the upper limb of a neonate

In this chapter, we will discuss the indications, technique of insertion and complications of epicutaneo-cava catheters (ECC) (Fig. 11.1). These central venous access devices have been often called 'PICCs' (peripherally inserted central catheters). Though this term is correct, it may yield confusion, since PICC is also the term commonly used for indicating central catheters inserted by ultrasound-guided puncture and cannulation of the deep veins of the arm in children and adults. ECCs and PICCs are completely different central devices: ECCs are small bore catheters (1–2.7Fr), made of silicone or old generation polyurethane, inserted via superficial veins of the limbs or scalp using direct vein visualization. PICCs are larger catheters (3Fr and more), made of new generation polyurethane, usually power-injectable, inserted into the deep veins of the arm (brachial, basilic, axillary) using ultrasound guidance.

There is a huge technological leap between these two devices, which translates in different performances: PICCs are appropriate for blood sampling, for high flow infusion (up to 1 ml/sec vs 1 ml/min of ECC), for hemodynamic monitoring (central venous pressure, central venous sampling for oxygen saturation in mixed venous blood, etc.) and for infusion of blood products; they have extended dwell time (even months); they can be secured with subcutaneously anchored sutureless systems, thus abolishing the risk of dislocation; their tip can be safely located using intracavitary ECG (difficult to use for ECC); an accurate diagnosis of PICC colonization or infection is consistently possible by the DTP method (Differential Time to Positivity), which is not applicable to ECC; and so on.

11.2 Indications

The most frequent indication of ECC in neonates are based on the type of infusion (solutions with pH <5 or > 9, emulsions with high osmolarity, such as parenteral nutrition, or irritant/vesicant solutions that might be associated—by different mechanisms—with endothelial damage), or on the expected duration of venous access (more than 6 days but less than 14 days), or on the venous patrimony of the neonate (difficult venous access).

The ECC, as any other central venous access, should be promptly removed as soon as a central line is not required any longer. Though there is uncertainty regarding the actual duration of an ECC, several reports show that—at least in preterm neonates—the risk of infective and mechanical complications of ECCs increases enormously after 14 days. Therefore, in many NICUs these devices are routinely replaced by new ones after two weeks. When the expected duration of intravenous infusion is beyond 2–3 weeks, a more appropriate option of central venous access is the placement of large bore polyurethane catheters (3-4Fr) by ultrasound-guided percutaneous puncture and cannulation of the internal jugular vein, of the brachiocephalic vein (CICC) or of the femoral vein (FICC).

11.3 Materials

ECCs are available in different caliber (from 1 to 2.7 Fr), single lumen or double lumen. Small ECC (1Fr) are more frequently used in preterm weighing less than 1000 g, while 2Fr catheters are used in neonates weighing >1000 g. According to the commonly accepted strategies of thrombosis prevention, the vein cannulated by the ECC should have an inner diameter at least three times the caliber of the catheter. In the case of ECC, this is not always possible, since often the superficial veins of the upper and lower limb have a diameter below 1 mm; this might explain the high incidence of thrombosis/phlebitis of ECC, particularly in the tract of the vein close to the exit site.

ECCs are available both in silicon and in polyurethane, though the latter are becoming more and more popular and should be preferred. Polyurethane ECCs are less fragile and associated with higher flow performances if compared to silicon ECCs. A new type of antimicrobial ECC coated with rifampicin (antibiotic) and miconazole (antifungal) is now available on the market. Randomized controlled trials are currently evaluating its effectiveness in reducing the risk of central line associated blood stream infection.

11.4 Choice of the Cannulation Site

The choice of the vein most suitable for the insertion of an ECC often relies upon an empiric decision, depending usually on the operator's preference and experience, after a non-systematic assessment of the main superficial veins (Fig. 11.2). This is not an optimal strategy, as it may be associated with an uncontrolled exploitation of the venous patrimony of the neonate. We strongly recommend adopting a protocol of systematic evaluation of all peripheral veins, such as the RaSuVA protocol (Rapid Superficial Veins Assessment), already described in Chap. 9. The RaSuVA consists

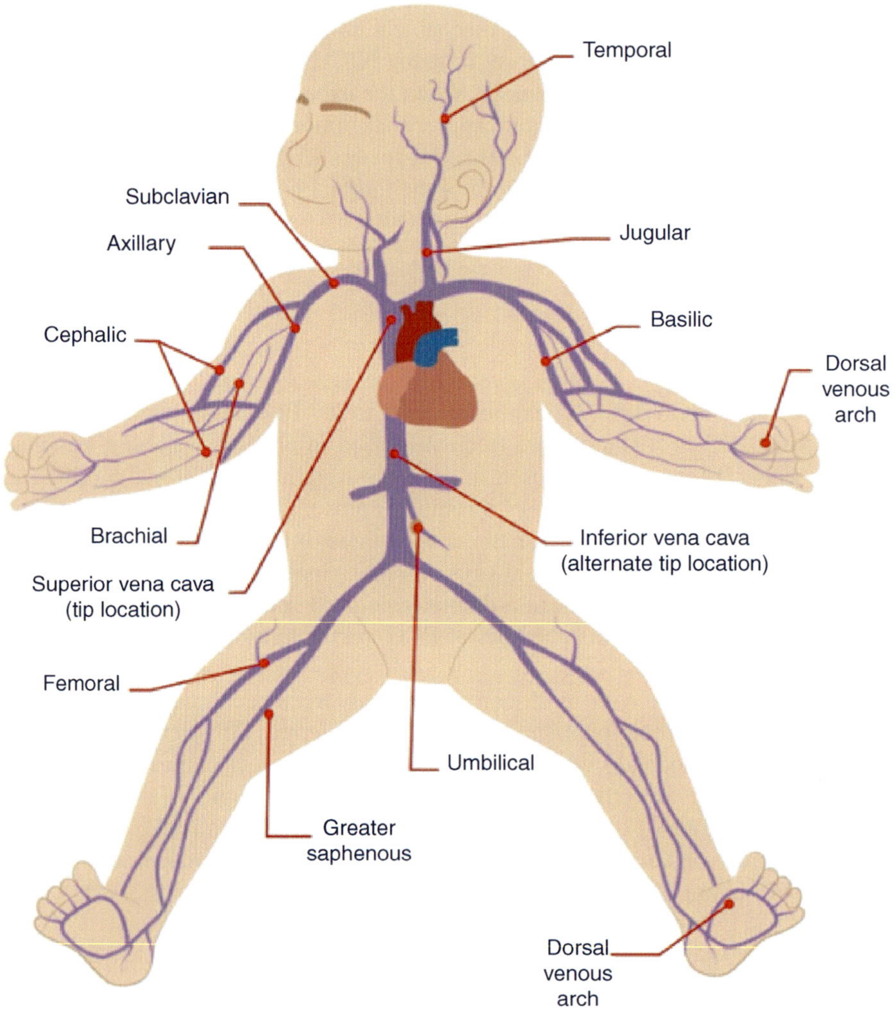

Fig. 11.2 Main veins that can be accessed for ECC insertion

in the sequential assessment of seven potential ECC sites, exploring the veins of the neonates ‘from foot to head’, first on the right and then on the left side: (1) medial malleolus, (2) lateral malleolus, (3) popliteal fossa, (4) back of the hand and wrist, (5) antecubital fossa, (6) anterior scalp veins, (7) posterior scalp veins. The exploration can be performed with direct eye visualization of the superficial veins, or by using NIR technology (see Chap. 5).

RaSuVA is an easy tool designed to build a detailed and complete map of the superficial veins of the neonate, through a rational and systematic approach, so to choose the best vein for cannulation and avoid unnecessary multiple venous punctures. Using the data derived from RaSuVA, it is possible to define a list of preferred veins in each patient, depending on the type of the venous device to insert (peripheral or central). For example, the insertion of peripheral cannulas is preferably performed in the lower limbs (excluding the saphenous vein) as a first option, or on the back of the hand and at the wrist as a second option. The insertion of an ECC is usually performed at the antecubital fossa (first option) or at the saphenous vein at the medial malleolus (second option). The puncture/cannulation of scalp veins is taken into consideration only in very selected cases.

11.5 Technique of Insertion

After choosing the cannulation site, the neonate is prepared to the procedure (proper immobilization, comfort-care, and sedation).

The next pre-procedural step is the estimation of the required length of the ECC, depending on the cannulation site and on the size of the patient (Fig. 11.3).

For cannulation site at the upper limb (Fig. 11.4) or on the scalp, length estimation is calculated as the distance from puncture site to the right sternoclavicular notch + the distance from the sternoclavicular notch to the third intercostal space.

For cannulation site at the lower limb, length estimation is calculated as the distance from puncture site to the groin + the distance between groin and navel + the distance between navel and xyphoid process.

Figure 11.2 summarizes the length estimation.

The procedure follows these steps:

- Hygiene of the hands (alcohol gel rub, as first option)
- Maximal barrier precautions (cap, mask, sterile gown, sterile gloves)
- Check of the content of the insertion pack (sterile drapes, sterile gauze, forceps, scissors, syringes, tourniquet, centimeter tape, etc.) and check of materials usually not included in the pack (saline, cyanoacrylate glue, chlorhexidine swab, etc.)
- Check of the content of the catheter kit: catheter (to be filled with saline) and introducer (usually, 20-24G breakable needle, or micro-introducer for modified Seldinger)
- Skin antisepsis with 2% chlorhexidine in alcohol, avoiding excessive amounts of antiseptic solution and friction movements (Fig. 11.5)

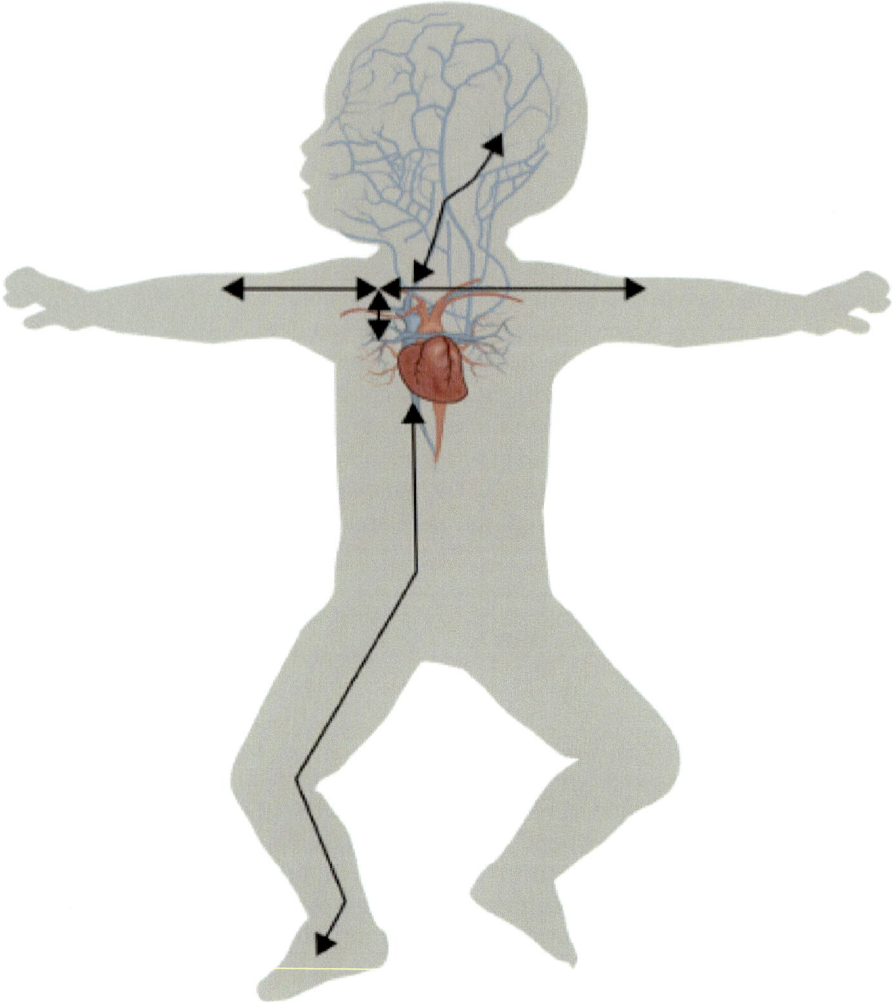

Fig. 11.3 Graphic representation of the methods for estimating the length of the ECC

- the antiseptic needs 30 seconds for reaching the maximal activity; after 30 seconds, the area is rinsed with saline
- wide sterile field, using fenestrated drapes (Fig. 11.6)
- placement of tourniquet (if cannulation site is on the limbs)
- direct puncture of the vein (Fig. 11.7), checking blood return (Fig. 11.8); the visualization, puncture and visualization of the vein may be facilitated by NIR devices (see Chap. 5)
- removal of the tourniquet
- insertion of the catheter through the needle or through the introducer

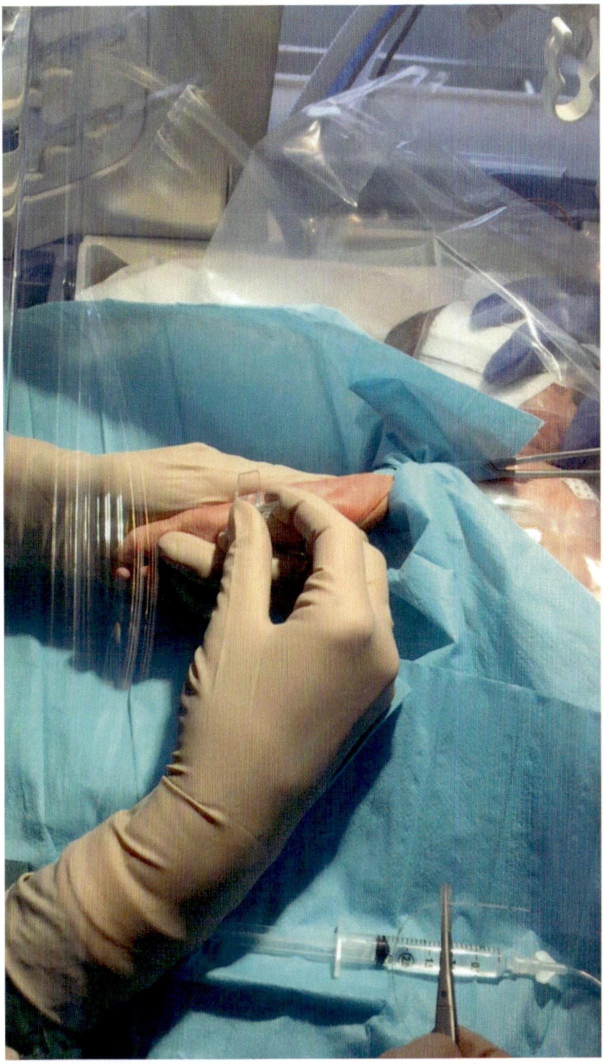

Fig. 11.4 Puncture at the upper limb

- as the catheter is inserted for the estimated length, the position of the tip is checked by real time ultrasound (see below)
- after checking the blood return by aspirating through the ECC, the needle/introducer is removed

the exit site is sealed with a minimal amount (< 0.25 ml) of cyanoacrylate glue; cyanoacrylate glue is safe, inexpensive, and easy to apply, and it yields the additional advantage of being very effective in preventing any bleeding/oozing at the puncture site; removal of cyanoacrylate glue is also consistently easy and harmless

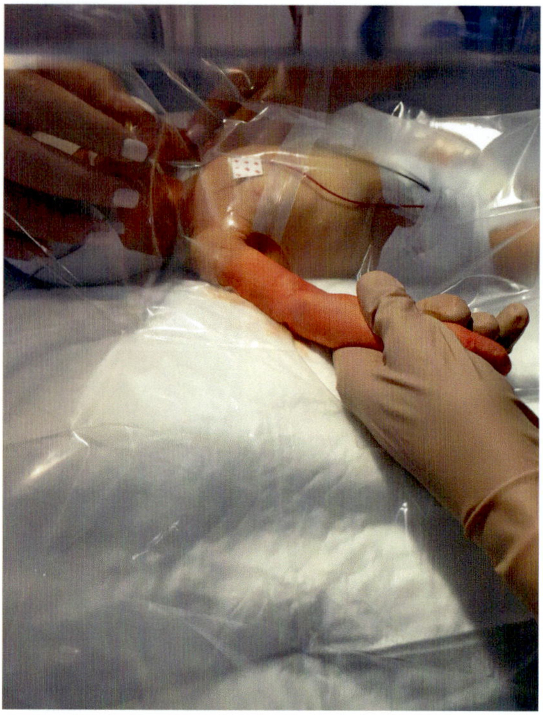

Fig. 11.5 Skin antisepsis with 2% chlorhexidine in alcohol

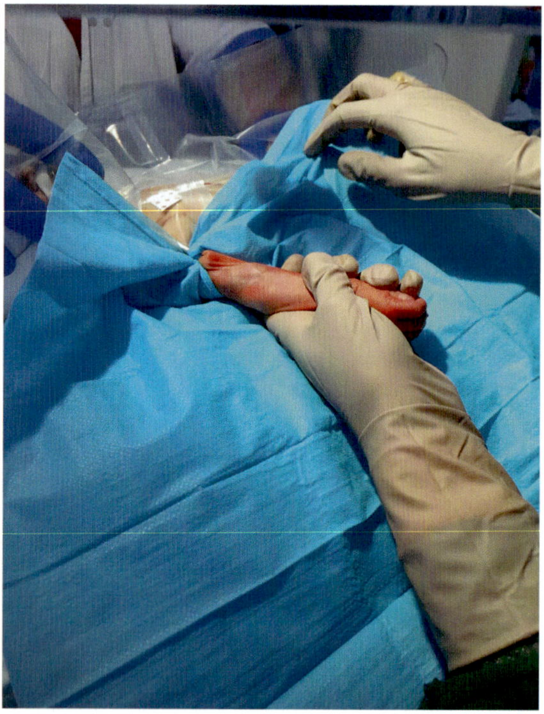

Fig. 11.6 Wide sterile field

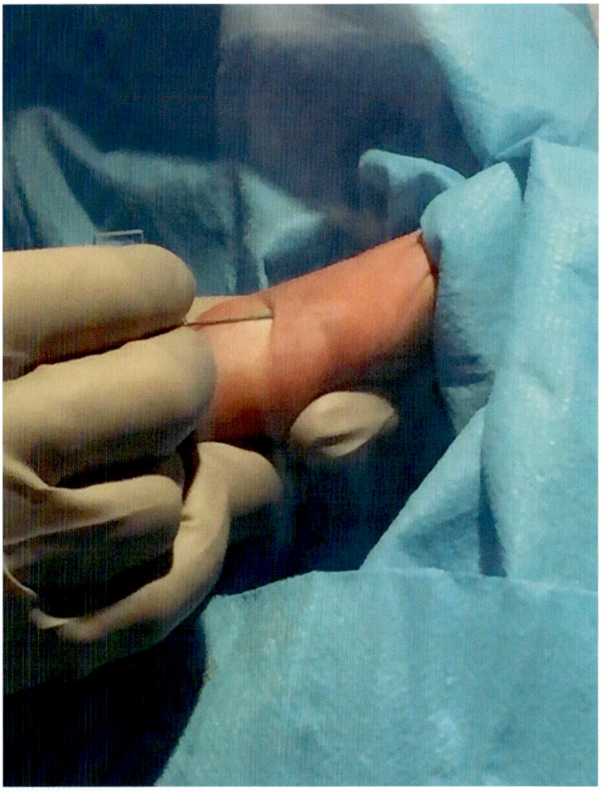

Fig. 11.7 Venipuncture

- if additional sterile strips are used, they should block the catheter on the skin at no less than 1 cm of distance from the exit site
- after cleaning the skin with saline, the area is wiped and then covered with semi-permeable transparent membranes with high permeability (high MVTR). (Fig. 11.9)

11.6 Insertion Complications

The most frequent complication during insertion is difficulty in the progression of the ECC, due to extravascular placement of the catheter or vascular abnormalities. When this happens, several maneuvers are used: changing the position of the limbs or the head, flushing the catheter with small amount of saline, etc.

The catheter should be left in place only after confirmation of the appropriate position of the tip by ultrasound and after verification of blood return.

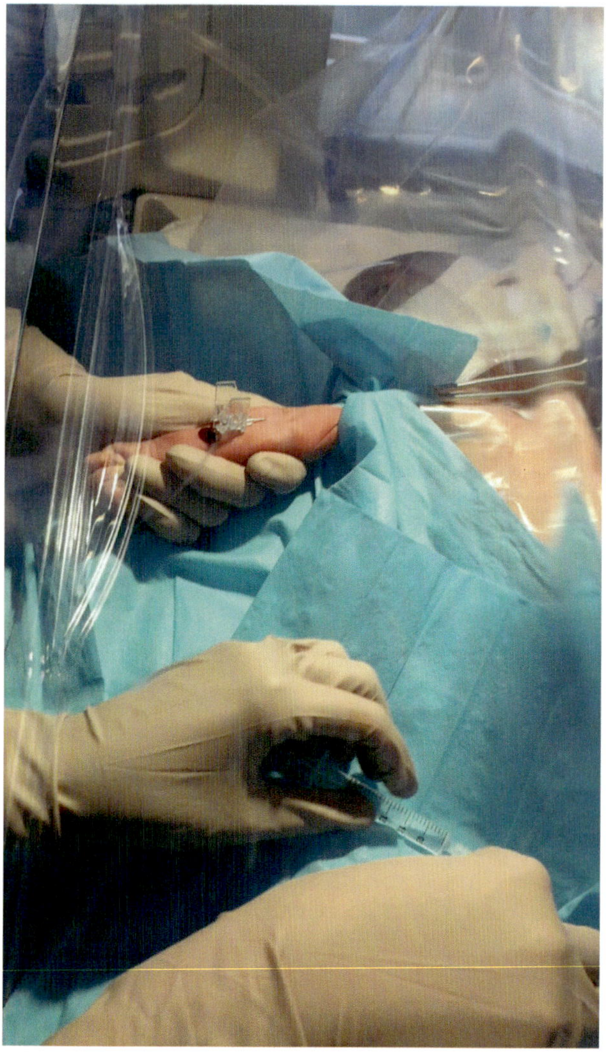

Fig. 11.8 Blood return from the needle

11.7 Tip Location

The old strategy for ECC placement, which unfortunately is still very popular, consists in the 'blind' placement of the catheter, based on the length estimation by surface landmarks, followed by a post-procedural radiological control by a chest/abdomen x-ray. Traditionally, an ECC inserted at the upper limb or on the scalp should have its tip radiologically projected at the level of the body of the fourth thoracic vertebra (T4), which corresponds, very approximately, to the SVC/RA junction; an ECC inserted at the lower limb should have its tip radiologically projected at the level of the body of the ninth thoracic vertebra (T9), which corresponds, very approximately, to the IVC/RA junction (Fig. 11.10). When the catheter

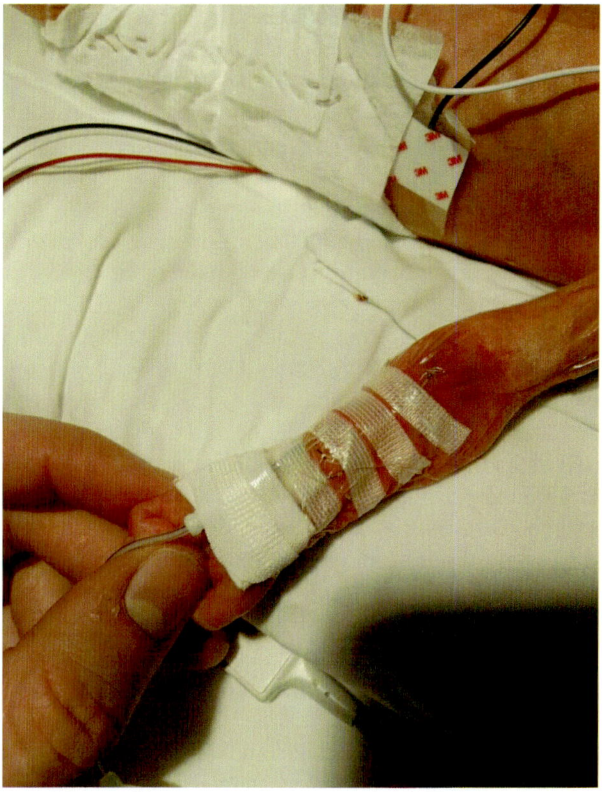

Fig. 11.9 Final dressing: cyanoacrylate glue, sutureless securement, sterile strips and transparent membrane with high permeability

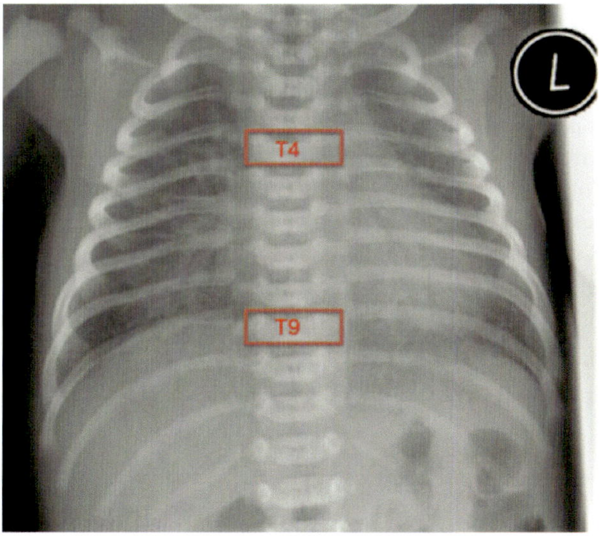

Fig. 11.10 Chest x-ray showing the fourth vertebral body (T4) and the ninth vertebral body (T9)

is difficult to visualize on x-ray, a small amount of contrast medium (0.3–0.5 ml) has been used to enhance visualization. This radiological method of tip location has many disadvantages: (a) it is quite inaccurate, since the SVC/RA junction and the IVC/RA junction are not directly seen on x-ray, but their location is indirectly inferred by radiological landmarks; (b) it is post-procedural, so that—if the tip position is not correct—it may be necessary to reposition the ECC; (c) it is not safe, since it implies x-ray exposure.

For these reasons, the method of tip location currently recommended is based on ultrasound: it is accurate, since both the catheter and the vascular structures can be easily visualized in the neonate; it is intraprocedural, so that the final position of the ECC can be verified immediately and the catheter can be secured immediately; it is safe, since exposure to ultrasound is harmless. Ultrasound has a role not only during the maneuver of placement, as a real-time method of verification of the correct direction of the catheter inside the vasculature (tip navigation) and of the final position of the tip (tip location), but also as an accurate and non-invasive post-procedural tool for the periodic verification of the position of the ECC, so to detect any secondary malposition or other catheter-related complications.

The use of ultrasound for tip navigation and tip location is described in detail in the Neo-ECHOTIP paper (see Bibliography). In short, when the ECC is inserted via veins of the scalp or the upper limbs, tip navigation is performed using a 10–14 MHz linear probe and assessing the progression of the catheter into the superior vena cava by a simple supraclavicular view (as the one described in the RaCeVA). When the ECC is inserted via the veins of the lower limbs, tip navigation is performed following the catheter inside the femoral vein and the external iliac vein, using a linear probe. In any case, tip location is performed using a subcostal longitudinal view that allows visualization of the right cavities of the heart, and/or a subcostal bi-caval view (Fig. 11.11) that allows visualization of SVC, RA and IVC (Fig. 11.12). The tip of the catheter is visualized directly, or indirectly by injecting a small flush of saline (0.5–1 ml).

In adults and in children, intracavitary ECG is nowadays the gold standard for the intra-procedural tip location, due to its great accuracy and feasibility. So far, few studies have investigated ECC placement with intracavitary ECG in neonates. The small number of patients enrolled and the poor quality of the signal, probably related to the small diameter of the catheter, make it impossible to draw a definite conclusion about the feasibility of this technique in the neonatal population. Though, this is an interesting field of research and in the next future intracavitary ECG may be an aid in tip location, together with ultrasound.

11.8 Maintenance

As for any vascular device, the adoption of proper strategies of maintenance of the ECC plays a pivotal role in minimizing complications and prolonging the life of the catheter. The implementation of dedicated teams for the management of central venous access is proven to be associated with successful clinical outcomes.

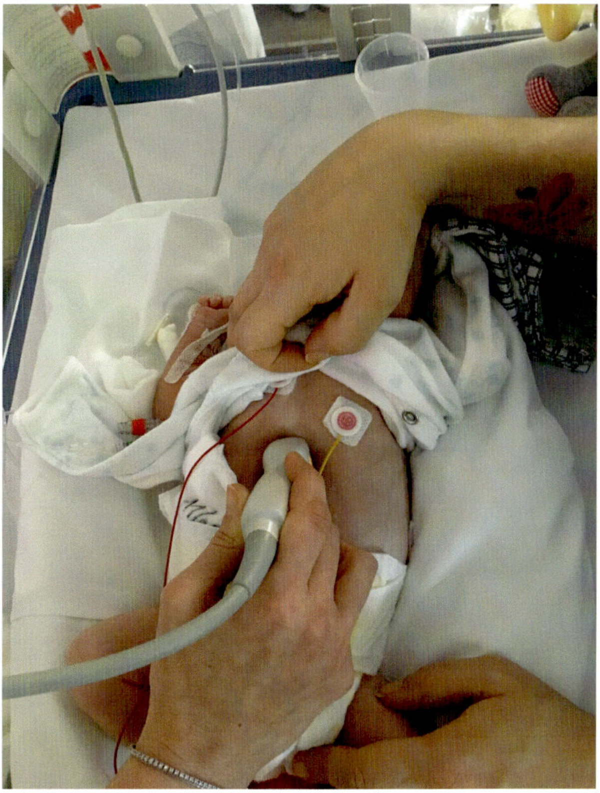

Fig. 11.11 Probe placed in the subcostal space

The most important recommendations are the following:

- proper hand hygiene before and after any procedure performed on the ECC
- sterile handling of the infusion lines and of the hubs
- maintenance of a constant flow (at least 0.5–1 ml/h for ECC < 2Fr) so to keep the lumen patent
- bolus infusions should be administered using 10 ml syringes, that exert low pressure (approximately 50 PSI), since no ECC is power injectable. Smaller syringes may be associated with higher pressure (100 PSI for 5 ml syringes and 200 PSI for 2 ml syringes) and risk of catheter rupture
- dressing change should be focused on the necessity of avoiding bacterial contamination of the exit site and catheter dislodgment and should be performed only in case of local problems (detachment of the membrane, bleeding, etc.). The cornerstones of a proper dressing of ECC are cyanoacrylate glue and semipermeable transparent dressings with high permeability (high MVTR—'moisture vapor transfer rate') (Fig. 11.13)

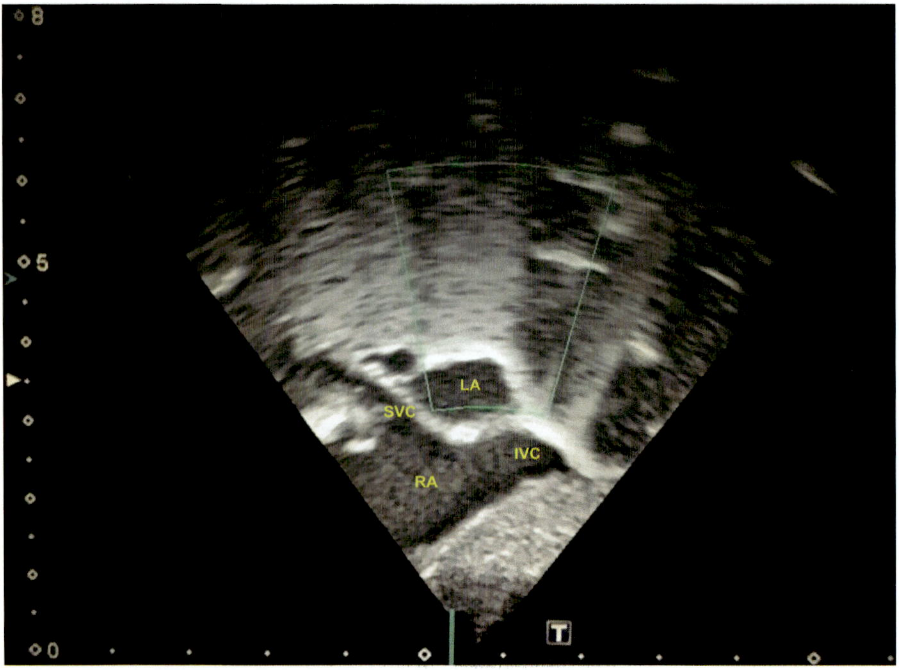

Fig. 11.12 Subcostal bi-caval view, showing right atrium (RA), superior vena cava (SVC) and inferior vena cava (IVC)

Fig. 11.13 Exit site of epicutaneo-cava catheter protected with glue and transparent membrane

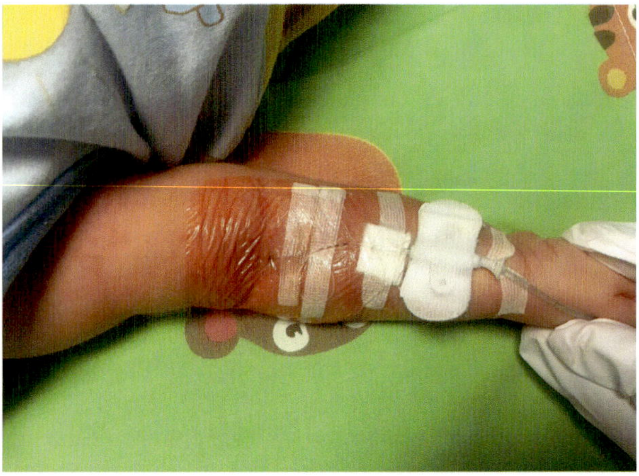

11.9 Removal

The removal of ECC must be done with sterile gloves and after proper skin antisepsis. The catheter should be removed very slowly. ECCs are fragile, even if in polyurethane, and minimal adhesions of the catheter to the vein wall (typically because of fibroblastic sleeve or phlebitis around the ECC) may offer resistance, and the catheter may fracture spontaneously. At the end of the procedure, the length of the catheter should be assessed, so to verify that no fragments have been lost in the vasculature.

When the catheter does not come away easily, several maneuvers are usually attempted, even if most of them are not expected to be effective. Probably, gentle slow traction, rotation of the catheter, and waiting are the best strategies. In some rare cases (catheter stuck inside a vein with phlebitis, or catheter rupture) surgery may be required.

11.10 Complications

11.10.1 Infection

The diagnosis of catheter-related blood stream infection (CRBSI) is not practical with ECCs, since the method of Differential Time to Positivity (DTP) cannot be applied since blood culture from an ECC is often impossible. Thus, the only feasible diagnosis is central line associated blood stream infection (CLABSI), which inevitably include not only ECC-related blood stream infections, but also blood stream infections secondary to other non-evident sources. The diagnosis of CLABSI implies a positive peripheral culture, with systemic signs of infection, in a neonate who had a central line for 48 h or more, in absence of other evident sources of infection. CLABSI is often the effect of a prolonged stay of the ECC (more than two weeks) and/or breakthrough of the aseptic technique during the maneuvers of insertion/maintenance. If CLABSI occurs, the ECC should be removed immediately, and proper antibiotic treatment started. An attempt at saving the central access might be considered only when (a) proper antibiotic treatment has begun, (b) the infection is not caused by S. Aureus, Candida, or Gram-negative germs, and (c) a second blood culture performed 48–72 h later is negative. After ECC removal because of infection, a new central access should not be inserted in the following 2–3 days.

11.10.2 Catheter Malfunction

Malfunction can be secondary to intraluminal obstruction (clots, drug precipitates, lipid aggregates, etc.) or extraluminal factors (catheter kinking, tip malposition, fibroblastic sleeve, venous thrombosis around the tip, etc.). If an intraluminal obstruction is suspected, the ECC should be flushed gently. The cause of the extraluminal obstruction can be assessed by ultrasound examination. Many of these causes eventually lead to ECC removal.

11.10.3 Catheter Dislodgment

This complication is usually secondary to accidental traction of the catheter during dressing change or general neonatal care. Few millimeters may not be clinically relevant but dislodgment of 1 cm or more are likely to be associated with important secondary malposition of the tip, so that the catheter cannot be considered central anymore. Assessment of the tip location can be easily performed by ultrasound. If tip malposition is detected, the options are (a) use of the catheter as peripheral line, or (b) removal.

11.10.4 Tip Migration

The tip of the ECC can migrate inside the vasculature even without any dislodgment of the catheter at the exit site, for instance because of variation of the intrathoracic pressure. The new location of the tip should be assessed by ultrasound. Treatment may include partial withdrawal of the catheter, or removal.

11.10.5 Local Phlebitis

Several factors may cause a local thrombophlebitis of the vein that has been cannulated for ECC insertion: mismatch between vein diameter and catheter caliber, trauma of the vein wall during cannulation, bacterial contamination due to poor skin antisepsis, chemical irritation of the vein caused by the powder inside the gloves, and so on. If the phlebitis does not recede in 48 h, the ECC must be removed.

11.10.6 Catheter-Related Venous Thrombosis

It is usually associated with an incorrect position of the tip. The diagnosis requires proper ultrasound exploration of the vasculature where the tip of the catheter appears to be located. Severe obstruction of the SVC or the IVC may require thrombolysis using alteplase (rTPA) or urokinase, preferably administered through the catheter, especially if the thrombosis is around the tip. Anticoagulant treatment should be started. When the thrombosis is associated with catheter malfunction and/or tip malposition, the ECC should be removed after a proper period of anticoagulant therapy (3–7 days).

11.10.7 Edema of the Limb

It is often secondary to a dressing that is too tight. Ultrasound should be used, so to assess that the edema is not secondary to catheter-related venous thrombosis.

11.10.8 Secondary Erosion of the Pericardium or of the Pleura

ECCs—if very thin, and/or very mobile, and/or if the tip is not properly located at the RA/SVC junction—may rarely cause an erosion of the vein wall with entrance of the tip of the catheter into the pleural space or into the pericardial space. In the first case, a pleural effusion occurs with respiratory distress; in the second case, a pericardial effusion with cardiac tamponade. Ultrasound plays a central role in the prevention of this complication (periodical assessment of tip location), in its diagnosis (detection of effusion by chest ultrasonography and echocardiography) and in its treatment (ultrasound-guided thoracentesis or pericardiocentesis) (Fig. 11.14).

11.11 Limitations of the ECCs

ECCs are extremely important in the management of the newborns: as central lines, they can be used for delivery of parenteral nutrition and of any solutions, even if irritant or vesicant to the vein wall. Though, they have many limitations:

- the flow is very slow (maximal flow 1 ml/min), so that may not be appropriate for critically ill neonates requiring transfusions or volume repletion
- as no ECC is power injectable, this venous access is particularly fragile and prone to rupture

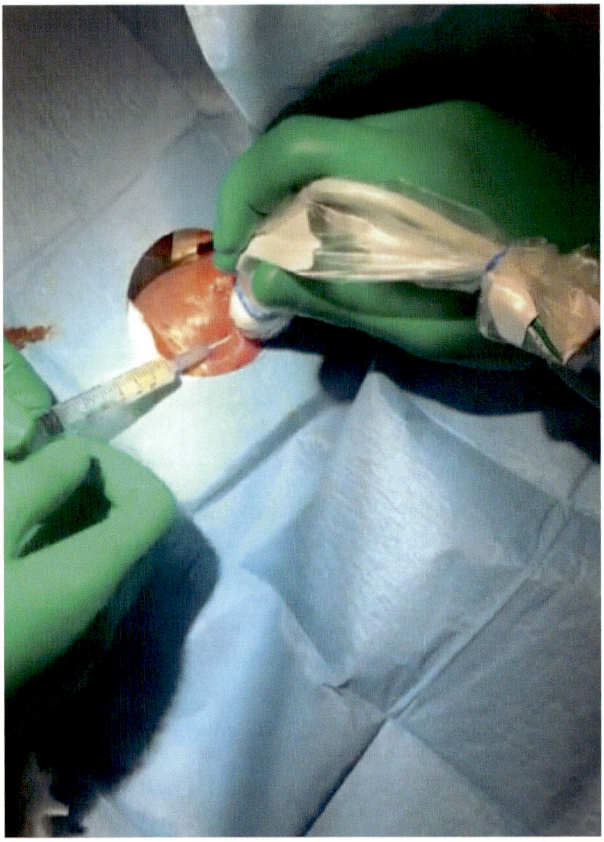

Fig. 11.14 Ultrasound-guided aspiration of pleural fluid effusion

- as blood withdrawal is difficult or impossible, blood samples must be obtained by additional punctures of peripheral veins; also, diagnosis of CRBSI by DTP is not possible, and measurement of oxygen saturation in mixed venous blood cannot be obtained
- due to the small caliber, measurement of central pressure is not possible
- their expected dwelling time is limited to few weeks (even less in preterm babies), because of the frequent complications.

This explains why ECCs may be appropriate in uncomplicated stable neonates requiring only hydration and parenteral nutrition, but not in critically ill neonates requiring surgery or aggressive intensive care treatments. In these latter cases, an ultrasound guided CICC will be more appropriate. Many papers of the last few years have suggested that ultrasound guided CICCs are feasible and safe even in very small neonates, with a high percentage of success and minimal risk, in experienced hands. CICCs and FICCs offer several advantages not only in term of performance (high flow, blood withdrawal, etc.) but also it is likely that they are associated with lower risk of complications (occlusion, secondary malposition, venous thrombosis, mechanical rupture, infection) if compared to ECC.

Bibliography

1. Barone G, D'Andrea V, Vento G, et al. A systematic ultrasound evaluation of the diameter of deep veins in the newborn: results and implications for clinical practice. Neonatology. 2019;115:335–40.
2. Barone G, Pittiruti M. Epicutaneo-caval catheters in neonates: new insights and new suggestions from the recent literature. J Vasc Access 2020 Nov;21(6):805–809. https://doi.org/10.1177/1129729819891546. Epub 2019 Dec 5. PMID: 31804149.
3. Brissaud O, Harper L, Lamireau D, et al. Sonography-guided positioning of intravenous long lines in neonates. Eur J Radiol. 2010;73:e18–21.
4. Çağlar S, Büyükyılmaz F, Bakoğlu İ, İnal S, Salihoğlu Ö. Efficacy of vein visualization devices for peripheral intravenous catheter placement in preterm infants: a randomized clinical trial. J Perinat Neonatal Nurs. 2019;33:61–7.
5. Capasso A, Mastroianni R, Passariello A, et al. The intra- cavitary electrocardiography method for positioning the tip of epicutaneous cava catheter in neonates: pilot study. J Vasc Access. 2018;19:542–7.
6. Costa P, Kimura AF, Brandon DH, et al. Predictors of nonelective removal of peripherally inserted central catheters in infants biological research for. Nursing. 2016;18(2):173–80.
7. Costa P, Kimura AF, Brandon DH, et al. The development of a risk score for unplanned removal of peripherally inserted central catheter in newborns. Rev Latino-Am Enfermagem. 2015;23(3):475–82.
8. D'Andrea V, Pezza L, Barone G, Prontera G, Pittiruti M, Vento G. Use of cyanoacrylate glue for the sutureless securement of epicutaneo-caval catheters in neonates. J Vasc Access 2021 Apr 8:11297298211008103. https://doi.org/10.1177/11297298211008103. Epub ahead of print. PMID: 33827329.
9. Erhard DM, Nguyen S, Guy KJ, et al. Dwell times and risk of non-elective removal of 1-French peripherally inserted central catheters according to catheter tip position in very preterm infants. Eur J Pediatr. 2017;176:407–11.
10. Escourrou G, De Luca D. Lung ultrasound decreased radiation exposure in preterm infants in a neonatal intensive care unit. Acta Paediatr. 2016;105:e237–9.
11. Gorski L, Hadaway L, Hagle ME, et al. Infusion therapy standards of practice. J Infus Nurs. 2016;39:S1–S159.
12. Mertens L, Seri I, Marek J, et al. Targeted neonatal echocardiography in the neonatal intensive care unit: practice guidelines and recommendations for training: writing group of the American Society of Echocardiography (ASE) in collaboration with the European association of echocardiography. Eur J Echocardiogr. 2011;45:131.
13. Gupta R, Drendel AL, Hoffmann RG, et al. Migration of central venous catheters in neonates: a radiographic assessment. Am J Perinatol. 2016;33:600–4.
14. Jain A, Deshpande P, Shah P. Peripherally inserted central catheter tip position and risk of associated complications in neonates. J Perinatol. 2013;33:307–12.
15. Jain A, McNamara PJ, Ng E, et al. The use of targeted neo- natal echocardiography to confirm placement of peripher-ally inserted central catheters in neonates. Am J Perinatol. 2012;29:101–6.
16. Katheria AC, Fleming SE, Kim JH. A randomized controlled trial of ultrasound-guided peripherally inserted central catheters compared with standard radiograph in neonates. J Perinatol. 2013;33:791–4.
17. Lamperti M, Pittiruti M II. Difficult peripheral veins: turn on the lights. Br J Anaesth. 2013;110:888–91.
18. Masilamani K, van der Voort J. The management of acute hyperkalemia in neonates and children. Arch Dis Child. 2012;97:376–80.
19. McCay AS, Cassady C. PICC placement in the neonate. N Engl J Med 2014 May 29;370(22):2154. https://doi.org/10.1056/NEJMc1404381. PMID: 24869737.

20. Mermel LA, Allon M, Bouza E, Craven DE, Flynn P, O'Grady NP, et al. Clinical practice guidelines for the diagnosis and management of intravascular catheter-related infection: 2009 update by the Infectious Diseases Society of America. Clin Infect Dis. 2009;49:1–45.
21. Milstone AM, Reich NG, Advani S, et al. Catheter dwell time and CLABSIs in neonates with PICCs: a multicenter cohort study. Pediatrics. 2013;132:e1609–15.
22. Nifong TP, McDevitt TJ. The effect of catheter to vein ratio on blood flow rates in a simulated model of peripherally inserted central venous catheters. Chest. 2011;140:48–53.
23. Ohki Y, Tabata M, Kuwashima M, et al. Ultrasonographic detection of very thin percutaneous central venous catheter in neonates. Acta Paediatr. 2010;89:1381–4.
24. Pettit J. Assessment of infants with peripherally inserted central catheters: part 2. Detecting less frequently occurring complications. Adv Neonatal Care. 2003;3:14–26.
25. Pettit J. Assessment of infants with peripherally inserted central catheters: part 1. Detecting the most frequently occurring complications. Adv Neonatal Care. 2002;2:304–15.
26. Phipps K, Modic A, O'Riordan MA, Walsh M. A randomized trial of the vein viewer versus standard technique for placement of peripherally inserted central catheters (PICCs) in neonates. J Perinatol. 2012;32:498–501.
27. Pittiruti M, Scoppettuolo G. Manuale Gavecelt Dei PICC E Dei Midline. 1st ed. Milan: EDRA S.p.A; 2016.
28. Pittiruti M. Central venous catheters in neonates: old territory, new frontiers. J Vasc Access. 2013;14:318–9.
29. Pittiruti M. The 'off-label' use of PICCs. In: Sandrucci S, Mussa B, editors. Peripherally inserted central venous catheters. Milan: Springer; 2014. p. 127–44.
30. Pittiruti M. Ultrasound guided central vascular access in neonates, infants and children. Curr Drug Targets. 2012;13:961–9.
31. Racadio JM, Doellman DA, Johnson ND, et al. Pediatric peripherally inserted central catheters: complication rates related to catheter tip location. Pediatrics. 2004;107:E28.
32. Sengupta A, Lehmann C, Diener-West M, et al. Catheter duration and risk of CLA-BSI in neonates with PICCs. Pediatrics. 2010;125:648–53.
33. Sharpe E, Pettit J, Ellsbury DL. A national survey of neonatal peripherally inserted central catheter (PICC) practices. Adv Neonatal Care. 2013;13:55–74.
34. Shekelle PG, Pronovost PJ, Wachter RM, et al. The top patient safety strategies that can be encouraged for adoption now. Ann Intern Med. 2013;158:365–8.
35. Spencer TR, Pittiruti M. Rapid central vein assessment (RaCeVA): a systematic, standardized approach for ultra- sound assessment before central venous catheterization. J Vasc Access. 2018;20:239–49.
36. Tauzin L, Sigur N, Joubert C, et al. Echocardiography allows more accurate placement of peripherally inserted central catheters in low birthweight infants. Acta Paediatr. 2013;102:703–6.
37. van den Berg J, Lööf Åström J, Olofsson J, et al. Peripherally inserted central catheter in extremely preterm infants: characteristics and influencing factors. J Neonatal Perinatal Med. 2017;10:63–70.
38. Wrightson DD. Peripherally inserted central catheter complications in neonates with upper versus lower extremity insertion sites. Adv Neonatal Care. 2013;13:198–204.
39. Zhou L, Xu H, Liang J, et al. Effectiveness of intracavitary electrocardiogram guidance in peripherally inserted central catheter tip placement in neonates. J Perinat Neonatal Nurs. 2017;31:E2.
40. Zhou LJ, Xua HZ, Xu MF, et al. An accuracy study of the intracavitary electrocardiogram (IC-ECG) guided peripherally inserted central catheter tip placement among neonates. Open Med. 2017;12:125–30.

Chapter 12
Ultrasound Guided Venous Access in Neonates

Christian Breschan and Mauro Pittiruti

12.1 Introduction

Ultrasound guidance permits the percutaneous placement of relatively large bore central venous catheters in extremely small weight infants. Such large bore catheters can be used for inotropes, parenteral nutrition, but also for transfusions, blood sampling, hemodynamic monitoring, and high flow infusions. This can have an impact on mortality and morbidity in critically ill, very small infants.

The recommended ultrasound-guided venous accesses in neonates are the brachio-cephalic vein and the common femoral vein. In the past, the short axis/out-of-plane cannulation of the internal jugular vein has been widely used; though, when adopting this access, the tip of the puncture needle is only poorly visible via sonography, and the vein collapses easily. On the contrary, the supraclavicular, long axis/in-plane cannulation of the non-compressible brachiocephalic vein displays the needle over the entire distance: this approach represents most likely the most appropriate access for the placement of a relatively large bore central venous catheter in neonates, the only potential limitations being local emphysema and non-availability of an ultrasound device.

C. Breschan
Klinikum Klagenfurt, Klagenfurt, Austria
e-mail: breschan.ch@chello.at

M. Pittiruti (✉)
Department of Surgery, Catholic University Hospital, Rome, Italy

D. G. Biasucci et al. (eds.), *Vascular Access in Neonates and Children*,
https://doi.org/10.1007/978-3-030-94709-5_12

12.2 Definitions

By definition, a central venous access device is a catheter that has its tip in the superior vena cava (SVC) or inferior vena cava (IVC) or in the right atrium (RA). CICCs (centrally inserted central catheters) are central lines inserted via large veins of the infra- or supraclavicular region. FICCs (femorally inserted central catheters) are central lines inserted in large veins of the groin.

12.3 Indications

Central venous catheters in neonates are required perioperatively as well as in intensive care treatment. The most important indications include:

- major surgery with potential hemodynamic instability
- measurement of the central venous pressure and oxygen saturation in mixed venous blood
- blood sampling
- transfusion
- need for rapid volume repletion
- infusion of vasoactive drugs and other potentially irritant/vesicant drugs
- parental nutrition
- inability to obtain a central venous access by UVC or ECC, due to technical reasons
- expected long duration of the need of central venous access (more than two weeks)

In all these situations, the ideal central venous access is a large bore polyurethane power injectable catheter placed by ultrasound guidance.

In the past, central lines have been inserted in neonates by venous cutdown. Such obsolete technique is currently discouraged, because of the high risk of early and late complications (bleeding, infection, venous thrombosis, etc.) and because it implies a permanent damage to the venous patrimony of the neonate. Also, percutaneous puncture guided by anatomical landmarks has been adopted; though, this 'blind' approach is associated with severe early complications (accidental arterial puncture, pneumothorax, hemothorax, etc.) and it is currently discouraged, too.

On the contrary, ultrasound guided placement of central catheters has been proven a safe and effective procedure, even in extremely premature infants. Catheters of different size can be inserted (from 2Fr to 4Fr, depending on the size of the vein). They can be tunneled or non-tunneled, and in either case they can remain in place for many weeks (even two months) with very low risk of complications. If used consistently for hydration, nutrition, and blood sampling, they could indirectly improve the neurocognitive outcome by avoiding many painful stimuli and by reducing the overall stress to the newborn. The ECCs usually used by neonatologists (Fig. 12.1) are too small for blood sampling and do not have such

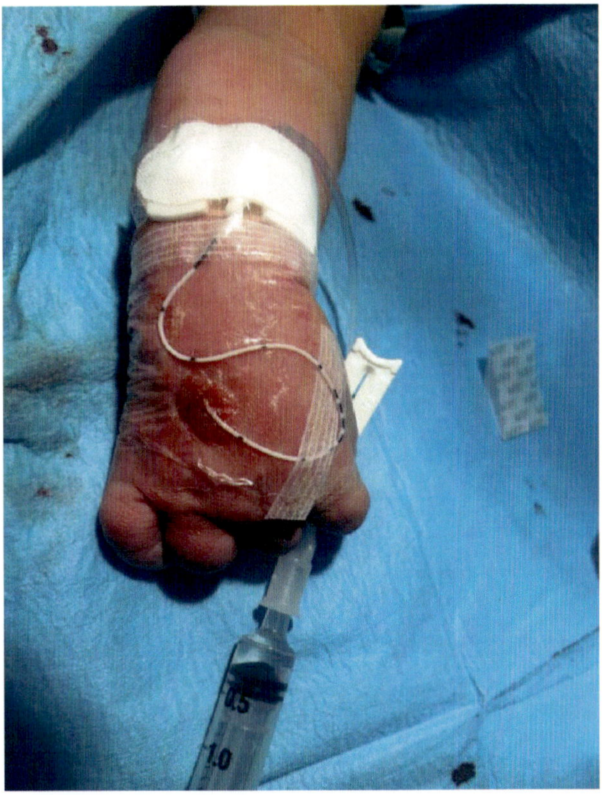

Fig. 12.1 Epicutaneo-cava catheter

advantage; also, especially in preterm babies, they often do not last more than 2 weeks.

The size and the age of the neonate are not a limit, since ultrasound guided approach to the brachio-cephalic vein has been described also in preterm infants weighing less than 500 g.

12.4 Venous Anatomy

Neonate's veins are small and - not surprisingly - cannulation success by the 'landmark technique' decreases with decreasing weight. Also, in low-birth-weight newborns, the muscle and bone landmarks are often difficult to palpate or locate, making the use of ultrasound absolutely necessary.

In neonates, internal jugular veins (IJV) and axillary veins (AxV) are particularly mobile, compressible, and they often collapse completely under the pressure of the approaching needle. A certain degree of immobilization of the IJV can be achieved by a hyperextension of the neck, when possible. As opposed to the IJV and AxV, the external jugular vein (EJV), the subclavian vein (SV) and the brachio-cephalic vein (BCV) are fixed to surrounding tissue structures making them non-compressible, non-collapsible, immobile, and patent even in most hypovolemic neonates. The IJV and BCV are significantly larger than EJV, SV or AxV in neonates. Figures 12.2 and 12.3 show the main veins of the supra/infra-clavicular area.

The deep veins of the upper limb (brachial, basilica, and axillary vein at the axilla) are too small for a safe ultrasound-guided cannulation (Fig. 12.4). As regards the deep veins of the lower limb, the common femoral vein (CFV) is of appropriate caliber only in neonates >2500 g. The saphenous vein and the superficial femoral vein are consistently very small. Figure 12.5 shows the CFV and the saphenous vein at the groin.

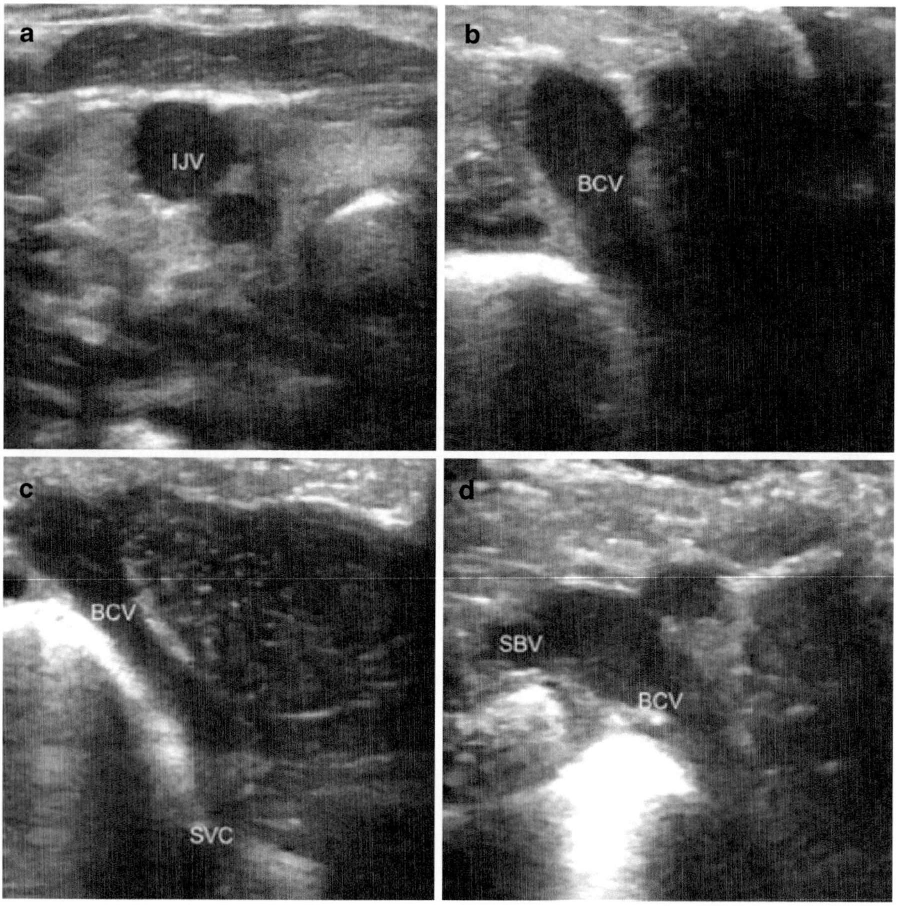

Fig. 12.2 Ultrasound imaging of the main central veins as visualized in the supraclavicular area with a linear probe. IJV = internal jugular vein (**a**); BCV = brachio-cephalic vein (**b–d**); SVC = superior vena cava (**c**); SBV = subclavian vein (**d**)

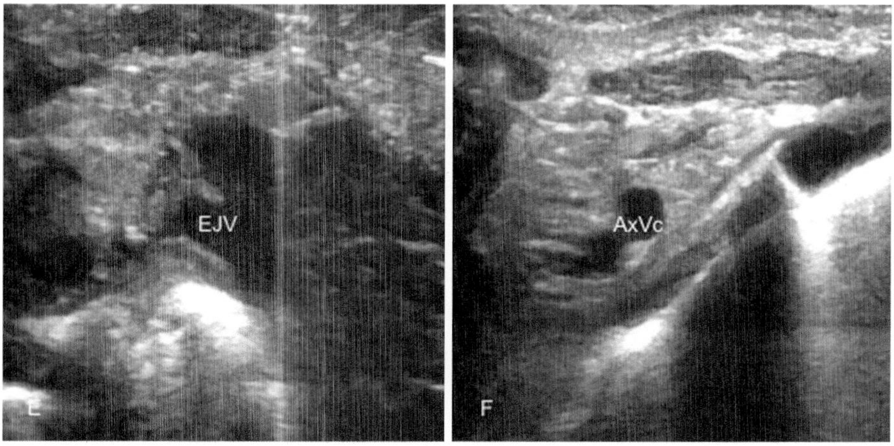

Fig. 12.3 Ultrasound imaging of two central veins rarely used for CICCs in neonates: EJV = external jugular vein; AxVc = axillary vein (in its thoracic tract)

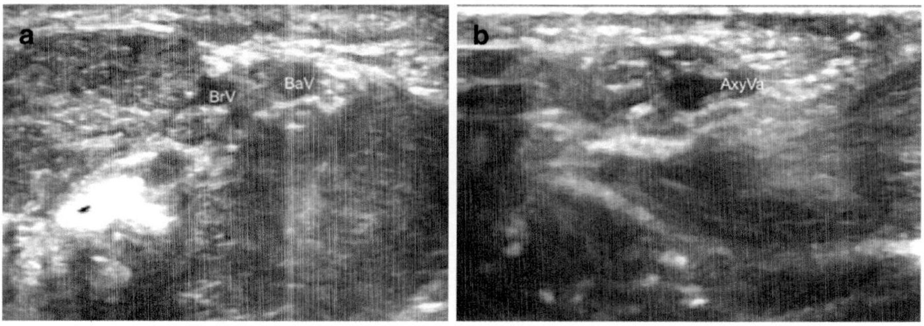

Fig. 12.4 Ultrasound imaging of deep veins at the arm: BrV = brachial vein and BaV = basilic vein (**a**); AxyVa = axillary vein (at axilla) (**b**)

In most cases, the BCV will be the largest vein available, and the easiest to puncture by ultrasound. The small caliber of the vessels, and the immaturity of the thrombolytic system make neonates particularly susceptible to catheter-related thrombosis. Therefore, it is of paramount importance to measure the size of the targeted vein by ultrasound prior to its cannulation: the outer diameter of the catheter should be equal or smaller than one third of the vessel lumen.

12.5 Material

Single, double, and triple lumen, 2–3-4 Fr catheters to be inserted via the direct Seldinger technique are available on the market and specifically designed for the use in neonates. Though, their use is not recommended for several reasons: (a) even

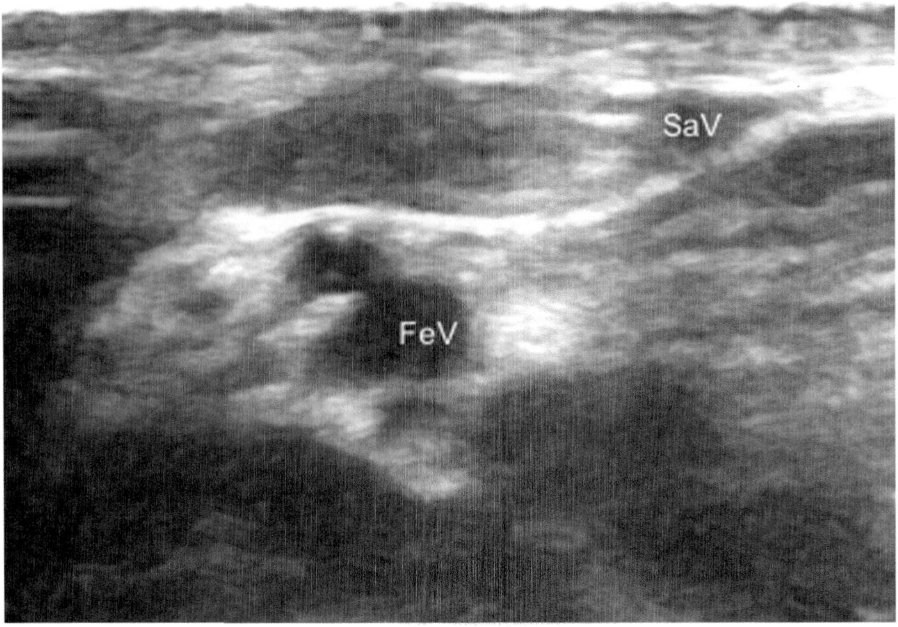

Fig. 12.5 Ultrasound imaging of the veins at the groin: FeV = common femoral vein; SaV = saphenous vein

when made in polyurethane, these catheters are not power injectable and so their flow performance is poor; (b) most of these catheters are provided in kits including large needles (20–19G) and J-shaped guidewires, which are unsuitable for neonates; (c) the direct Seldinger technique is not ideal in neonates, since it may be quite traumatic and does not allow tunnelling; (d) all of these catheters are not trimmable, so that a specific catheter of specific length must be chosen case by case.

On the contrary, we recommend the 'off-label' use of central venous catheters marketed as peripherally inserted central catheters (PICCs) for children and adults. Figure 12.6 shows a 3Fr single lumen catheter and Fig. 12.7 a double lumen 4 Fr catheter: both are PICCs used 'off label' as CICCs. These catheters have many advantages:

- They are of new generation, high quality polyurethane
- They are power injectable, so that even a 3Fr catheter will allow high flow (1 ml/sec)
- They are provided with a state-of-the-art high quality micro-insertion kit including echogenic 21G needle, soft straight tip 0.018-inch nitinol micro-guidewire, and 3.5–4.5Fr micro-introducer-dilator
- Because of the insertion by modified Seldinger technique, they can be easily tunneled
- They are available as single lumen 3Fr or 4Fr and as double lumen 4Fr, covering most requirements of critically ill neonates

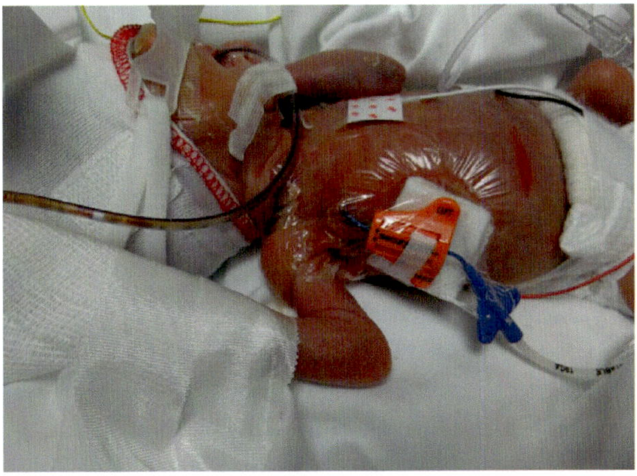

Fig. 12.6 3Fr single lumen polyurethane power injectable PICC used as tunneled CICC in a neonate

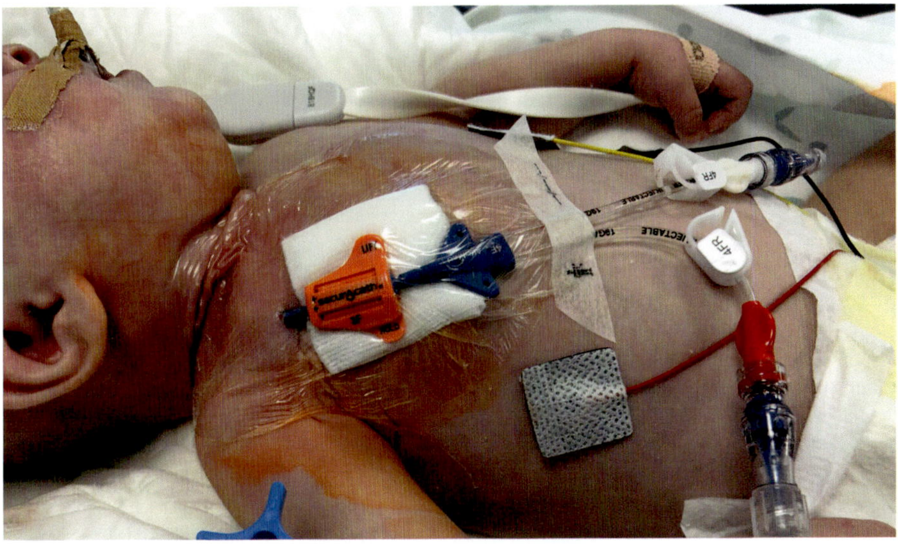

Fig. 12.7 4Fr double lumen polyurethane power injectable PICC used as tunneled CICC in a neonate

- Their length can be adjusted taking into consideration the site of insertion, the length of tunneling and the planned extravascular tract
- They can be secured by subcutaneous anchorage.

The same catheters can be used 'off label' as FICCs (Fig. 12.8). Their only limit is that the smallest caliber available is 3Fr (1 mm of external diameter: approximately 20G as internal area). This implies that if a BCV or a CFV is smaller than 3Fr, 22G or 24G should be used (Fig. 12.9). This can be done by off-label use of short peripheral venous cannulas or short peripheral arterial cannulas (available in polyurethane and in poly-ether-bloc-amide).

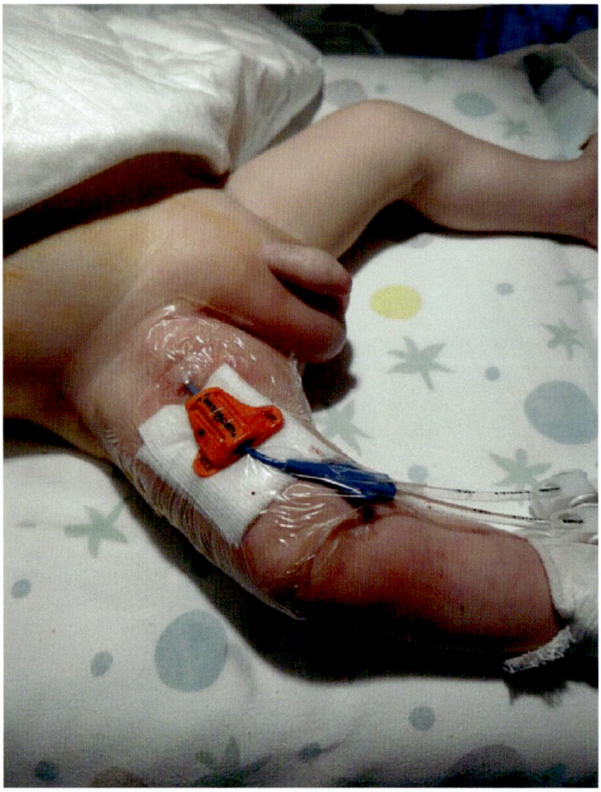

Fig. 12.8 3Fr single lumen polyurethane power injectable PICC used as FICC in a neonate

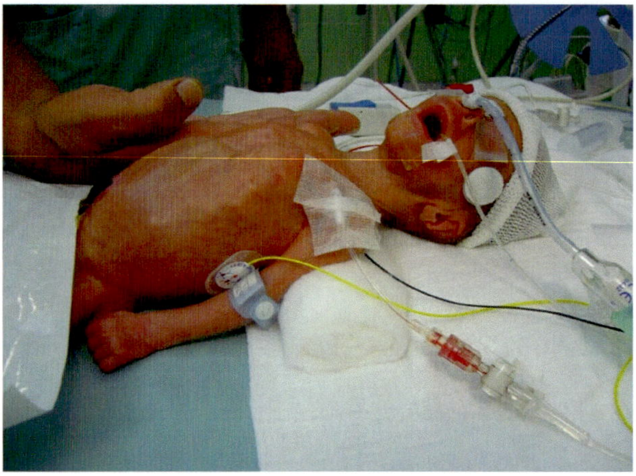

Fig. 12.9 Short venous cannula used as CICC in a neonate

Also, high quality ultrasound machines are needed. Linear transducers with high resolution (10–13 MHz) and short footprint (26 mm) must be used for ultrasound-guided puncture and cannulation of the vein. A 'hockey stick' shape will be particularly useful when accessing the BCV, so to facilitate the tilting of the probe. Tip location will require a micro-sectorial probe or a micro-convex probe.

12.6 Pre-Procedural Maneuvers

In order to avoid pain-response related movements of the neonate, CICCs and FICCs are inserted under general anesthesia or deep sedation. Hypovolemia should be corrected before the procedure, as feasible.

Before the preparation of the sterile field, a proper ultrasound examination of the local veins should be performed, using a systematic standardized protocol as the RaCeVA (before CICC insertion) or the RaFeVA (before FICC insertion), so to carefully choose the vein and the site to be punctured. The need for tunneling will be based on the RAVESTO protocol: in most elective punctures of the BCV, a tunnel to the infraclavicular area is strongly recommended, so to achieve an ideal exit site in terms of management; in most elective FICCs, a tunneling to mid-thigh will be useful, so to move the exit site away to the groin area.

Sterile precautions are mandatory, including hand hygiene (preferably using alcohol-based gel rub), proper skin antisepsis with 2% chlorhexidine in alcohol and maximal barrier precautions (cap, mask, sterile gown, sterile gloves, wide sterile drapes all over the patient and sterile cover for the ultrasound probe).

A towel roll is preferably placed under the shoulder of the baby and the head turned to the contralateral side, whenever a CICC must be placed. In FICC placement, the lower limb is fixed in extension and slight abduction.

The operator is always standing on one side of the patient, while the display of the ultrasound device is placed contralaterally.

12.7 Ultrasound-Guided Venipuncture

Any ultrasound-guided puncture can be defined describing (a) the spatial relationship between the vein and the probe (short axis, oblique axis, or long axis) and (b) the spatial relationship between the needle and the probe (in-plane, out-of-plane). In-plane techniques are safer and should be preferred for CICC insertion: their major advantage is the visibility of the advancing needle over the entire distance, so that the surrounding structures and their relation to the needle can be easily recognized. Though, the in-plane technique is not easy, since it requires an exact alignment of probe, vessel, and needle. Optimal hand-eye coordination is mandatory. The out-of-plane technique is easier and gives a good anatomical overview. However, the major disadvantage is the poor visibility of the needle tip, so that there is risk of accidental perforation of the vessel and injuries to underlying structure. For this reason, the out-of-plane approach should not be adopted for CICC insertion.

12.8 Tip Navigation

Soon after venipuncture and after insertion of the micro-guidewire, the intravascular location of the wire and its direction should be checked, using the same linear probe utilized for venipuncture. In the case of CICC insertion, the guidewire must be seen entering the SVC (visualized in long axis, placing the probe in the supraclavicular region, and tilting so to visualize the mediastinum). In the case of FICC insertion, the wire should be visualized inside the external iliac vein (visualized in long axis). The maneuver can be repeated—if needed—so to also visualize the micro-introducer and the catheter itself, after insertion. Ultrasound-based tip navigation will allow to immediately detect wrong direction of the wire (for example, into the contralateral BCV).

12.9 Tip Location

Ideally, the tip of a CICC should be located at the junction between RA and SVC, while the tip of a FICC may be located either in the IVC or in the RA, depending on the indication for central venous access (need for hemodynamic monitoring will imply a tip inside the RA). The easiest, safest, and most cost-effective methods of tip location are ultrasound and intracavitary electrocardiography (IC-ECG), which also have the great advantage of being intraprocedural. The old-fashioned method of 'blind' guess of the length of the catheter during the procedure, followed by a post-procedural chest x-ray should be abandoned. Radiological tip location (a) it is less accurate than either ultrasound or IC-ECG, particularly in neonates; (b) it is unsafe, since it implies x-ray exposure; (c) it is expensive; (d) being post-procedural, it may be associated with the necessity of repositioning the catheter (performing a new procedure and—what is worst—a new anesthesia/sedation of the neonate).

Intracavitary ECG (IC-ECG), though not recommended for UVC and ECC, because of some logistic problems, is particularly easy and rapid with CICC and FICC with caliber 3Fr or larger. It only requires a sterile cable for the connection between the catheter and the ECG monitor (see Chap. 6). Decades of clinical studies have demonstrated that IC-ECG is highly accurate and almost 100% applicable and feasible in neonates and children.

Ultrasound-based tip location is also easy and rapid in neonates, with almost 100% applicability and feasibility in neonates. A 7–8 MHz small sectorial probe placed in the subcostal area will allow to visualize the SVC, the IVC and the RA; when the catheter cannot be directly visualized, a rapid injection of a small amount of saline (0.5–1 ml) will enhance its visualization (so called 'bubble test').

As both methods are easy and inexpensive, the most reasonable strategy is to use both together. Considering that both methods are more accurate than radiology, a post-procedural chest-x-ray will be useless. In the rare case of suspected pleura-pulmonary damage, ultrasound scan of the pleura will be far more accurate and more cost-effective than radiological control (see Chap. 7).

12.10 Options for Venous Access

CICC can be inserted by ultrasound-guided approach of several veins of the supra-clavicular area (IJV, EJV, SV, BCV) and of the infraclavicular area (AxV). In clinical practice, the easiest and safest approach is the BCV.

The IJV has been the most popular vein because it is relatively large and easy to scan; though, due to its compressibility, it may not be easy to puncture; also, the progression of the catheter inside the vein before entering the BCV may be difficult. The EJV is punctured by ultrasound-guidance only in its distal tract, where it runs parallel, posterior, and superior to the SV; it is a rather easy and safe vein to cannulate, but its main limit is the small caliber. The SV can be punctured by a supra-clavicular approach or by a mixed infra-supraclavicular approach (see below); it is not compressible, but its puncture and cannulation is less safe than other accesses, due to its intimate contact with the pleura. On the other hand, the supraclavicular approach to the BCV will rapidly become the first choice for ultrasound-guided central venous access in neonates. The BCV is relatively large, easy to scan and non-compressible as is the SV; however, as opposed to the SV, the full visualization of the BCV is easier. The ultrasound-guided infraclavicular approach to the AxV has never been described in neonates, mostly because of its compressibility and the very small caliber in this age group (Fig. 12.10).

FICC can be inserted by ultrasound-guided approach of the common femoral vein (CFV), the external iliac vein, the superficial femoral vein, and the saphenous vein. In clinical practice, most FICCs in the neonate are inserted puncturing the CFV.

12.10.1 Internal Jugular Vein

The highly unpredictable and variable course of the IJV and its relationship to the carotid artery are not issues any more when using ultrasound (US). A short axis/out-of-plane approach is potentially dangerous (perforation of the posterior wall of the IJV, with resulting injury to the underlying subclavian vein). A short-axis/in-plane or an oblique axis/in-plane approach should be preferred. In either case, the IJV should be visualized and punctured as low as possible, close to its confluence with the BCV. The US probe is placed perpendicular to the skin so to visualize the IJV in short-axis or slight oblique-axis. The needle enters the skin laterally to the probe, so to be visualized in all its trajectory. As the needle is visualized inside the vein, the micro-guidewire is threaded inside the vein. An oblique-axis approach may facilitate the progression of the wire, if compared to the short-axis.

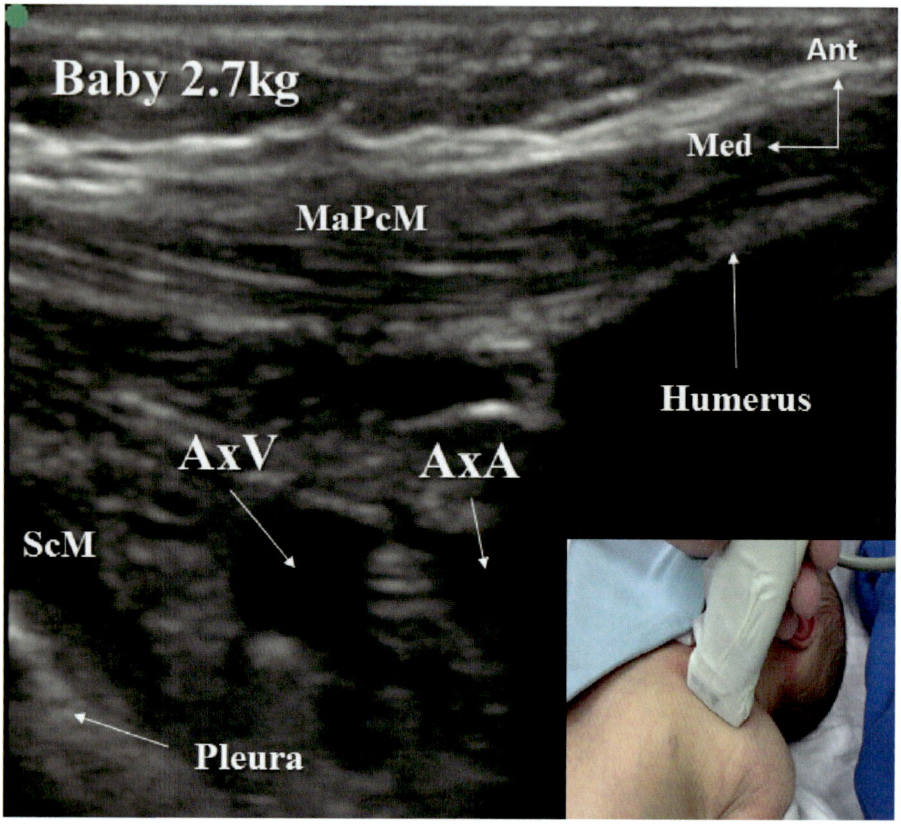

Fig. 12.10 Infraclavicular region in a neonate: AxV = axillary vein; AxA = axillary artery; MaPcM = major pectoral muscle; ScM = scalene muscle

12.10.2 Brachio-Cephalic Vein

The BCV is relatively large (the largest vein that can be accessed by ultrasound in the neonate) and fixed to surrounding tissue structures, so that it is non-compressible and patent even in hypovolemic patients. A short 10–14 MHz linear probe is used, preferably with 'hockey stick' shape. The BCV is localized using the RaCeVA protocol: by placing the ultrasound probe perpendicular to the skin at the level of the cricoid cartilage, a short-axis view of the IJV is obtained initially (RaCeVA, position 1); the probe is then moved caudally following the IJV until it crosses the subclavian artery (RaCeVA, position 2). The probe is then turned slightly medially and tilted behind the clavicle until the optimum sonographic long-axis view of the BCV is obtained (RaCeVA, position 3) (Fig. 12.11). The trajectory of the right BCV is

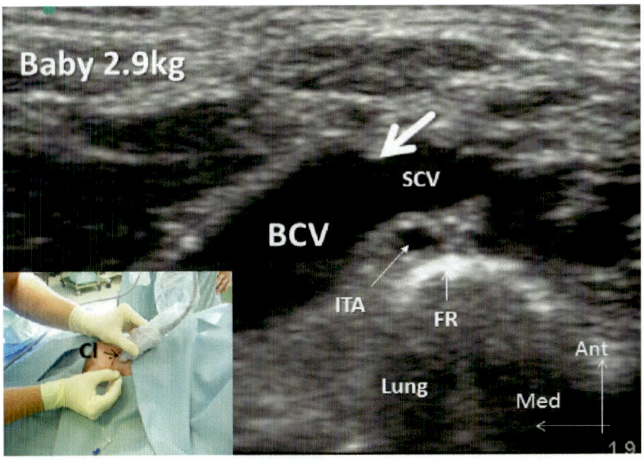

Fig. 12.11 Ultrasound imaging of the left brachio-cephalic vein (BCV) and of the subclavian vein (SCV), both in long axis

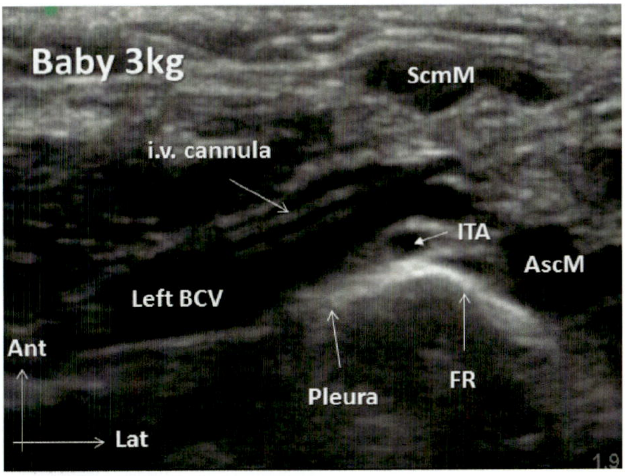

Fig. 12.12 Intravenous cannula entering the left brachio-cephalic vein (BCV)

vertical or oblique, while the left BCV is more horizontal; nonetheless, on both sides, the BCV is easily visualized in long axis in any neonate.

Using the in-plane approach, the echogenic needle is then advanced from lateral to medial, strictly under the long axis of the ultrasound probe until visualized on the ultrasound screen. The tip of the needle is then guided under real-time ultrasound control into the BCV (Fig. 12.12). When then needle is visualized inside the vein, the micro-guidewire is threaded into the needle.

The left BCV may be easier to cannulate because of its horizontal orientation. Though, when threading the catheter into the vasculature, some difficulty may be encountered when the confluence between left and right BCV is T-shaped; in these situations, the access to the right BCV (Fig. 12.13) allows an easier progression of the catheter from the BCV to the SVC.

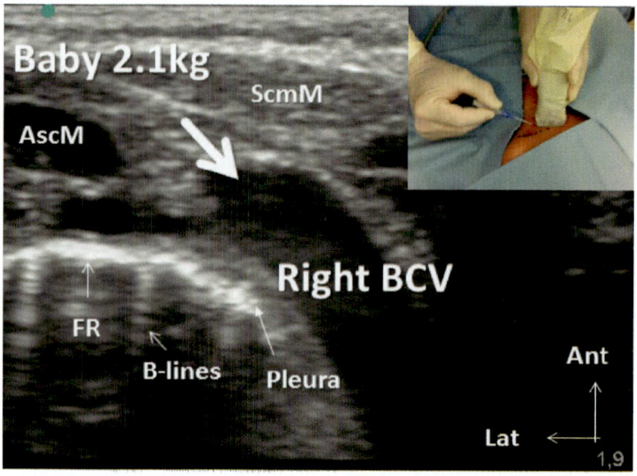

Fig. 12.13 Ultrasound imaging of the right brachio-cephalic vein (BCV) in long axis

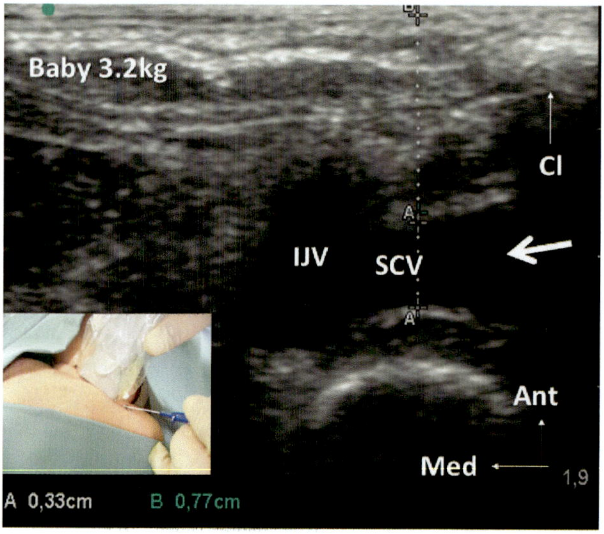

Fig. 12.14 Ultrasound access to the left subclavian vein (SCV), close to its confluence into the internal jugular vein (IJV)

12.10.3 Subclavian Vein

Like the BCV, the SV is also fixed to the surrounding tissue making it likewise non-compressible, and patent in hypovolemia. However, the SCV is much smaller than the BCV. Also, the risk of accidental injury to the pleura is higher.

Two different in-plane approaches have been described. The first is a completely supraclavicular approach, like the BCV approach but with the needle entering more laterally (care must be adopted to avoid any damage to the subclavian artery and to the pleura) (Fig. 12.14). The second is a combined infra/supraclavicular approach: the probe is placed over the clavicle, and it follows the needle while it enters the AxV/SV, visualized in long-axis in the infraclavicular area. When the clavicle is still echo-transparent, as in very small neonates, the maneuver is relatively safe.

Nonetheless, the main reason for not puncturing the SV is related to its smaller caliber if compared to the BCV. When the goal is to insert a catheter of good performance (3Fr, power injectable), a vein of at least 3 mm should be chosen, so to minimize the thrombotic risk. While most neonates >500 g may have a BCV of 3 mm, this does not occur for the SV.

12.10.4 Common Femoral Vein

The CFV is usually accessed with a short-axis/out-of-plane approach since a potential perforation of the posterior wall of the vein is not associated with relevant damages. Also, the short-axis approach allows a panoramic view of the surrounding structures and allows to avoid accidental arterial injury. After the puncture, though, a long axis visualization of the CFV and of the external iliac vein is useful for the proper visualization of the guidewire (ultrasound-based tip navigation). In fact, as the angle between CFV and external iliac vein is quite sharp, there is some risk that the needle (or the guidewire) may damage the anterior wall of the external iliac vein, placing the catheter in the pelvic space in extravascular position.

12.11 Tunneling

As already mentioned, according to the RAVESTO protocol, the choice of the ideal puncture site should be completed by the choice of the exit site. The two most common puncture sites for CICCs and FICCs in neonates (the supraclavicular area and the groin) cannot be regarded as optimal as exit site, because of the high risk of contamination. For this reason, tunneling is almost always recommended. When accessing the BCV, the catheter is tunneled caudally, so to get the exit site in the infraclavicular area (Fig. 12.15). When puncturing the CFV, the catheter is tunneled so to locate the exit site at mid-thigh. The rationale and the technique of tunnelling are discussed in Chap. 8.

Tunneling is always technically feasible for 3–4Fr polyurethane catheters inserted by modified Seldinger technique. It may be difficult or impossible for catheters inserted by simple Seldinger technique.

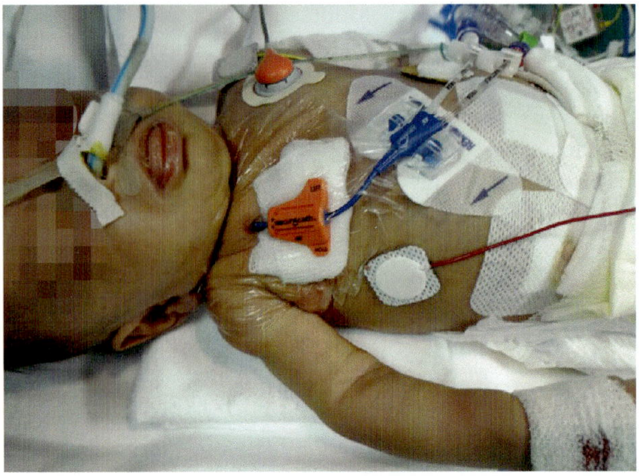

Fig. 12.15 CICC inserted into the brachio-cephalic vein and then tunneled to the infraclavicular area

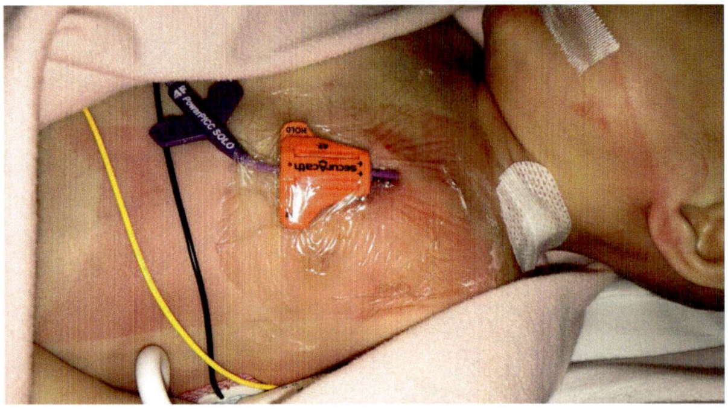

Fig. 12.16 Tunneled CICC secured with subcutaneous anchorage

12.12 Securement

As for other central venous access devices, the cornerstone of catheter securement and protection of the exit site are cyanoacrylate glue, sutureless devices and transparent membranes. The great advantage of using 3–4Fr polyurethane catheters is that they can be secured with the best securement method currently available, subcutaneous anchorage (Fig. 12.16). On the contrary, catheter <3Fr can only be secured by skin adhesive sutureless systems, which are less effective (see Chap. 8).

12.13 Complications

12.13.1 Immediate Complications

Puncture-related complications, such as pneumothorax, hemothorax and accidental arterial puncture have been described during 'blind' insertion of CICC and FICC, but they are apparently very rare or exceptional using ultrasound guidance. The best methods of prevention are (a) pre-procedural correction of hypovolemia, (b) optimal sedation/anesthesia, (c) choice of the largest and easiest vein (the BCV, in most cases), (c) use of appropriate material (ultrasound device, needles, guidewires, catheters, etc.), and—finally—(d) proper training of the operator. All puncture-related complications can be ruled out or detected early by ultrasound (see Chap. 7).

12.13.2 Early Complications

Late cardiac tamponade and pleural effusions due to vessel perforation have been described for ECC but not for CICC and FICC. As these complications are often secondary to primary or secondary malposition, the best prevention strategies are (a) the use of a proper intraprocedural method of tip location (IC-ECG or ultrasound) and (b) proper securement of the catheter.

12.13.3 Late Complications

The most frequent late complications include infection, venous thrombosis and lumen occlusion.

The risk of a catheter-related infection in neonates is inversely proportional to gestational age and directly proportional to the duration of catheterization. Other risk factors include the use of parenteral nutrition, catheter type, and altered integrity of skin and gastrointestinal barriers. The best prevention strategies are a proper protection of the exit site (tunneling, glue, subcutaneous anchorage, transparent membranes) and an appropriate protocol of maintenance of the infusion line (frequent saline flushes, use of needle free connectors with disinfecting caps, etc.).

Lumen occlusion is frequent with ECC, but less frequent with power injectable CICCs and FICCs; prevention consists in proper maintenance of the line (see above).

Venous thrombosis seems to be quite rare for CICCs and FICCs, as long as the proper match between catheter caliber and vein diameter is adopted, and a proper intraprocedural method of tip location (ultrasound and/or IC-ECG) is used.

12.14 Conclusion

Ultrasound guided CICCs and FICCs are the ideal central venous access in critically ill neonates requiring surgery, intensive care treatments, transfusions, frequent blood sampling and hemodynamic monitoring.

For minimizing complications, an appropriate insertion bundle should be adopted:

1. Preprocedural ultrasound examination of the venous patrimony (RaCeVA, RaFeVA)

2. Determination of the size of the targeted vessel via ultrasound
3. Proper planning of the puncture site and of the exit site
4. Hand hygiene, skin antisepsis with 2% chlorhexidine and maximal barrier precautions
5. Puncture/cannulation of the vessel under real-time ultrasound guidance, ruling out immediate puncture-related complications by ultrasound
6. Tip navigation = ultrasound control of the course of the guidewire and of the catheter
7. Intraprocedural tip location by ultrasound and/or intra-cavitary ECG
8. Tunneling, as required
9. Protection of the exit site with cyanoacrylate glue
10. Catheter securement with sutureless devices (preferably, subcutaneously anchored)
11. Coverage of the exit site with transparent membranes with high permeability

Bibliography

1. Ahn Y. The relationship between behavioral states and pain responses to various NICU procedures in premature infants. J Trop Pediatr. 2006;52:201–5.
2. Alderson PJ, Burrows FA, Stem LI, Holtby HM. Use of ultrasound to evaluate internal jugular vein anatomy and to facilitate central venous cannulation in paediatric patients. Br J Anaesth. 1993;70:145–8.
3. Agricola E, Arbelot C, Blaivas M, et al. Ultrasound performs better than radiographs. Thorax. 2011;66:828–9.
4. Araujo CL, Lima MC, Talbo GM. Percutaneous subclavian central venous catheterization in children and adolescents: success, complications and related factors. J Pediatr. 2007;83:64–70.
5. Arul GS, Livingstone H, Bromley P, Bennett J. Ultrasound-guided percutaneous insertion of 2.7 Fr tunnelled Broviac lines in neonates and small infants. Pediatr Surg Int. 2010;26(8):815–8.
6. Al Hamod DA, Zeidan S, Al Bizri A, Baaklini G, Nassif Y. Ultrasound-guided central line insertion and standard peripherally inserted catheter placement in preterm infants: comparing results from prospective study in a single-center. N Am J Med Sci. 2016;8(5):205–9.
7. Barone G, D'Andrea V, Vento G, Pittiruti M. A systematic ultrasound evaluation of the diameter of deep veins in the Newborn: results and implications for clinical practice. Neonatology 2019;115(4):335–340. https://doi.org/10.1159/000496848. Epub 2019 Mar 15. PMID: 30878998.
8. Barone G, Pittiruti M, Ancora G, Vento G, Tota F, D'Andrea V. Centrally inserted central catheters in preterm neonates with weight below 1500 g by ultrasound-guided access to the brachio-cephalic vein. J Vasc Access 2021a May;22(3):344–352. https://doi.org/10.1177/1129729820940174. Epub 2020 Jul 10. PMID: 32648811.
9. Barone G, Pittiruti M, Biasucci DG, Elisei D, Iacobone E, La Greca A, Zito Marinosci G, D'Andrea V. Neo-ECHOTIP: a structured protocol for ultrasound-based tip navigation and tip location during placement of central venous access devices in neonates. J Vasc Access 2021b Apr 5:11297298211007703. https://doi.org/10.1177/11297298211007703. Epub ahead of print. PMID: 33818191.
10. Blum LV, Abdel-Rahman U, Klingebiel T, Fiegel H, Gfroerer S, Rolle U. Tunneled central venous catheters in children with malignant and chronic diseases: a comparison of open vs. percutaneous implantation. J Pediatr Surg. 2017;52:810–2.
11. Breschan C, Kraschl R, Krenn R, Krumpholz R, Jost R, Likar R. Anaesthetic management of liver haemorrhage during laparotomy in a premature infant with necrotizing enterocolitis. Pediatr Anesth. 2000;10(4):425–8.

12. Breschan C, Platzer M, Jost R, Schaumberger F, Stettner H, Likar R. Comparison of catheter-related infection and tip colonization between internal jugular and subclavian central venous catheters in surgical neonates. Anesthesiology. 2007;107(6):946–53.
13. Breschan C, Platzer M, Jost R, Stettner H, Likar R. Size of internal jugular vs subclavian vein in small infants: an observational, anatomical evaluation with ultrasound. Br J Anaesth. 2010;105(2):179–84.
14. Breschan C, Platzer M, Jost R, Stettner H, Beyer AS, Feigl G, Likar R. Consecutive, prospective case series of a new method for ultrasound-guided supraclavicular approach to the brachiocephalic vein in children. Br J Anaesth. 2011;106(5):732–7.
15. Breschan C, Platzer M, Jost R, Stettner H, Feigl G, Likar R. Ultrasound-guided supraclavicular cannulation of the brachiocephalic vein in infants: a retrospective analysis of a case series. Pediatr Anesth. 2012;22(11):1062–7.
16. Breschan C, Graf G, Jost R, Stettner H, Feigl G, Goessler A, Neuwersch S, Koestenberger M, Likar R. Ultrasound-guided supraclavicular cannulation of the right brachiocephalic vein in small infants: a consecutive, prospective case series. Pediatr Anesth. 2015;25(9):943–9.
17. Breschan C, Graf G, Jost R, Stettner H, Feigl G, Neuwersch S, Stadik C, Koestenberger M, Likar R (2017). A retrospective analysis of the clinical effectiveness of supraclavicular, ultrasound-guided brachiocephalic vein cannulations in preterm infants. Anesthesiology in press.
18. Brescia F, Pittiruti M, Ostroff M, Biasucci DG. Rapid femoral vein assessment (RaFeVA): a systematic protocol for ultrasound evaluation of the veins of the lower limb, so to optimize the insertion of femorally inserted central catheters. J Vasc Access 2020 Oct 16:1129729820965063. https://doi.org/10.1177/1129729820965063. Epub ahead of print. PMID: 33063616.
19. Crawford M, Soukup SM, Woods SS, Deisch P. Peripherally inserted central catheter program. Nurs Clin North Am. 2000;35:349–60.
20. Cruzeiro PC, Camargos PA, Miranda ME. Central venous catheter placement in children: a prospective study of complications in a Brazilian public hospital. Pediatr Surg. 2006;22:536–40.
21. D'Andrea V, Barone G, Pezza L, Prontera G, Vento G, Pittiruti M. Securement of central venous catheters by subcutaneously anchored suturless devices in neonates. J Matern Fetal Neonatal Med 2021 May 9:1–4. https://doi.org/10.1080/14767058.2021.1922377. Epub ahead of print. PMID: 33969783.
22. Eifinger F, Brisken K, Roth B, Koebke J. Topographical anatomy of central venous system in extremely low-birth weight neonates less than 1000 grams and the effect of central venous catheter placement. Clin Anatomy. 2011;24(6):711–6.
23. Goldstein SD, Pryor H, Salazar JH, Dalesio N, Stewart FD, Abdullah F, Colombani P, Lukish JR. Ultrasound-guided percutaneous central venous access in low birth weight infants: feasibility in the smallest of patients. J Laparoendosc Adv Surg Tech A. 2015;25(9):767–9.
24. Groff DB, Ahmed N. Subclavian vein catheterization in the infant. J Pediatr Surg. 1974;9(2):171–4.
25. Hsu CC, Kwan GN, Evans-Barns H, Rophael JA, van Driel ML. Venous cutdown versus the Seldinger technique for placement of totally implantable venous access ports. Cochrane Database Syst Rev. 2016;8:CD008942.
26. Janik JE, Conlon SJ, Janik JS. Percutaneous central access in patients younger than 5 years: size does matter. J Pediatr Surg. 2004;39:1252–6.
27. Johnson EM, Saltzman DA, Suh G, Dahms RA, Leonard AS. Complications and risks of central venous catheter placement in children. Surgery. 1998;124(5):911–6.
28. Kim H, Jeong CH, Byon HJ, Shin HK, Yun TJ, Lee JH, Park YH, Kim JT. Predicting the optimal depth of left-sided central venous catheters in children. Anaesthesia. 2013;68(10):1033–7.
29. Lichtenstein DA, Meziere G, Lascols N, et al. Ultrasound diagnosis of occult pneumothorax. Crit Care Med. 2005;33:1231–8.
30. Marhofer P. Needle guidance techniques. In: Marhofer P, ed. Ultrasound guidance for nerve blocks. Principles and practical implementation. Oxford: Oxford University Press, 2008: 45–47, ISBN 978–0–19-954756-2.

31. Montes-Tapia F, Rodríguez-Taméz A, Cura-Esquivel I, Barreto-Arroyo I, Hernández-Garduño A, Rodríguez-Balderrama I, Quero J, de la O-Cavazos M (2016). Efficacy and safety of ultrasound-guided internal jugular vein catheterization in low birth weight newborn. J Pediatr Surg; 51(10):1700–1703.
32. Morita M, Sasano H, Azami T, Sasano N, Fujita Y, Ito S, Sugiura T, Sobue K. A novel skin-traction method is effective for real-time ultrasound-guided internal jugular vein catheterization in infants and neonates weighing less than 5 kilograms. Anesth Analg. 2009;109(3):754–9.
33. Ostroff MD, Moureau N, Pittiruti M. Rapid assessment of vascular exit site and Tunneling options (RAVESTO): a new decision tool in the management of the complex vascular access patients. J Vasc Access 2021 Jul 21:11297298211034306. https://doi.org/10.1177/11297298211034306. Epub ahead of print. PMID: 34289721.
34. Oulego-Erroz I, Alonso-Quintela P, Domínguez P, Rodríguez-Blanco S, Muñíz-Fontán M, Muñoz-Lozón A, López-Blanco G, Rodríguez-Nuñez A. Ultrasound-guided cannulation of the brachiocephalic vein in neonates and infants. Ann Pediatr Barc. 2016;84(6):331–6.
35. Pandit PB, Pandit FA, Govan J, O'Brien K. Complications associated with surgically placed central venous catheters in low birth weight neonates. J Perinatol. 1999;19:106–9.
36. Pinelli F, Pittiruti M, Van Boxtel T, Barone G, Biffi R, Capozzoli G, Crocoli A, Elli S, Elisei D, Fabiani A, Garrino C, Graziano U, Montagnani L, Prato AP, Scoppettuolo G, Zadra N, Zanaboni C, Zerla P, Konstantinou E, Jones M, Rosay H, Simcock L, Stas M, Pepe G. GAVeCeLT-WoCoVA consensus on subcutaneously anchored securement devices for the securement of venous catheters: current evidence and recommendations for future research. J Vasc Access. 2020 Jul 2:1129729820924568. https://doi.org/10.1177/1129729820924568. Epub ahead of print. PMID: 32613887.
37. Pirotte T, Veyckemans F. Ultrasound-guided subclavian vein cannulation in infants and children: a novel approach. Br J Anaesth. 2007;98:509–14.
38. Pirotte T. Vascular access in the perioperative period. In: Asuto M, Ingelmo PM, editors. Perioperative medicine in Pediatric Anesthesia. Springer international Publishing Switzerland; 2016. p. 285–340. isbn:978-3-319-21960-8.
39. Pittiruti M, Pelagatti F, Pinelli F. Intracavitary electrocardiography for tip location during central venous catheterization: a narrative review of 70 years of clinical studies. J Vasc Access 2020 Jun 24:1129729820929835. https://doi.org/10.1177/1129729820929835. Epub ahead of print. PMID: 32578489.
40. Pittiruti M, Scoppettuolo G, Dolcetti L, Celentano D, Emoli A, Marche B, Musarò A. Clinical experience of a subcutaneously anchored sutureless system for securing central venous catheters. Br J Nurs 2019 Jan 24;28(2):S4-S14. https://doi.org/10.12968/bjon.2019.28.2.S4. PMID: 30673323.
41. Rhondali O, Attof R, Combet S, Chassard D, de Queiroz SM. Ultrasound-guided subclavian vein cannulation in infants: supraclavicular approach. Pediatr Anesth. 2011;21:1136–41.
42. Sasano H, Morita M, Azami T, Ito S, Sasano N, Kato R, Hirate H, Ito H, Takeuchi A, Sobue K. Skin-traction method prevents the collapse of the internal jugular vein caused by an ultrasound probe in real-time ultrasound-assisted guidance. J Anesth. 2009;23(1):41–5.
43. Sener M. Supraclavicular subclavian vein approach for central venous catheterization is a safe and preferable method also in pediatric patients. Pediatr Anesth. 2012;22(5):506–7.
44. Spencer TR, Pittiruti M. Rapid central vein assessment (RaCeVA): a systematic, standardized approach for ultrasound assessment before central venous catheterization. J Vasc Access 2019 May;20(3):239–249. https://doi.org/10.1177/1129729818804718. Epub 2018 Oct 4. PMID: 30286688.
45. Stevens B, Johnston C, Franck L, Petryshen P, Jack A, Foster G. The efficacy of developmentally sensitive interventions and sucrose for relieving procedural pain in very low birth weight neonates. Nurs Res. 1999;48(1):35–43.
46. Wu J, Mu D. Vascular catheter-related complications in newborns. J Paediatr Child Health. 2012;48:E91–5.

Part III
Venous Access in Children

Chapter 13
Peripheral Venous Access: Short Cannulas, Mini-Midlines, Midlines

Davide Celentano and Mauro Pittiruti

Peripheral venous access devices are the most commonly used vascular access devices in pediatric patients. They are inexpensive and relatively safe, even if—in not used properly—may be associated with severe complications. If compared with adult patients, peripheral venous access in children has some peculiarities in terms of indication, choice of material, technique of insertion and maintenance, which all will be discussed in this chapter.

13.1 Classification

Several peripheral venous access devices are available, with different cost, different performance and different indications, though all of them should be strictly used only for infusion of peripherally compatible solutions.

1. *Steel needles with butterfly wing set*. They have been largely replaced by plastic cannulas, but they are still used for blood sampling and for bolus infusion. Their utilization for continuous infusion is not appropriate, since steel needles are associated with a very high risk of local complications (phlebitis, infiltration, infection).
2. *Short peripheral cannulas*. According to the 2021 Standards of the Infusion Nursing Society and to the 2021 ERPIUP Consensus (ERPIUP = European

D. Celentano
Pediatric Intensive Care Unit, Fondazione Policlinico Universitario "A. Gemelli" IRCCS, Rome, Italy
e-mail: Davide.celentano@policlinicogemelli.it

M. Pittiruti (✉)
Department of Surgery, Catholic University Hospital, Rome, Italy

D. G. Biasucci et al. (eds.), *Vascular Access in Neonates and Children*,
https://doi.org/10.1007/978-3-030-94709-5_13

Recommendations for the Proper Indication and Use of Peripheral venous access), short cannulas are catheters of length <6 cm, either in polyurethane or in poly-tetra-fluoroethylene (Teflon), to be inserted in superficial veins (less than 7 mm of depths) with the technique called 'cannula over needle'. Polyurethane should be preferred since Teflon is associated with increased risk of phlebitis. They are available in different calibers: the calibers most frequently used in children are 22G (code color: blue) and 24G (code color: yellow). Larger cannulas (20G—code color: pink) should be used for rapid fluid infusion in hypovolemic patients or for transfusions. Smaller cannulas (26G—code color: purple) may be useful in very small infants but are utilized mainly in neonates. According to all guidelines, the caliber of the cannula should be as small as possible, but still compatible with the clinical needs. Short cannulas may have several characteristics, which are associated with different profiles of safety, different costs, and different clinical performance. One additional feature is whether the short cannula is "ported" or "non-ported." The presence of a port enables the intravenous administration of drugs without disconnecting the infusion; on the other hand, the port is very difficult to decontaminate and often it is not possible to close it with needle-free connectors, so that a ported cannula is easily exposed to bacterial contamination (Fig. 13.1). A 'ported' cannula should be used only in emergency and removed as soon as possible. Most short cannulas have mechanisms that protect the operator from accidental needle puncture ('no-stick' or 'safety' mechanisms) or from accidental contamination with the patient's blood ('blood-stop' mechanisms or 'closed systems'). Most short cannulas are also provided with wings for improving the stabilization of the device over the skin ('winged' cannulas). Some winged cannulas are provided with a preassembled extension and a preassembled needle-free connector ('integrated' cannulas); these cannulas seem to be associated with prolonged dwelling time, since the exit site is continuously protected by the transparent membrane and is not manipulated during the change of the infusion line (Fig. 13.2). While a standard short cannula

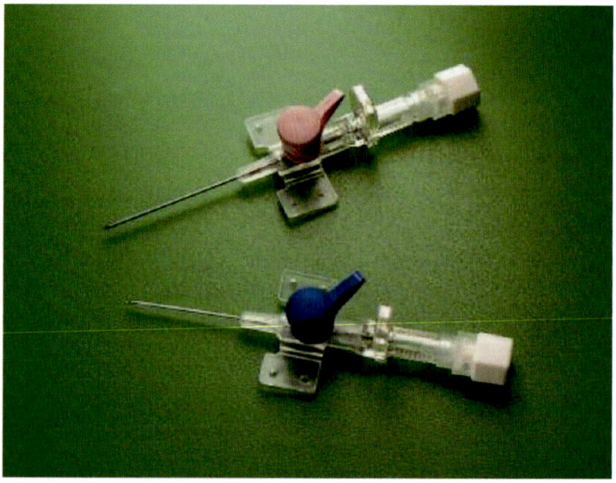

Fig. 13.1 'Ported' short cannulas

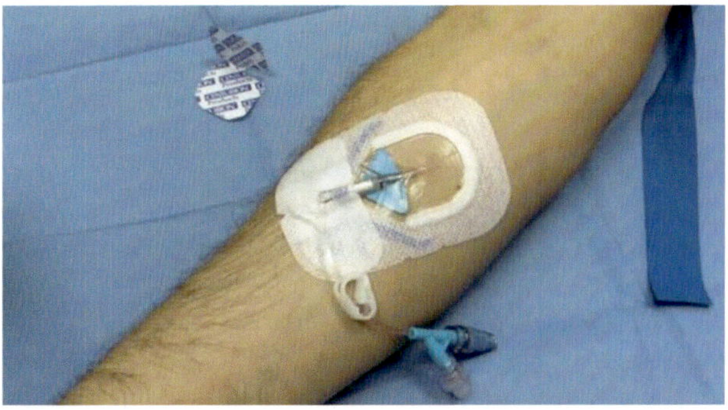

Fig. 13.2 'Integrated' short cannula

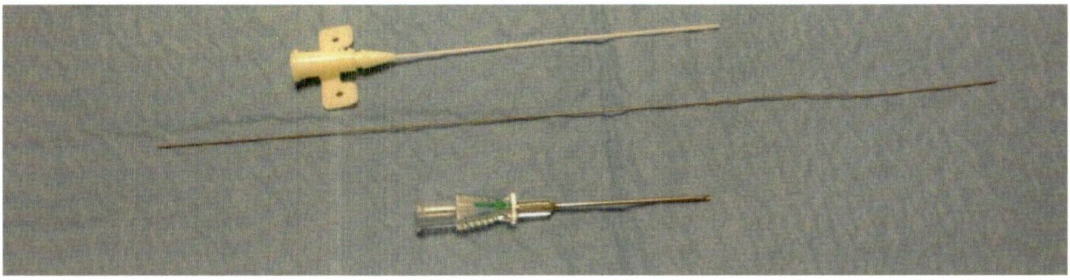

Fig. 13.3 Long peripheral catheter (3Fr—8 cm long—in polyurethane) plus accessories for the simple Seldinger technique (micro-guidewire and 21G needle)

may have an expected dwelling time of 48–72 hours, an 'integrated' short cannula may stay in place for several days, even for one week.

3. *Long peripheral catheters* (also known as 'mini-midline' or 'short midline' catheters). According to INS 2021 and ERPIUP 2021 (see above), these catheters are longer than 6 cm but shorter than 15 cm. They are available in different materials (polyurethane, polyethylene, poly-ether-bloc-amide) and in different external diameter (3Fr, with an internal area of approximately 20G; 4Fr, with an internal area of approximately 18G) (Fig. 13.3). Most mini-midlines currently available are power injectable. Polyethylene catheters should not be routinely used for venous access, since they are associated with increased risk of phlebitis/thrombosis. The choice of the caliber of catheter is depending on the inner diameter of the vein, as measured by ultrasound: ideally, 3Fr (= 1 mm) cannulas should be inserted only in veins of 3 mm or larger, so to reduce the risk of thrombosis; 4Fr cannulas require veins of 4 mm or larger. Three different types of long peripheral cannulas are available: (a) catheters to be inserted with the 'cannula over needle' technique; (b) catheters to be inserted by simple Seldinger technique ('catheter over guidewire'); (c) catheters to be inserted by simple Seldinger technique but provided as an 'all-in-one' device containing needle, guidewire, and cannula, arranged coaxially, and maneuvered by appropriate mechanisms. The main limitation of 'cannula over needle' mini-midlines is that insertion may be difficult because of problems in the progression of the cannula into the vein. The main limitations of the 'all-in-one' mini-midlines are that they are quite difficult to

operate, and that they are very expensive. In pediatric patients, we strongly recommend preferring 3Fr mini-midline catheters inserted with simple Seldinger technique—by ultrasound guidance—in superficial or deep veins of the forearm or of the arm. Their expected dwelling time is longer than short cannulas (2–3 weeks, with proper maintenance). Also, long peripheral catheters have the advantage of being inserted—if needed—even in children with difficult intravenous access (DIVA), since they can be inserted in deep veins by ultrasound guidance.

4. *Midline catheters*. According to the ERPIUP consensus, midline catheters (also known as 'midclavicular') are venous cannulas longer than 15 cm (usually 20–25 cm). The caliber range between 3Fr and 5Fr. They are available also as double lumen. The material may be polyurethane or silicon, and the catheter may be valved or non-valved. We strongly recommend using exclusively non-valved, power injectable, polyurethane catheters, since silicon midline catheters are prone to rupture and other mechanical complications, while valved catheters are consistently associated with catheter malfunction. Some polyurethane midline catheters are coated with antimicrobials (chlorhexidine), but there is no evidence that this coating may be effective in reducing infective complications for these devices. Midline catheters are different from 'mini-midline' catheters not only because of their length, but also because of the technique of insertion (modified Seldinger technique, or 'catheter through introducer'). Also, the tip of the catheter is not inside a vein of the arm (as for mini-midlines) but inside the thoracic tract of the axillary vein of even inside the subclavian vein. Midline catheters are not commonly used in small children, but they may be indicated when prolonged peripheral venous access is required in non-hospitalized teen-agers: for example, for outpatient antimicrobial treatments (OPAT), for periodic administration of blood components, or for palliative care.

13.2 Indication

Peripheral venous access devices are indicated exclusively for administration of peripherally compatible solutions; infusion of solutions non-peripherally compatible (parenteral nutrition, irritant drugs, vesicants, etc.) and/or the need for hemodynamic monitoring or repeated daily blood sampling are well-defined indication for a central venous access.

Insertion of a short cannula by direct venipuncture of a superficial vein is the first option for a child needing intravenous support in emergency. If the superficial veins are not clearly visible, NIR technology (see Chap. 5) may facilitate the visualization and the puncture of the vein (Fig. 13.4). If superficial veins are difficult to puncture and cannulate (so called DIVA patients), as it may happen in presence of edema, obesity, hypovolemia, dark color of the skin, etc., then ultrasound guidance is required (Fig. 13.5). The incidence of children with 'DIVA' (difficult intravenous access) in emergency room may be as high as 20–24%. Though short cannulas can

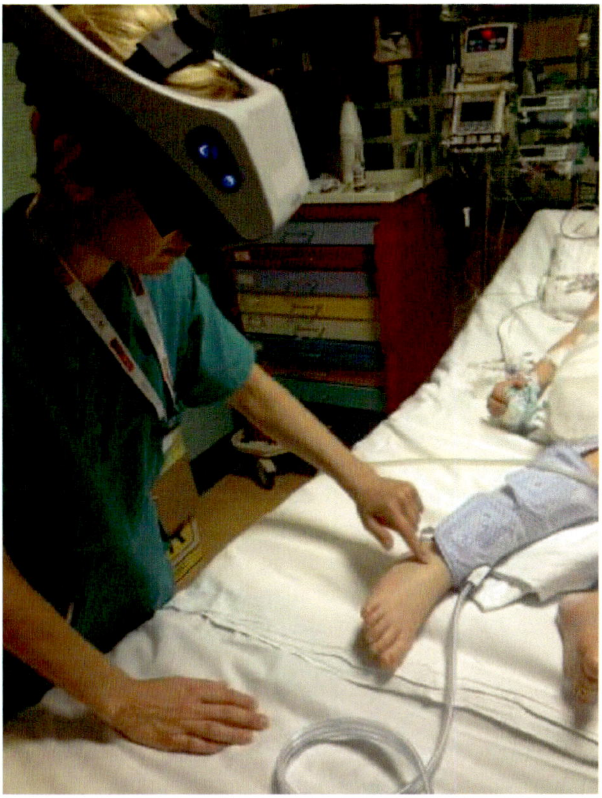

Fig. 13.4 Near Infra Red technology for visualization of superficial vein

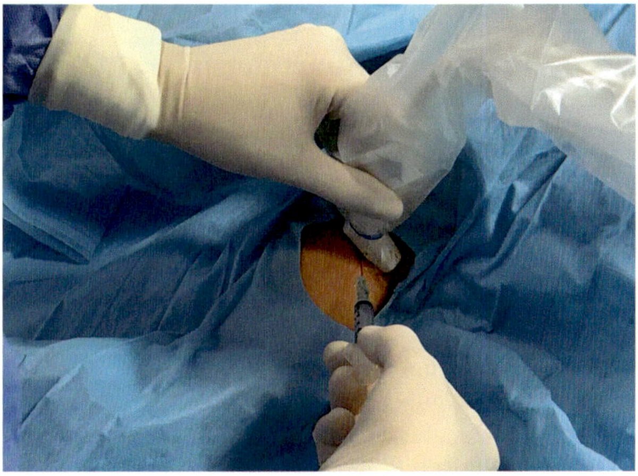

Fig. 13.5 Ultrasound-guided access to a deep vein

be inserted by ultrasound guided venipuncture of deep veins, they are associated with a high risk of early dislodgment; therefore, if an ultrasound-guided peripheral venous access is needed, it is recommended to use long peripheral catheters. In some emergencies, when a venous access is immediately and urgently required as a lifesaving maneuver, intraosseous access should be considered (see Chap. 20).

Short cannulas also have indication in non-emergency intravenous treatments for pediatric patients, if only peripherally compatible solutions are to be administered. If the required dwelling time is longer than 48 hours, an 'integrated' short cannula should be preferably used. If the required dwelling time of the peripheral access is more than one week, a long peripheral catheter should be preferred. For any expected dwelling time, short or long, if access to the superficial veins is difficult (DIVA patients), we recommend using a long peripheral catheter inserted by ultrasound-guided puncture and cannulation of a deep vein of the arm.

Short cannulas are not appropriate in non-hospitalized children: if peripheral venous access is appropriate, in these patients a long peripheral catheter (expected dwelling time: weeks) or a midline catheter (expected dwelling time: months) should be used.

The main pediatric indications for long peripheral catheters, as mentioned above, are (a) need of peripheral venous access in a DIVA patient, and (b) expected need of peripheral venous access for more than one week and less than one month. In fact, 8–10 cm cannulas placed in the veins of the arm are not likely to stay in place with optimal function for more than four weeks; even with proper maintenance and in absence of infective or thrombotic complications, sooner or later malfunction occurs, due to the occlusion of the tip (probably secondary to formation of fibroblastic sleeve). Considering this time limit, long peripheral cannulas can nonetheless be used also in non-hospitalized children.

Midline catheters are seldom used in children, though they might have indication in older children requiring peripheral venous access in the extra-hospital setting.

13.3 Insertion of Short Peripheral Cannulas

The basic recommendations for insertion of short cannulas are thoroughly discussed in the recent ERPIUP document. Though this consensus is focused on peripheral venous access in adults, most recommendations are also valid for pediatric patients. In the insertion of a short cannula, we should consider the following steps:

- Appropriate indication: short cannulas should be inserted only when peripheral venous access is required for few days (<7 days) and when there are visible/palpable superficial veins.
- Choice of the puncture site: cannulas inserted on the back of the hand (Fig. 13.6) or at the antecubital fossa are at high risk of early dislodgment and have a shorter dwelling time than cannulas inserted at the forearm or soon above the antecubital fossa; the wrist should always be avoided as insertion site, because of the high risk of accidental damage to nerves or arteries; cannulas inserted at the neck in the superficial tract of the external jugular vein or inserted in superficial veins of the lower limb (collateral of the saphenous veins) are acceptable only in emer-

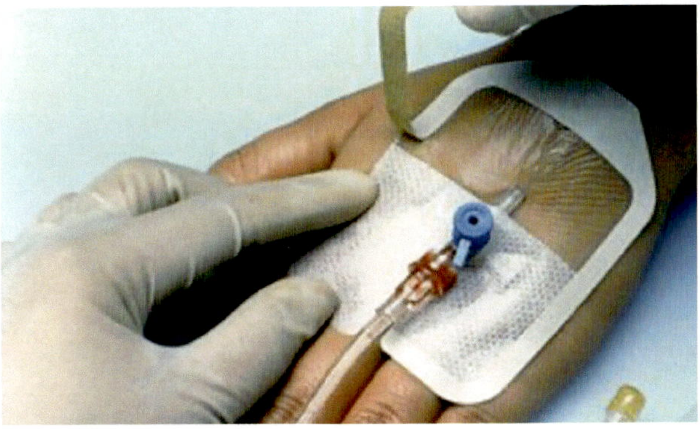

Fig. 13.6 'Ported' cannula inserted on the back of the hand (to be removed as soon as possible)

gency, and should be replaced as soon as possible with a definitive venous access device.

- Hand hygiene (preferably with alcohol-based gel rub).
- Non-sterile gloves.
- Proper skin antisepsis with 2% chlorhexidine in 70% isopropyl alcohol (apply for 30 seconds and let dry for 30 seconds).
- Choice of the short cannula: 22G or 24G, depending on the size of the vein; 20G only in special situation (emergency) and in older children. Prefer polyurethane catheters with 'no-stick' and 'blood stop' mechanisms. Prefer 'integrated' cannulas for expected dwelling time >48 hours.
- Placement of the tourniquet.
- Direct insertion on the cannula into the vein, paying attention at not touching the puncture site with the non-sterile gloves.
- As backflow of blood is visualized inside the cannula, the needle is withdrawn.
- Removal of the tourniquet.
- Connection of the cannula with an extension closed with a needle-free connector (unless it is an 'integrated' cannula, already preassembled to an extension and a needle-free connector).
- Connection to the infusion line.
- Whenever available, protect the exit site with a small amount (0.15–0.25 ml) of cyanoacrylate glue. The glue will (a) stop any bleeding and oozing, (b) reduce bacterial contamination, and (c) improve the stabilization of the device.
- Cover and protect the exit site with semipermeable transparent membranes with high permeability (high MVTR = high moisture vapor transfer rate); the skin of children has high transpiration and if the membrane is not permeable enough, maceration can occur below the dressing. Bordered membranes will allow a better stabilization of the device (Fig. 13.7).
- In some situations, joint stabilization devices are used, in particular for short cannulas placed in unstable areas such as the back of the hand or the antecubital fossa. If used, they must not harm the patient (they must be padded, and they must not cause pressure damage to nerves or arteries) and they must allow visual inspection of the exit site.

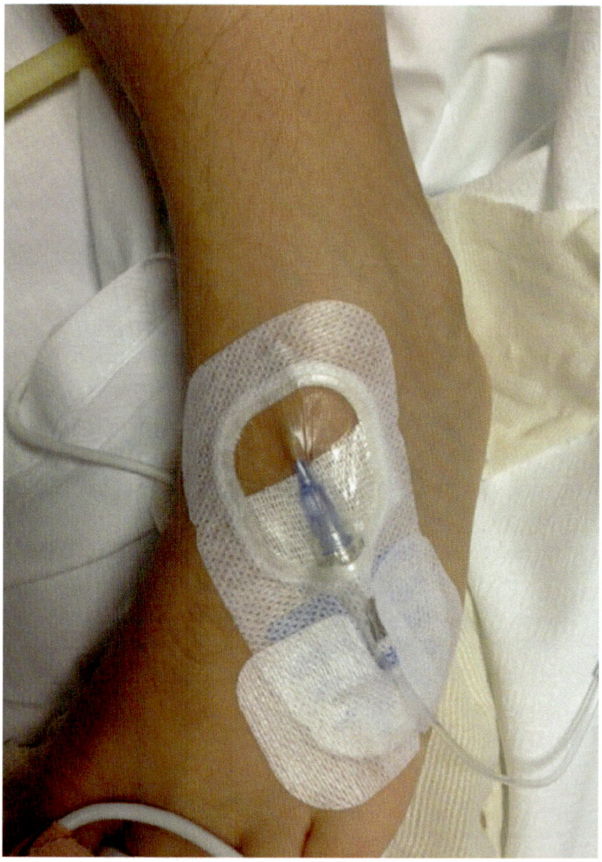

Fig. 13.7 Short cannula secured and protected with glue and bordered transparent membrane

Depending on the age and the degree of collaboration of the child, the insertion of a short cannula may be performed with or without light sedation and with or without the use of topical anesthetic cream.

13.4 Insertion of Long Peripheral Catheters (Mini-Midline)

In the insertion of a long peripheral catheter, we should consider the following steps:

- Appropriate indication: long peripheral catheters should be inserted only when peripheral venous access is required for at least one week and no more than 3–4 weeks, or whenever a peripheral venous access is required but there are no visible/palpable superficial veins (DIVA patients).

- Choice of the puncture site: long peripheral catheters must be preferably inserted in the cephalic vein or basilic vein at the forearm or in the cephalic vein at the upper arm. Basilic vein and brachial veins at the upper arm are a second choice, since—ideally—they should be saved for PICC insertion. The puncture site must be planned so that the length of the catheter is completely in the forearm or in the upper arm, and not crossing the antecubital fossa.
- Hand hygiene (preferably with alcohol-based gel rub).
- Sterile gloves and maximal barrier precautions (sterile gown, wide sterile field over the child, long sterile cover for the ultrasound probe) are recommended. If maximal barrier precautions are not adopted (as it may occur in emergency), the long peripheral catheter must be removed as soon as possible (within 48 hours).
- Proper skin antisepsis with 2% chlorhexidine in 70% isopropyl alcohol (apply for 30 seconds and let dry for 30 seconds).
- Choice of the long peripheral cannula: prefer 8–10 cm polyurethane or PEBA catheters; prefer long peripheral catheters to be inserted with simple Seldinger technique; choose between 3Fr and 4Fr, according to the inner diameter of the vein, as evaluated by ultrasound (3Fr catheters require veins of 3 mm or larger; 4Fr catheters require veins of 4 mm or larger).
- Placement of the tourniquet.
- Ultrasound guided puncture and cannulation of the vein.
- As the needle is visualized inside the vein and blood withdrawal is possible, the guidewire is threaded inside the needle and the needle removed.
- Removal of the tourniquet.
- The presence of the guidewire inside the vein can be assessed by ultrasound scan in long axis.
- The catheter is inserted over the guidewire and the guidewire removed.
- Connection of the catheter with an extension closed with a needle-free connector (unless it is a device with preassembled extension and preassembled needle-free connector).
- Flush of the catheter with saline.
- Seal the exit site with a small amount (0.15–0.25 ml) of cyanoacrylate glue. The glue will (a) stop any bleeding and oozing, (b) reduce bacterial contamination, and (c) improve the stabilization of the device.
- Secure the catheter with skin-adhesive sutureless device (Fig. 13.8).
- Cover and protect the exit site with semipermeable transparent membranes with high permeability (high MVTR = high moisture vapor transfer rate); the skin of children has high transpiration and if the membrane is not permeable enough, maceration can occur below the dressing. Bordered membranes will allow a better stabilization of the device.

Depending on the age and the degree of collaboration of the child, the insertion of a long peripheral catheter may be performed under light sedation or with local infiltration of anesthetic (0.75% ropivacaine).

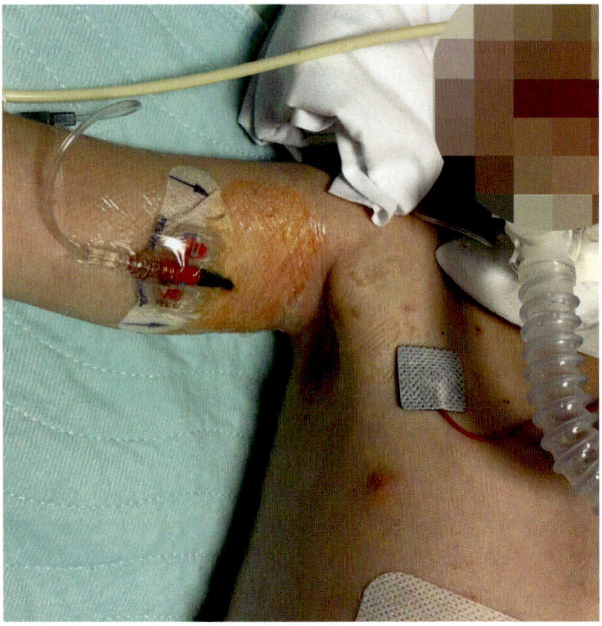

Fig. 13.8 Long peripheral catheter secured and protected with glue, skin-adhesive sutureless device, and transparent membrane

13.5 Insertion of Midline Catheters

In the insertion of a midline catheter, we should consider the following steps:

- Appropriate indication: midline catheters should be inserted only when peripheral venous access is required for more than 3–4 weeks, in non-hospitalized children.
- Choice of the puncture site: midline catheters must be preferably inserted in the basilic vein and brachial veins at the upper arm. The cephalic vein at the upper arm is a second choice. The exit site must be planned in the middle third of the upper arm (Dawson's green zone). If the most appropriate puncture site is in the upper third (Dawson's yellow zone), the midline catheters can be tunneled, so to obtain a puncture site in the yellow zone and an exit site in the green zone.
- Hand hygiene (preferably with alcohol-based gel rub).
- Sterile gloves and maximal barrier precautions (sterile gown, wide sterile field over the child, long sterile cover for the ultrasound probe) are mandatory.
- Proper skin antisepsis with 2% chlorhexidine in 70% isopropyl alcohol (apply for 30 seconds and let dry for 30 seconds).
- Choice of the midline catheter: prefer power injectable, non-valved polyurethane catheters; choose between 3Fr and 4Fr, according to the inner diameter of the vein, as evaluated by ultrasound (3Fr catheters require veins of 3 mm or larger; 4Fr catheters require veins of 4 mm or larger). Adjust the length of the catheter so that the tip may be located in the axillary tract of the axillary vein, before the clavicle.
- Tourniquet should be used only if needed. Most venipunctures of the deep veins of the upper arm can be performed safely without tourniquet.

- Ultrasound guided puncture and cannulation of the vein.
- As the needle is visualized inside the vein and blood withdrawal is possible, the guidewire is threaded inside the needle and the needle removed.
- The presence of the guidewire inside the vein can be assessed by ultrasound scan in long axis.
- The micro-introducer dilator is inserted over the guidewire.
- After removal of the dilator and of the guidewire, the catheter is inserted into the peel-away micro-introducer.
- The introducer is removed.
- The position of the tip is assessed by ultrasound scan of the axillary vein in the infra-clavicular area (with the same linear probe used for ultrasound-guided venipuncture): the catheter tip is visualized by short axis or long axis view of the axillary vein. An insufficient visualization of the tip can be enhanced by rapid flush of saline inside the catheter (bubble test)
- Lock of the catheter with saline.
- Seal the exit site with a small amount (0.15–0.25 ml) of cyanoacrylate glue. The glue will (a) stop any bleeding and oozing, (b) reduce bacterial contamination, and (c) improve the stabilization of the device.
- Secure the catheter with skin-adhesive sutureless device or with subcutaneous anchorage (Fig. 13.9) (if subcutaneous anchorage is used, the glue must be applied after the securement).
- Cover and protect the exit site with semipermeable transparent membranes with high permeability (high MVTR = high moisture vapor transfer rate); the skin of children has high transpiration and if the membrane is not permeable enough, maceration can occur below the dressing. Bordered membranes will allow a better stabilization of the device.

Depending on the age and the degree of collaboration of the child, the insertion of a short cannula may be performed under sedation, general anesthesia, or with local infiltration of anesthetic (0.75% ropivacaine).

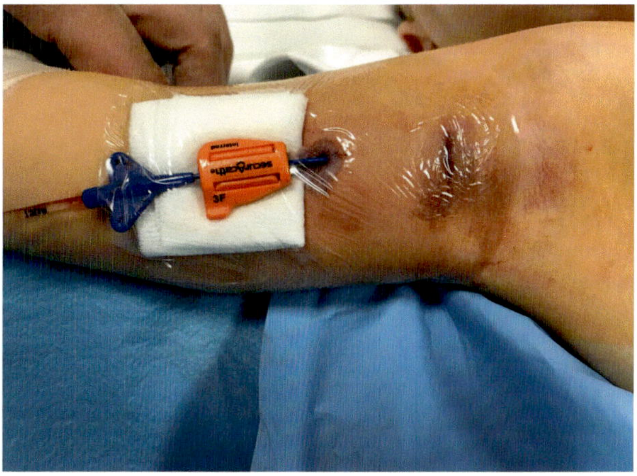

Fig. 13.9 Midline catheter secured and protected with subcutaneous anchorage, glue and transparent membrane

13.6 Maintenance

The basic recommendations for the proper maintenance of a peripheral venous access are (1) appropriate care of catheter at the exit site, (2) appropriate care of the infusion lines.

1. The care of the exit site is focused on the prevention of dislodgment and on the prevention of bacterial contamination by the extraluminal route. For short cannulas, no scheduled dressing change is needed since transparent dressing are meant to stay in place for one week and very few short cannulas would resist so long. The combined use of cyanoacrylate glue and transparent dressing will significantly reduce the occurrence of unscheduled dressing change. On the other hand, long peripheral catheters (mini-midline) and midline catheters require weekly dressing changes, which include: (1) after hand hygiene, wearing non-sterile gloves, removal of the old transparent dressing and of the skin-adhesive sutureless securement (if present); (2) skin antisepsis with 2% chlorhexidine in 70% isopropyl alcohol (apply for 30 seconds and let dry for 30 seconds); (3) placement of new sutureless securement (if needed) and of new transparent dressing. An important role is played by surveillance and more specifically by periodic visual inspection of the exit site (2–3 times/day) for an early detection of local complications.
2. The care of the infusion line is focused on the prevention of lumen occlusion and on the prevention of bacterial contamination by the intraluminal route. The main strategies for reducing the risk of contamination and of lumen occlusion are: for peripheral venous devices use intermittently, adoption of needle-free connectors with neutral displacement, covered by passive disinfection caps (so-called "port protectors"); routine change of continuous administration sets (used for other than lipid solutions or blood or blood products) not more frequently than every 96 hours; change of intermittent administration sets every day; change of administration sets for blood products at the end of every unit or every four hours; change of needle-free connectors with the administration sets; flush with 2–5 ml of normal saline before and after each infusion; lock the peripheral venous access devices, if used intermittently, with saline only.

13.7 Complications

Though peripheral venous access devices are commonly regarded as safe if compared to central venous access devices, they are nonetheless associated with a high incidence of minor local complications, which all concur eventually to the same outcome, "catheter failure", that is, forced, unscheduled removal of the VAD. Its pathogenesis is often difficult to define, especially for short cannulas, since the reasons for catheter failure include: "phlebitis" (i.e., "thrombophlebitis") of superficial veins, secondary to bacterial contamination and/or chemical injury and/or

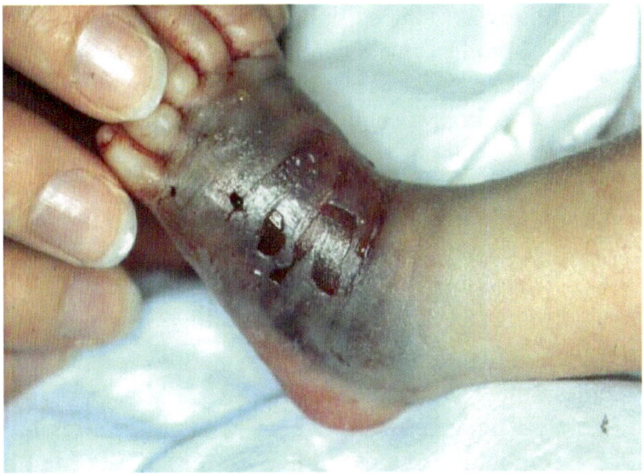

Fig. 13.10 Extravasation

mechanical injury and/or local obstruction of the blood flow; partial dislodgment of the catheter with associated infiltration/extravasation of the infusate in the surrounding tissues (Fig. 13.10); occlusion of the catheter lumen. The differentiation between these complications may be difficult, since the clinical picture is identical: local pain or tenderness, swelling, redness, obstruction to flow. Furthermore, more recently, peripheral venous devices have also been related to more severe systemic complications such as bloodstream infections.

1. Infection. The incidence of systemic infections (catheter-related bloodstream infections) due to peripheral devices is quite low, probably below 0.5 episodes/1000 catheter days. On the other hand, the rate of local infection is difficult to define since it may be difficult to differentiate from other causes of 'catheter failure'. Probably, infection of the exit site due to inappropriate antisepsis at the time of insertion is a major cause of 'catheter failure'. The best prevention is the adoption of the strategies described above in the paragraph about maintenance, plus a strict policy of visual inspection of the exit site (to be performed 2–3 times per day). According to the Visual Exit Score suggested by the 2021 Standards of the Infusion Nursing Society, the presence of redness *or* tenderness of the exit site is not a sufficient reason for removing the device, while the simultaneous evidence of redness *and* tenderness (with or without other local signs such as secretions, swelling, etc.) is an indication for removal.
2. Lumen occlusion. This complication is not frequent for short cannulas, but it is a frequent cause of 'catheter failure' for long peripheral catheters and midline catheters. An intraluminal occlusion may be secondary to drug precipitates or blood clots; an extraluminal obstruction of the tip is often secondary to venous thrombosis or to formation of fibroblastic sleeve. The preventive strategies include: avoidance of simultaneous infusion of incompatible drugs; saline flush before and after each infusion; use of the device exclusively for peripherally compatible solutions.

3. Dislodgment. This complication is a very frequent cause of catheter failure for short cannulas, but not for mini-midlines and midline catheters. In fact, short cannulas are more prone to be inserted in unstable areas (back of the hand, antecubital fossa, etc.) and are typically secured only by the transparent dressing. In pediatric patients, there is an additional risk related to the possible lack of collaboration of the patient. The prevention of dislodgment includes both the proper choice of the puncture site and an appropriate securement and coverage. As regards securement/protection, we recommend cyanoacrylate glue + bordered transparent membrane for short cannulas, cyanoacrylate glue + skin adhesive sutureless securement + transparent membrane for long peripheral catheters, and subcutaneous anchorage + cyanoacrylate glue + transparent membrane for midline catheters.
4. Phlebitis/thrombosis. Different types of injuries may cause an inflammation of the vein wall and a disruptive damage of the endothelial integrity, which is followed by the local formation of a thrombus. These pathophysiological events are variously described as "phlebitis" or "thrombophlebitis" or "thrombosis", though there is little pathological evidence to differentiate the prevalence of the inflammation of the vein from the local venous thrombosis. Furthermore, the same phenomena may be elicited by a mechanical injury, by bacteria or by chemical substances contained in the infused solution. The local changes may be self-limiting, or they may be associated with a loss of the integrity of the vein wall, with resulting infiltration or extravasation. Prevention of bacterial phlebitis has been discussed above. Prevention of mechanical and chemical phlebitis is based on the following recommendations: (1) if the short cannula is inserted on the hand, in the external jugular vein and in veins of the lower limb, remove it within 24–48 hours; (2) use the smallest practical size of venous access device, still compatible with the infusion required; long peripheral catheters and midline catheters should be chosen respecting the 1:3 catheter/vein ratio; (3) use appropriate stabilization (see above) to avoid micro-motion of the catheter, which is known to be associated with the risk of mechanical phlebitis; (4) do not use a peripheral venous access device for repeated or prolonged administration of solutions that are not peripherally compatible (chemical irritants, vesicant drugs, parenteral nutrition with osmolality >850 mOsm/L, etc.).

Bibliography

1. Cellini M, Bergadano A, Crocoli A, Badino C, Carraro F, Sidro L, Botta D, Pancaldi A, Rossetti F, Pitta F, Cesaro S. Guidelines of the Italian Association of Pediatric Hematology and Oncology for the management of the central venous access devices in pediatric patients with onco-hematological disease. J Vasc Access. 2020;10:1129729820969309. https://doi.org/10.1177/1129729820969309.
2. Crocoli A, Tornesello A, Pittiruti M, Barone A, Muggeo P, Inserra A, Molinari AC, Grillenzoni V, Durante V, Cicalese MP, Zanazzo GA, Cesaro S. Central venous access devices in pediatric

malignancies: a position paper of Italian Association of Pediatric Hematology and Oncology. J Vasc Access. 2015;16(2):130–6. https://doi.org/10.5301/jva.5000314.

3. Elli S, Pittiruti M, Pigozzo V, Cannizzo L, Giannini L, Siligato A, Rondelli E, Foti G, Lucchini A. Ultrasound-guided tip location of midline catheters. J Vasc Access. 2020 Sep;21(5):764–8. https://doi.org/10.1177/1129729820907250.
4. Gorski L, Hadaway L, Hagle M, et al. Infusion therapy standards of practice. J Infus Nurs. 2021;44(1S Suppl 1):S1–S224.
5. Lamperti M, Pittiruti M II. Difficult peripheral veins: turn on the lights. Br J Anaesth. 2013 Jun;110(6):888–91. https://doi.org/10.1093/bja/aet078.
6. Paladini A, Chiaretti A, Sellasie KW, Pittiruti M, Vento G. Ultrasound-guided placement of long peripheral cannulas in children over the age of 10 years admitted to the emergency department: a pilot study. BMJ Paediatr Open. 2018;2(1):e000244. https://doi.org/10.1136/bmjpo-2017-000244.
7. Pinelli F, Pittiruti M. The integrated short peripheral cannula: a new peripheral venous access device? J Vasc Access. 2021;19:11297298211034023. https://doi.org/10.1177/11297298211034023.
8. Pinelli F, Pittiruti M, Van Boxtel T, Barone G, Biffi R, Capozzoli G, Crocoli A, Elli S, Elisei D, Fabiani A, Garrino C, Graziano U, Montagnani L, Prato AP, Scoppettuolo G, Zadra N, Zanaboni C, Zerla P, Konstantinou E, Jones M, Rosay H, Simcock L, Stas M, Pepe G. GAVeCeLT-WoCoVA consensus on subcutaneously anchored securement devices for the securement of venous catheters: current evidence and recommendations for future research. J Vasc Access. 2020;2:1129729820924568. https://doi.org/10.1177/1129729820924568.
9. Pittiruti M, Van Boxtel T, Scoppettuolo G, Carr P, Konstantinou E, Ortiz Miluy G, Lamperti M, Goossens GA, Simcock L, Dupont C, Inwood S, Bertoglio S, Nicholson J, Pinelli F, Pepe G. European recommendations on the proper indication and use of peripheral venous access devices (the ERPIUP consensus): a WoCoVA project. J Vasc Access. 2021;4:11297298211023274. https://doi.org/10.1177/11297298211023274.
10. Qin KR, Pittiruti M, Nataraja RM, Pacilli M. Long peripheral catheters and midline catheters: insights from a survey of vascular access specialists. J Vasc Access. 2020;20:1129729820966226. https://doi.org/10.1177/1129729820966226.
11. Ullman AJ, Bernstein SJ, Brown E, Aiyagari R, Doellman D, Faustino EVS, Gore B, Jacobs JP, Jaffray J, Kleidon T, Mahajan PV, McBride CA, Morton K, Pitts S, Prentice E, Rivard DC, Shaughnessy E, Stranz M, Wolf J, Cooper DS, Cooke M, Rickard CM, Chopra V. The Michigan appropriateness guide for intravenous catheters in pediatrics: miniMAGIC. Pediatrics. 2020 Jun;145(Suppl 3):S269–84. https://doi.org/10.1542/peds.2019-3474I.
12. Vallecoccia MS, De Pascale G, Taraschi C, De Angelis DR, Dolcetti L, Pittiruti M, Scoppettuolo G. Closed vs open systems: when should short peripheral intravenous catheters be the first choice? J Hosp Infect. 2015;89(1):72–3. https://doi.org/10.1016/j.jhin.2014.09.010.

Chapter 14
Peripherally Inserted Central Catheters (PICC) in Children

Massimo Lamperti and Mauro Pittiruti

The use of Peripherally Inserted Central Catheters (PICCs) in pediatric patients is not new. Since many years, these catheters have been used to deliver intravenous therapy, especially when required for prolonged periods. Their use began first in Pediatric Intensive Care Units (PICU) and in oncological wards but, in the recent years, with the introduction of new materials and techniques, PICCs have been widely adopted as first-option central venous access for both hospitalized children and for children on homecare therapy.

14.1 Definition

For many years, the term PICC has been confusing in the pediatric vascular world, being used for peripherally inserted central catheters both in children and in neonates.

A "pediatric" PICC is a medium-long term, tunneled or non-tunneled, central venous access device inserted into deep veins of the upper arm with a cross-sectional diameter greater or equal to 3 mm (Fig. 14.1). These catheters must be inserted by ultrasound guided venipuncture, and the final position of the tip must be assessed either by intracavitary ECG or by ultrasound-based tip location (ECHOTIP-Ped protocol) (see below). Pediatric PICCs are only available with caliber equal or larger than 3Fr and most of them are power-injectable and in polyurethane; they can

M. Lamperti
Anesthesiology Institute, Cleveland Clinic, Abu Dhabi, UAE
e-mail: lamperm@clevelandclinicabudhabi.ae

M. Pittiruti (✉)
Department of Surgery, Catholic University Hospital, Rome, Italy

D. G. Biasucci et al. (eds.), *Vascular Access in Neonates and Children*,
https://doi.org/10.1007/978-3-030-94709-5_14

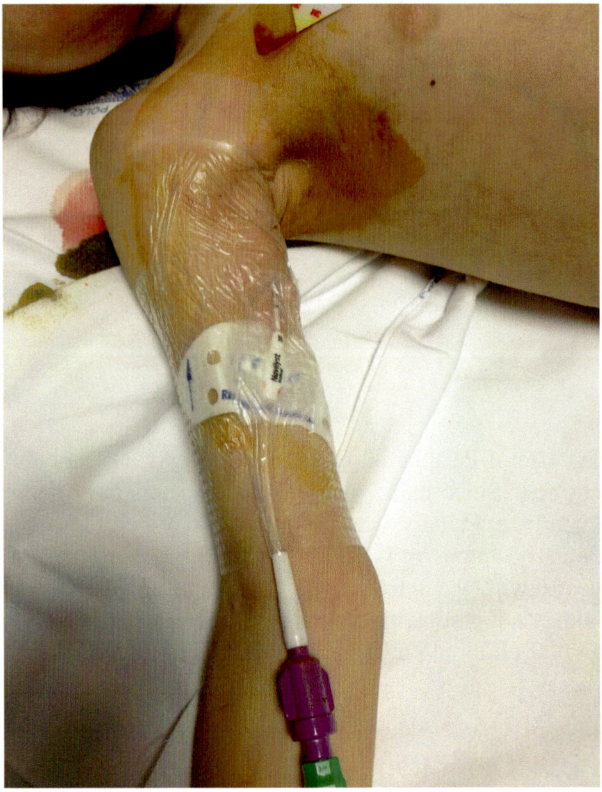

Fig. 14.1 Non-tunneled PICC

be used for standard infusion but also for transfusion or blood sampling or hemodynamic monitoring. As their minimal caliber is 3Fr (= 1 mm), they should be inserted only in veins with an inner diameter of 3 mm or larger; in fact, a catheter occupying more than 30% of the inner diameter of the vein would be associated with venous stasis, increasing the risk of thrombosis. PICC insertion is safe, as insertion-related complications are very rare; late non-infective complications are rare.

On the other hand, "neonatal" PICCs—which should be preferably called epicutaneo-cava catheters (ECCs)—are short-term, non-tunneled central venous access devices inserted into superficial veins of upper limbs, of lower limbs or at the scalp. They are the most used central venous catheters in Neonatal Intensive Care Units (NICU). They have a very small size (from 1 to 2.7 Fr), so that they cannot be used for transfusion or blood sampling or hemodynamic monitoring, but only for infusion. They are inserted by direct percutaneous visualization, with or without the aid of Near Infra-Red devices, and the final position of the tip is assessed by ultrasound-based tip location (Neo-ECHOTIP protocol). ECCs are usually made of polyurethane but are not power-injectable. They have a minor risk of life-threatening complications, as early or late pericardial tamponade.

Table 14.1 Main differences between PICCs and ECCs

Pediatric PICCs	Epicutaneo-cava catheters (ECCs)
Only in children	Only in neonates
Vein with cross sectional diameter >3 mm	Any small vein
Deep veins of the arm	Superficial veins of limbs and scalp
3–4–5 Fr catheters, power injectable	1–2.7 Fr catheters
Ultrasound-guided venipuncture	Direct or NIR-guided venipuncture
Tip location by IC-ECG or ultrasound	Tip location by ultrasound
Appropriate for transfusions	Not appropriate for transfusions
Hemodynamic monitoring	Hemodynamic monitoring impossible
Appropriate for blood sampling	Infusion only
Appropriate for medium-long term treatments	Appropriate for short term treatments

In short, Peripherally Inserted Central Catheters (PICCs) are different from Epicutaneo-cava catheters (ECC) and the two devices should not be confused. Table 14.1 summarizes the main differences between PICCs and ECCs.

14.2 Indications

Indications for PICC insertion in pediatric patients are the same general indications for a central venous access:

- Prolonged infusion of solutions potentially associated with endothelial damage (parenteral nutrition, drugs with osmolarity >600 mOsm/L or pH <5 or >9, as well as any irritant or vesicant solution)
- Requirement for multiple blood samplings during the hospital staying
- Rapid infusion of fluids for volume replacement (power injectable PICCs can infuse fluids at 1–2 ml/sec for each lumen)
- Need for hemodynamic monitoring (central venous pressure, oxygen saturation in mixed venous blood)
- Needle-phobic children

They should be preferred to centrally inserted central catheters in some specific situations:

- low platelet count or high bleeding risk for any other reason
- tracheostomy
- high risk of venous catheterization through central veins of the supra/infra-clavicular area
- need for prolonged intravenous treatment (typically, in non-hospitalized children).

This last indication has made PICCs one of the most used long-term central venous catheters for pediatric homecare in the last decade, as they have advantages over ports (no need of puncture when the system is accessed) and over both ports and tunneled-cuffed CICCs (once the treatment is concluded, PICCs are easily removed without surgical procedure).

For these reasons, PICC has become very popular not only in acute care settings (PICU) but also as a valid option for any medium/long term intravenous treatment in pediatric patients. In non-hospitalized children, a long-term dwelling of the PICC can be obtained by tunneling the catheter (as this will reduce the risk of infection) and securing with subcutaneous anchorage (as this will reduce the risk of dislodgement).

Contraindications to PICC insertion are:

- absence of veins of proper caliber at the arm
- pathological abnormalities of the arm (fracture, ankylosis, venous thrombosis, skin infections, paresis, etc.)
- chronic renal failure of grade 3b–4–5 (present or future need for arterial-venous fistula).

14.3 Technique of Insertion

As for PICCs in adults, the successful insertion of a PICC is guaranteed by the adoption of a proper insertion bundle, such as the SIP protocol (Table 14.2) Before PICC insertion, an accurate assessment of the venous patrimony of the patient is essential. The protocol of Rapid Peripheral Vein Assessment (RaPeVA) (Fig. 14.2). The main steps of the protocol are described in Figs. 14.3, 14.4, 14.5, 14.6, 14.7; RaPeVA includes an ultrasound examination of all main vessels of the mid-arm,

Table 14.2 The SIP protocol (SIP = Safe insertion of PICCs)

1. Bilateral ultrasound scan of all veins at arm and neck using the RaPeVA (Rapid Peripheral Vein Assessment)
2. Proper policy of hand hygiene, skin antisepsis with 2% chlorhexidine in alcohol, maximal barrier precautions
3. Choice of the appropriate vein: inner diameter of the vein must be at least 3 times the external caliber of the catheter; puncture site must be in Dawson's green zone, but if puncture site is in the yellow zone, tunnel the catheter so to get an exit site in the green zone
4. Clear identification of median nerve and brachial artery before venipuncture
5. Ultrasound guided venipuncture with micro-introducer kit (including 21G needle and floppy straight tip nitinol guidewire)
6. US-based tip navigation during introduction of the PICC
7. Tip location by intracavitary ECG and/or ultrasound
8. Securement of the catheter with sutureless device (prefer subcutaneous anchorage) and protection of the exit site with cyanoacrylate glue and transparent dressing

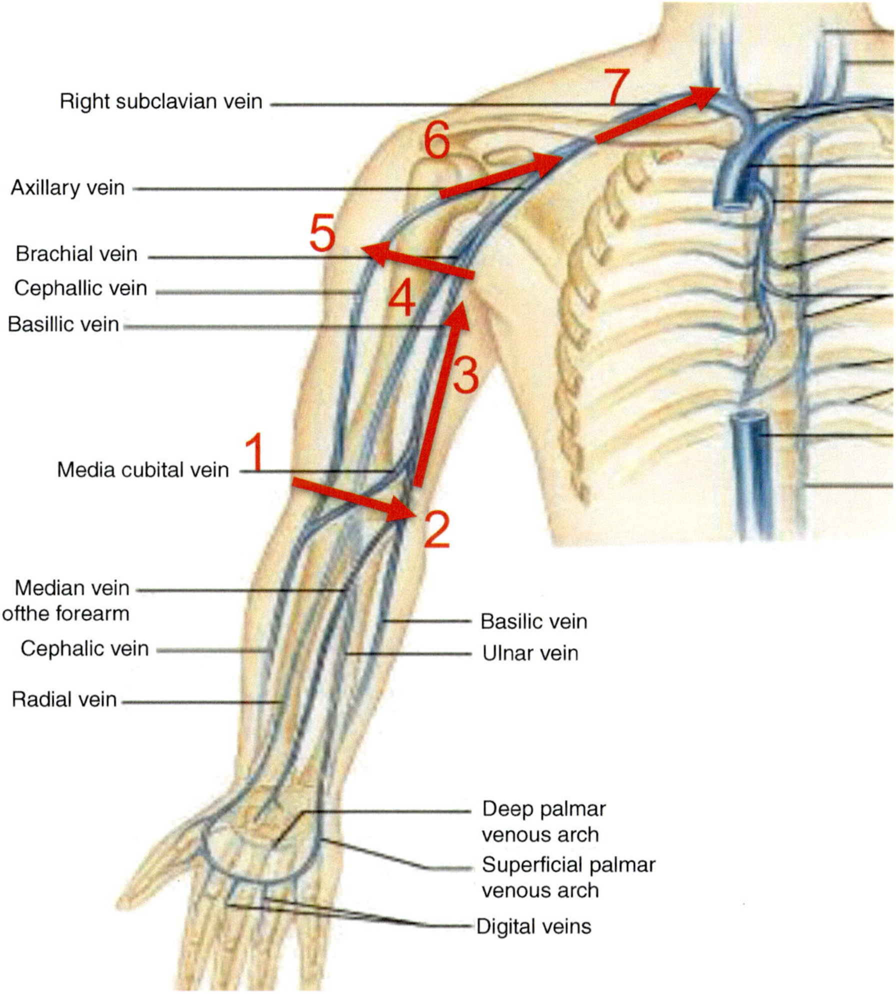

Fig. 14.2 Summary of the RaPeVA protocol

upper arm, axilla, and infra and supra-clavicular area. This assessment allows to verify the possibility of PICC insertion, the best puncture site, the best exit site, and the need for tunneling (according to the RAVESTO protocol) (Table 14.3). The best exit site for PICC is in the middle third of the upper arm, in the so-called 'green zone' according to Dawson's Zone Insertion Method; if the best puncture site (i.e., a vein of appropriate size), is only available in the 'yellow zone' (medial third of the upper arm), tunneling is an option (see below).

As regards the choice of the PICC, we strongly recommend using only power injectable, polyurethane, non-valved catheters. Silicon PICCs are associated with high risk of mechanical complications, while valved PICCs are associated with high risk of malfunction. The caliber should be chosen after measurement of the vein

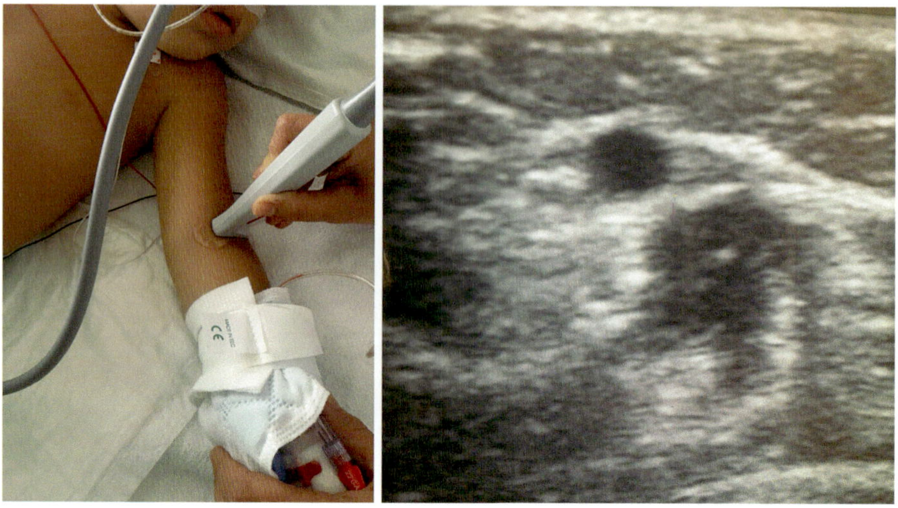

Fig. 14.3 Venous examination according to the RaPeVA protocol: cephalic vein at the antecubital fossa

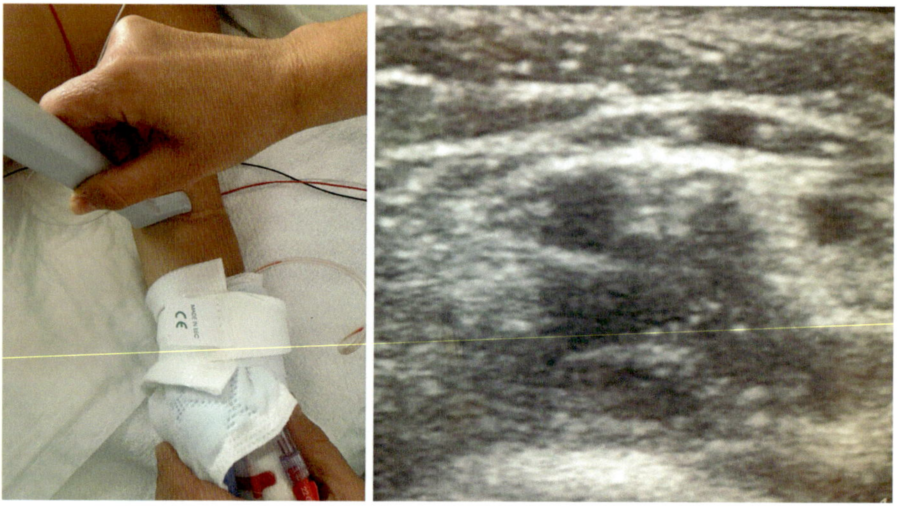

Fig. 14.4 Brachial artery and veins at the antecubital fossa

chosen for cannulation; 3 Fr catheters will adapt to 3 mm veins (or larger), 4 Fr catheters to 4 mm veins (or larger), and so on. The number of lumen (single, double, or triple) will be dictated by the expected clinical use; double and triple lumen PICCs have an important role in PICU; single lumen PICCs should be preferred for home care and for long term use.

Another important issue is related to the setting where the PICC insertion is performed. These procedures are commonly performed at bedside when the child is in

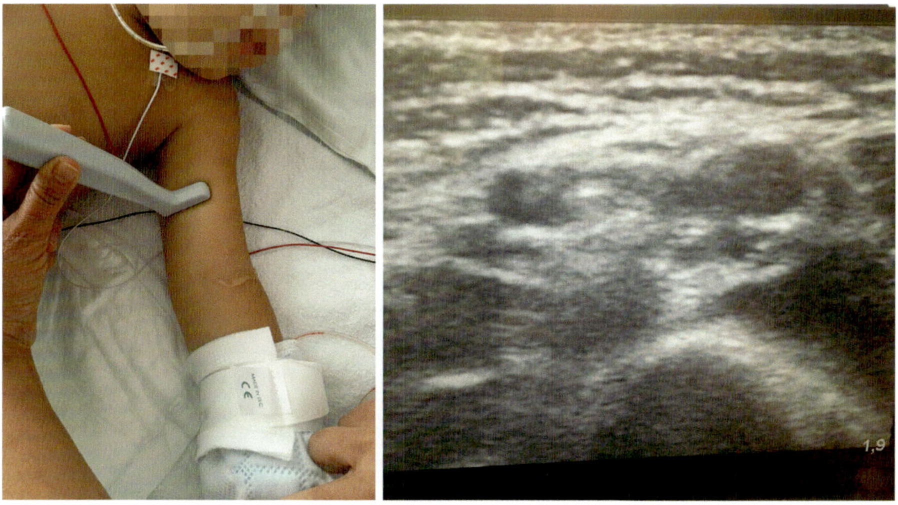

Fig. 14.5 Basilic vein, brachial artery and veins, median nerve at the middle third of upper arm

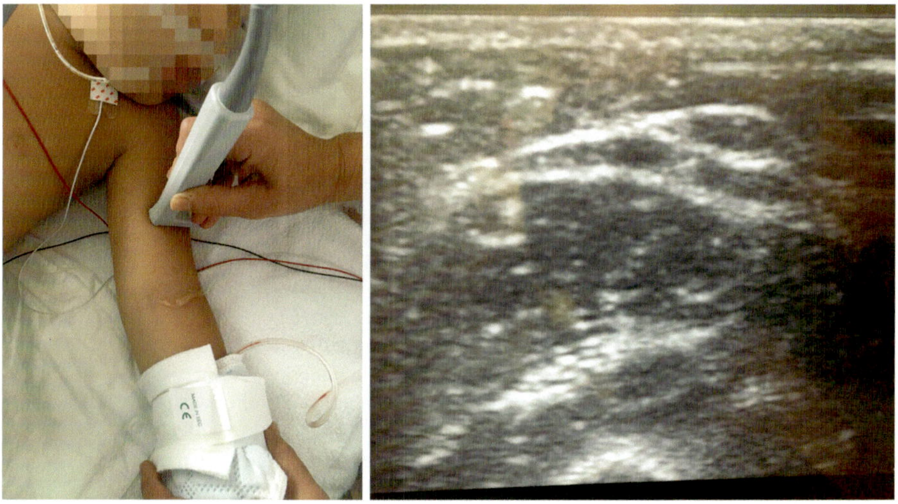

Fig. 14.6 Cephalic vein at the middle third of upper arm

the PICU. For pediatric patients who are not in an intensive care unit, the best option is to insert PICCs in a dedicated area of the hospital equipped with all proper materials (PICCs, micro-introducers, ultrasound device with pediatric probes, ECG monitor, etc.) and with dedicated personnel expert in pediatric procedures. In most of these insertions, some type of procedural sedation and analgesia is required; the personnel should be trained in PALS (pediatric advanced life support). The physician dedicated to the sedation and care of the child should be different from the

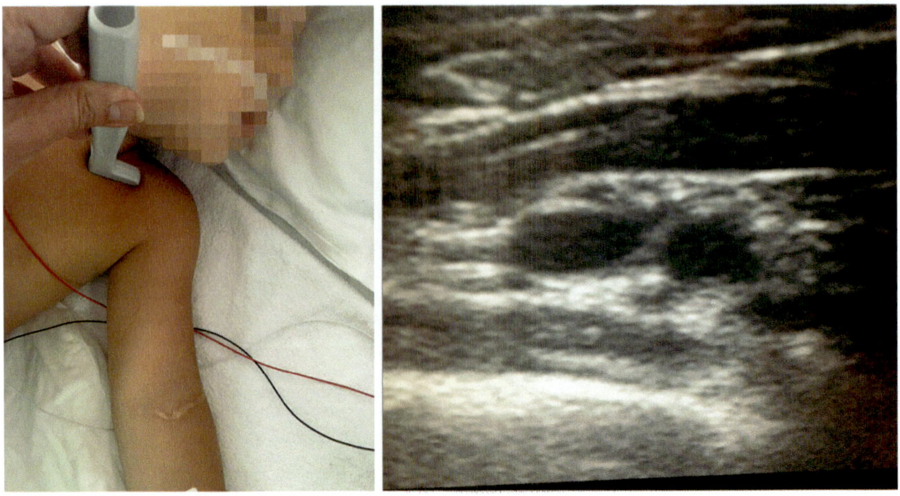

Fig. 14.7 axillary vein and artery in the infraclavicular area

Table 14.3 The RAVESTO protocol (RAVESTO = Rapid Assessment of Venous Exit Site and Tunneling Options)

Central venous access device	Type and path of tunnel	Indications for tunneling
PICC	Tunnel to Dawson's green area	Puncture site in Dawson's yellow area; non-hospitalized patients with expected long intravenous treatment
CICC (supraclavicular puncture)	Tunnel to infraclavicular area	Long term intravenous treatment in non-hospitalized patients (antibiotics, parenteral nutrition, chemotherapy); expected difficulties in management of the exit site in hospitalized patients (beard, humidity, tracheostomy, instability, etc.)
	Tunnel to arm	Compromised skin integrity of the chest area; oral or endotracheal secretions over chest; implanted device on ipsilateral chest; chest surgery; contracted shoulder; etc.
	Tunnel to back	Cognitive disorder resulting in device removal; contraindication to chest or arm exit site
CICC (infraclavicular puncture)	Tunnel to lower chest	Long term intravenous treatment in non-hospitalized patients (antibiotics, parenteral nutrition, chemotherapy); expected problems in management of the exit site in hospitalized patients (tracheostomy, etc.)
	Tunnel to arm	Compromised skin integrity of the chest area; oral or endotracheal secretions over chest; implanted device on ipsilateral chest; chest surgery; contracted shoulder; etc.
	Tunnel to back	Cognitive disorder resulting in device removal; contraindication to chest or arm exit site

Table 14.3 (continued)

Central venous access device	Type and path of tunnel	Indications for tunneling
FICC (puncture at the groin)	Tunnel to the abdomen	Non-emergency line in walking patients with contraindication to PICC/CICC
	Tunnel to mid-thigh	Non-emergency line in bedridden patients with contraindication to PICC/CICC
FICC (puncture at mid-thigh)	Tunnel to the abdomen	Non-emergency line in walking patients with contraindication to PICC/CICC
	Tunnel to distal thigh	Long term intravenous treatment in bedridden patients with contraindication to PICC/CICC

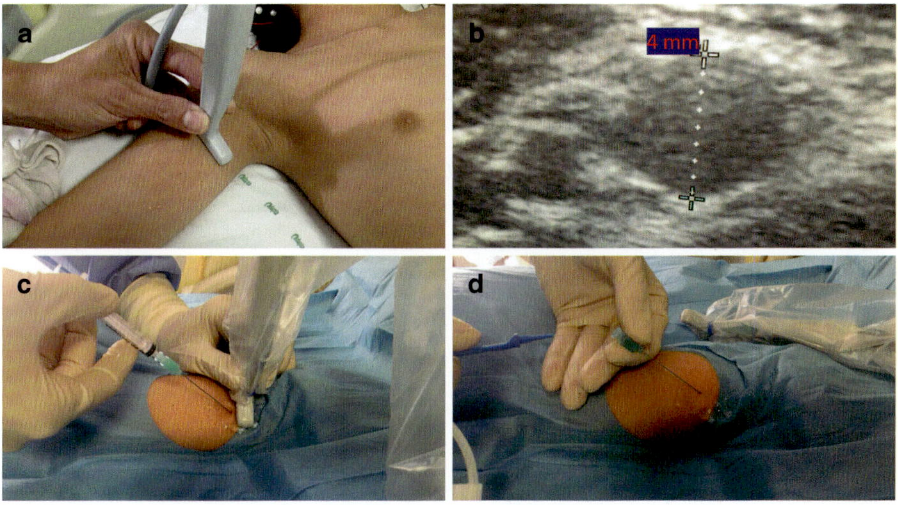

Fig. 14.8 Tunneled PICC insertion: RaPeVA (**a**); measurement of the vein (**b**); ultrasound guided venipuncture (**c**); introduction of the guidewire (**d**)

clinician performing the insertion. Even in case of requirement of general anesthesia (usually for smaller patients or agitated patients), the operating room is not strictly necessary, if a proper dedicated procedural room is available. The most appropriate combination of local anesthesia, sedation, analgesia, intravenous or gaseous anesthesia depends on the age and the clinical conditions of the child.

The insertion of the PICC starts with an accurate placement of the arm so to avoid any movement during the venipuncture. The operator should have the screen of the ultrasound device in front of his/her eyes and have the possibility to put the elbows on the operating table so to handle comfortably the ultrasound probe and the needle while performing the venipuncture.

The main steps of PICC insertion are illustrated in Figs. 14.8, 14.9, 14.10. Once the vein has been punctured and the guidewire inserted, it is recommended to check

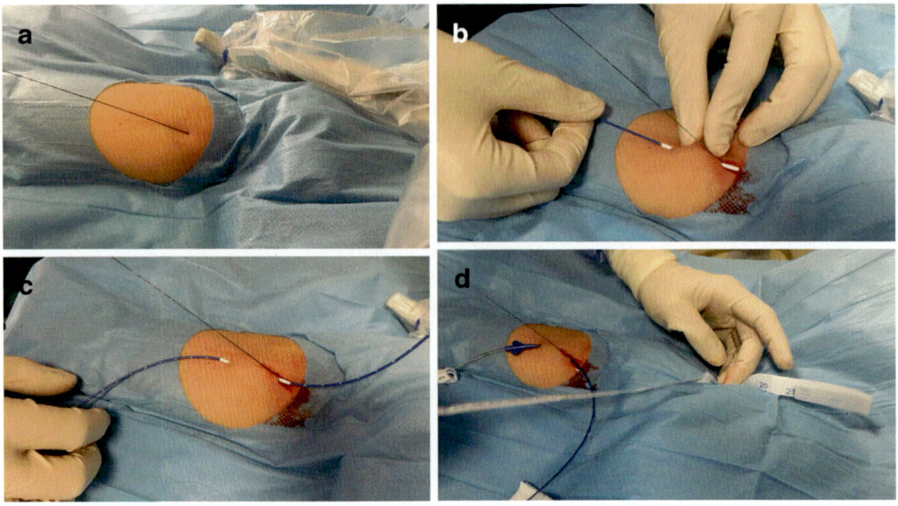

Fig. 14.9 Puncture site with guidewire (**a**); tunneling through a 14G cannula (**b**); the catheter is threaded through the cannula (**c**); length estimation (**d**)

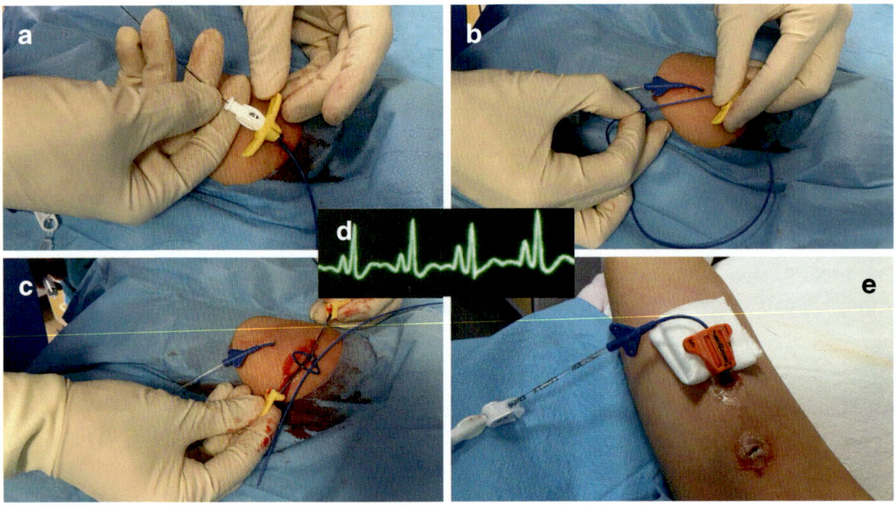

Fig. 14.10 Insertion of the micro-introducer-dilator over the guidewire (**a**); insertion of the trimmed catheter into the introducer (**b**); removal of the introducer by peel-away (**c**); verification of the proper tip location by intracavitary ECG (**d**); subcutaneous anchorage (for securement of the catheter); (**e**) application of cyanoacrylate glue (for sealing the exit site and closing the puncture site)

its presence in the vein of the upper arm by ultrasound. According to the modified Seldinger technique, the needle is removed, and the micro-introducer-dilator is inserted over the guidewire. After removing the dilator and the guidewire, the PICC is inserted into the micro-introducer, and the operator use ultrasound to assess that the catheter enters the subclavian and then the brachio-cephalic vein ('tip

Table 14.4 Ultrasound-based tip navigation/location of PICCs according to the ECHOTIP-Ped protocol

	Protocol	Probe	Windows
PICC	Tip navigation	Linear 'hockey stick' probe, 10–14 MHz	Same acoustic windows as in RaPeVA and RaCeVA
	Tip location	Micro-convex probe, 4–8-MHz, or small sectorial probe, 3–7 MHz	Subcostal bi-caval view (recommended) or 4-chambers apical view (as alternative option)

navigation', as described in the ECHOTIP-Ped protocol) (Table 14.4). The correct location of the catheter tip can be verified by intracavitary ECG (IC-ECG) or by ultrasound. Tip location by IC-ECG has been validated in children since a decade; this method is very accurate, safe, inexpensive, intraprocedural, rapid, and easy to perform. If the heart rate is high, it is recommended to increase the speed of the ECG monitor from 25 mm/sec to 50 mm/sec, for a better interpretation of the ECG trace. The old-fashioned method of tip location (approximate length estimation followed by post-procedural chest x-ray) is not recommended by current guidelines, since it is inaccurate, expensive, and time-consuming. Another acceptable option for tip location is ultrasound-based tip location, with the adjunct of the 'bubble test', as described by the ECHOTIP-Ped protocol (Table 14.4). This technique has been validated in adults, and it is even easier to perform in children, since the ultrasound visualization of the inferior vena cava, right atrium and the junction between superior vena cava and atrium, by subcostal window, is optimal in these patients.

Once the PICC is inserted and the tip location is verified, it is mandatory to secure it so that it cannot be pulled out accidentally, considering that children and toddlers are sometimes very active and restless. Securement must be obtained either by skin-adhesive sutureless devices (Fig. 14.11) or by subcutaneous anchorage. In both cases, we recommend sealing the exit site with cyanoacrylate glue, for the purpose of improving the stabilization of the catheter, avoiding any bleeding/oozing, and reducing bacterial contamination. Subcutaneous anchorage (Fig. 14.12) is extremely effective in avoiding the risk of accidental dislodgment or removal of the PICC, events that are quite frequent in the pediatric population. The securement of the catheter and the protection of the exit site is completed by covering with a semi-permeable transparent membrane, to be removed after 7 days. The traditional strategy of protecting the exit site with a temporary dressing with sterile gauzes in the first 24 hours, so to absorb any possible minimal local bleeding, and then applying the definitive dressing, is not justified anymore when cyanoacrylate glue is used. The safest and most cost-effective strategy is to apply directly glue, sutureless device and transparent membrane at the time of insertion. One week later, the dressing is changed: if securement is obtained by subcutaneous anchorage, it must not be replaced; on the other hand, skin-adhesive sutureless devices must be replaced weekly. After the first week, protection of the exit site can be achieved either replacing the sealing with cyanoacrylate glue or applying locally a chlorhexidine-releasing sponge dressing. The safety of repeated local applications of glue is not demonstrated, so that it is currently recommended to use the sponge dressing, after the first week; if the PICC is tunneled (see below), the cost-effectiveness of the

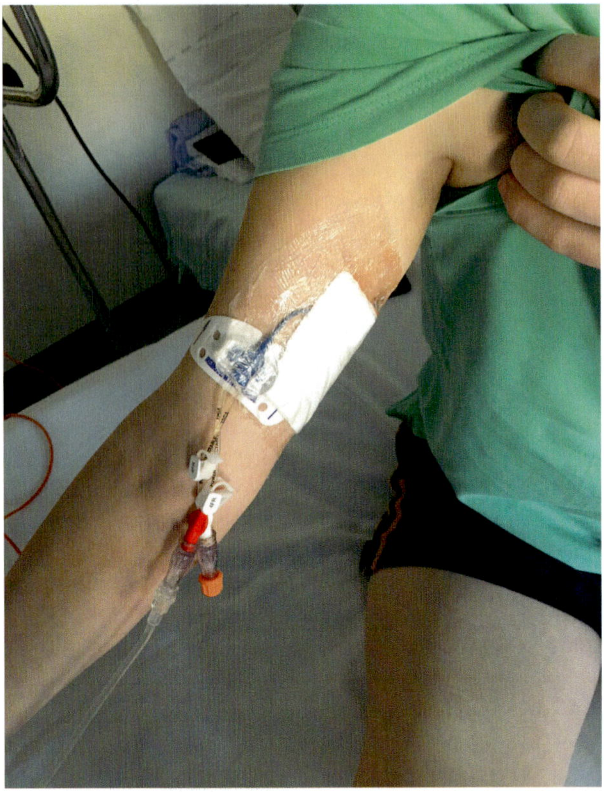

Fig. 14.11 Non-tunneled PICC secured with a skin-adhesive sutureless device

chlorhexidine-releasing sponge dressing is questionable. At any case, the semipermeable transparent dressing must be replaced weekly. In pediatric patients, transparent membranes must have high permeability (high MVTR = high moisture vapor transfer rate) since the skin of children is characterized by high transpiration. An MVTR >1500 is recommended. Transparent membranes with chlorhexidine-releasing gel should always be avoided because the gel pad has no permeability does not allow a proper transpiration, increasing the risk of MARSI (skin maceration + local irritation due to chlorhexidine, amplified by the local humidity).

14.4 Tunneling

As already mentioned, insertion of a 3Fr (or 4Fr) PICC usually requires the visualization of a vein 3 mm or larger (or 4 mm or larger) in Dawson's green zone. In children, the deep veins of the arm are often quite small, so that a vein of appropriate caliber may be detected only in the yellow zone (which is not considered optimal as location of the exit site). In this situation, which occurs frequently in the pediatric patient, tunneling is a simple, safe, and inexpensive technique that allows to have

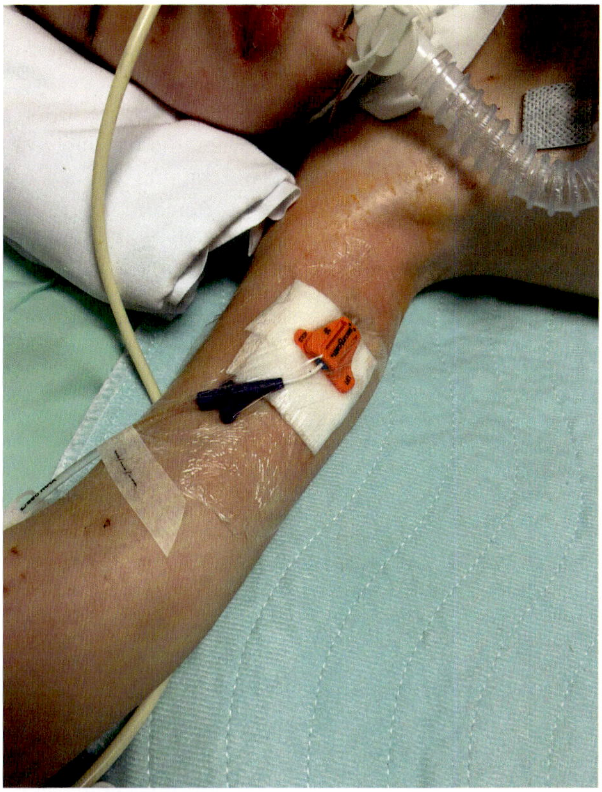

Fig. 14.12 Non-tunneled PICC secured with subcutaneous anchorage

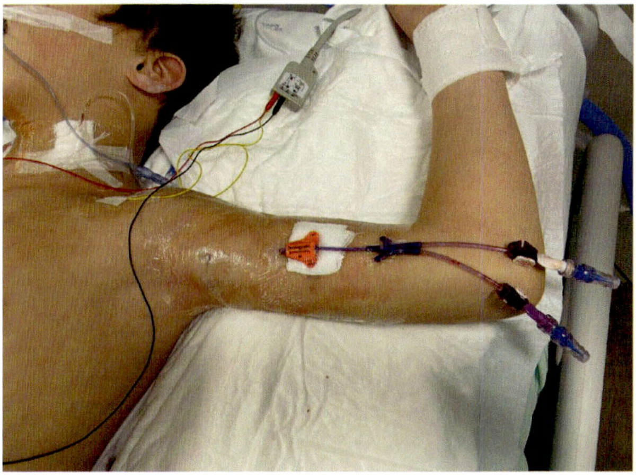

Fig. 14.13 Tunneled PICC

the puncture site where the vein has the best caliber (the yellow zone) and the exit site in the ideal location (the green zone) (Fig. 14.13).

The technique is quite easy: after ultrasound guided venipuncture and insertion of the guidewire, the exit site is planned so to be located in the upper portion of the green zone. A blunt dissection of the subcutaneous tissue between the exit site and the puncture site is obtained, injecting saline or local anesthetic (depending on the overall strategy of sedation/anesthesia adopted in each case). The catheter is passed into the subcutaneous tissue, from the exit site to the puncture site ('anterograde' tunneling) either using dedicated metallic tunnelers or intravenous cannulas; a 3Fr catheter can be threaded into a 16G cannula, while a 4–5 Fr PICC will require a 14G cannula. As the catheter gets to the puncture site, it can be inserted into the vein by the modified Seldinger technique ('catheter through introducer'). At the end of the maneuver, cyanoacrylate glue is used both for closing the exit site and for sealing the puncture site (Fig. 14.10e).

14.5 Maintenance

As for any other central access device, the goal of maintenance is to protect the PICC from infective and non-infective complications.

The care of the exit site is focused on the prevention of dislodgment and of extraluminal bacterial contamination; for this purpose, the main recommended strategies are: proper frequency of dressing change (every 7 days or more frequently, if the dressing is loose or wet or detached), skin antisepsis with 2% chlorhexidine in alcohol, weekly replacement of the skin-adhesive sutureless securement (if the catheter is not secured by subcutaneous anchorage), weekly replacement of chlorhexidine-releasing sponge dressing (in non-tunneled catheters), and weekly replacement of the semipermeable transparent dressing.

The care of the infusion lines is focused on the prevention of lumen occlusion and of intraluminal bacterial contamination, and the main recommended strategies are: saline flushing with normal saline—using a push-stop technique—before and after each infusion, and at least every week if the PICC is not used; adoption of neutral displacement needle free connectors, covered with disinfecting caps (so called 'port protectors'); in specific cases at high risk for infection, periodic prophylactic lock of the catheter with 2% taurolidine.

As far as the PICC is still indicated and there are no complications requiring removal, the device can be left in place for an unlimited period. The main limitation is related to the fact the child grows, so that a catheter with the tip properly located at the time insertion may become too short with the passing of time.

14.6 Complications

As already mentioned, insertion-related complications are rare if adopting a proper insertion bundle as the SIP protocol. On the other hand, late complications may occur.

- *Infection*—Infection may occur as infection of the exit site, infection of the tunnel or catheter-related blood stream infection (CRBSI). The latter is a severe and

possibly life-threatening complication, which may occur especially in immunocompromised children and/or in PICCs used for parenteral nutrition. The diagnosis is made by simultaneous blood cultures from peripheral vein and from the catheter, using the method of the Differential Time to Positivity (DTP). The standard treatment of CRBSI is the removal of the PICC and antibiotic therapy. The prevention relies on proper policies of care of the exit site and of the infusion line. CRBSI should not be confused with catheter colonization (at DTP: catheter blood culture is positive, but peripheral blood culture is negative): the standard treatment of colonization is PICC removal, though in some cases a de-colonization using lock with 2% taurolidine should be considered.
- *Venous thrombosis*—Catheter-related thrombosis (CRT) may be symptomatic or asymptomatic and is usually caused by a mismatch between vein diameter and catheter caliber (a catheter that occupies >33% or >45% of the venous lumen), and/or by relevant damage of the vein during repeated attempts of venipuncture, and/or by an inappropriate location of the tip (i.e., far from the cavo-atrial junction), and/or by thrombophilia of the child. When adopting the SIP protocol, the occurrence of CRT is minimized, both in adults and in children, and it may be expected to be 0–3% (slightly more frequent in children with leukemia). Diagnosis is based on ultrasound examination of the veins occupied by the PICC. The standard treatment is anticoagulation with low molecular weight heparin; the PICC is removed only if there is concomitant malfunction or infection. At the ultrasound examination, asymptomatic CRT should not be confused with fibroblastic sleeve (FS), a very common physiological phenomenon associated with vascular devices (much more frequent than CRT), which consists in a sleeve of connective tissue enwrapping the catheter in some segments. FS is a benign event that does not require treatment.
- *Lumen occlusion*—Malfunction due to lumen occlusion is a complication of PICCs somehow more frequent in children than in adults, because of the smaller caliber of the catheter, but completely preventable by a proper policy of flushing with saline (before starting the infusion, in between different infusions, at the closing of the PICC). It may occur after blood sampling or after infusion of viscous solutions (blood, blood derivatives, lipids, contrast media, etc.), if the catheter is not properly flushed. Heparinization of the catheter has no role in preventing lumen occlusion, and—as a matter of fact—may cause lumen occlusion by facilitating the precipitation of lipids and/or drugs with high pH.
- *Dislodgment*—Dislodgment used to be a very frequent cause of accidental PICC removal. Today, it can be successfully prevented by subcutaneous anchorage.

14.7 Conclusion

PICCs are medium-long term central venous access devices, and they should be considered the first option for any central venous access, both in hospitalized and in non-hospitalized children, as long as the deep veins of the arm are of appropriate caliber. The preservation of the venous patrimony is of paramount importance in children: therefore, proper indication of the device, proper technique of insertion and accurate protocols of maintenance and care should be implemented systematically, so to avoid unscheduled removal of the PICC. The care of the child and his family - together with the care for the PICC - are the key to success to grant a good clinical outcome.

Bibliography

1. Cellini M, Bergadano A, Crocoli A, Badino C, Carraro F, Sidro L, Botta D, Pancaldi A, Rossetti F, Pitta F, Cesaro S. Guidelines of the Italian Association of Pediatric Hematology and Oncology for the management of the central venous access devices in pediatric patients with onco-hematological disease. J Vasc Access. 2020;10:1129729820969309. https://doi.org/10.1177/1129729820969309.
2. Chiaretti A, Pittiruti M, Sassudelli G, Conti G, Rossi M, Pulitanò SM, Mancino A, Pusateri A, Gatto A, Tosi F. Comparison between sedation room and operating room in central venous catheter positioning in children. J Vasc Access. 2021;22(2):184–8. https://doi.org/10.1177/1129729820932415.
3. Crocoli A, Cesaro S, Cellini M, Rossetti F, Sidro L, Pinelli F, Pittiruti M. In defense of the use of peripherally inserted central catheters in pediatric patients. J Vasc Access. 2021;22(3):333–6. https://doi.org/10.1177/1129729820936411.
4. Crocoli A, Martucci C, Sidro L, Delle Donne D, Menna G, Pittiruti M, De Pasquale MD, Strocchio L, Natali GL, Inserra A. Safety and effectiveness of subcutaneously anchored securement for tunneled central catheters in oncological pediatric patients: a retrospective study. J Vasc Access. 2021;4:11297298211009364. https://doi.org/10.1177/11297298211009364.
5. Crocoli A, Tornesello A, Pittiruti M, Barone A, Muggeo P, Inserra A, Molinari AC, Grillenzoni V, Durante V, Cicalese MP, Zanazzo GA, Cesaro S. Central venous access devices in pediatric malignancies: a position paper of Italian Association of Pediatric Hematology and Oncology. J Vasc Access. 2015;16(2):130–6. https://doi.org/10.5301/jva.5000314.
6. Galloway S, Bodenham A. Long-term central venous access. Br J Anaesth. 2004;92:722–34.
7. Gorski L, Hadaway L, Hagle M, et al. Infusion therapy standards of practice. J Infus Nurs. 2021;44(1S Suppl 1):S1–S224.
8. Iacobone E, Elisei D, Gattari D, Carbone L, Capozzoli G. Transthoracic echocardiography as bedside technique to verify tip location of central venous catheters in patients with atrial arrhythmia. J Vasc Access. 2020;21(6):861–7. https://doi.org/10.1177/1129729820905200.
9. Lamperti M, Biasucci DG, Disma N, Pittiruti M, Breschan C, Vailati D, Subert M, Traškaitė V, Macas A, Estebe JP, Fuzier R, Boselli E, Hopkins P. European Society of Anaesthesiology guidelines on peri-operative use of ultrasound-guided for vascular access (PERSEUS vascular access). Eur J Anaesthesiol. 2020;37(5):344–76. https://doi.org/10.1097/EJA.0000000000001180. Erratum in: Eur J Anaesthesiol. 2020;37(7):623
10. Nifong TP, McDevitt TJ. The effect of catheter to vein ratio on blood flow rates in a simulated model of peripherally inserted central venous catheters. Chest. 2011;140:48–53.
11. Ostroff MD, Moureau N, Pittiruti M. Rapid assessment of vascular exit site and tunneling options (RAVESTO): a new decision tool in the management of the complex vascular access patients. J Vasc Access. 2021;21:11297298211034306. https://doi.org/10.1177/11297298211034306.
12. Pinelli F, Pittiruti M, Van Boxtel T, Barone G, Biffi R, Capozzoli G, Crocoli A, Elli S, Elisei D, Fabiani A, Garrino C, Graziano U, Montagnani L, Prato AP, Scoppettuolo G, Zadra N, Zanaboni C, Zerla P, Konstantinou E, Jones M, Rosay H, Simcock L, Stas M, Pepe G. GAVeCeLT-WoCoVA consensus on subcutaneously anchored securement devices for the securement of venous catheters: current evidence and recommendations for future research. J Vasc Access. 2020;2:1129729820924568. https://doi.org/10.1177/1129729820924568.

13. Pittiruti M, Lamperti M. Late cardiac tamponade in adults secondary to tip position in the right atrium: an urban legend? A systematic review of the literature. J Cardiothorac Vasc Anesth. 2015;29:491–5.
14. Pittiruti M, Pelagatti F, Pinelli F. Intracavitary electrocardiography for tip location during central venous catheterization: a narrative review of 70 years of clinical studies. J Vasc Access. 2020;24:1129729820929835. https://doi.org/10.1177/1129729820929835.
15. Rossetti F, Pittiruti M, Lamperti M, et al. The intracavitary ECG method for positioning the tip of central venous access devices in pediatric patients: results of an Italian multicenter study. J Vasc Access. 2015;16:137–43.
16. Vezzani A, Brusasco C, Palermo S, et al. Ultrasound localization of central vein catheter and detection of postprocedural pneumothorax: an alternative to chest radiography. Crit Care Med. 2010;38:533–8.
17. Zito Marinosci G, Biasucci DG, Barone G, D'Andrea V, Elisei D, Iacobone E, La Greca A, Pittiruti M. ECHOTIP-Ped: a structured protocol for ultrasound-based tip navigation and tip location during placement of central venous access devices in pediatric patients. J Vasc Access. 2021;13:11297298211031391. https://doi.org/10.1177/11297298211031391.

Chapter 15
Centrally and Femorally Inserted Central Catheters (CICC and FICC) in Children

Mauro Pittiruti

15.1 Definition

As already mentioned in previous chapter, the current definition of central venous access device (VAD) implies that the tip of the catheter must be located in the superior vena cava (SVC), or in the inferior vena cava (IVC) or in the right atrium (RA). Any catheter with the tip in any of these locations is to be considered a central access, even if some special performance may require a specific position of the tip. For example, monitoring of central venous pressure requires that the tip is in the SVC or RA; monitoring of oxygen saturation in mixed venous blood requires that the tip is in the RA. In general, the most appropriate positions are the lower third of the SVC or the SVC/RA junction (for PICCs and CICCs), and the IVC/RA junction or the middle portion of the IVC (for FICCs).

In pediatric patients, central VADs may be placed by percutaneous cannulation of superficial veins (epicutaneo-cava catheters = ECC), or direct cannulation of the umbilical vein (umbilical venous catheter = UVC), or ultrasound guided cannulation of deep veins in the supra/infra-clavicular area (centrally inserted central catheter = CICC), or at the arm (peripherally inserted central catheter = PICC), or at the groin (femorally inserted central catheter = FICC). The old-fashioned technique of central venous cannulation by venous cutdown (of the internal or external jugular vein, of the cephalic vein, or of the saphenous vein) is not acceptable anymore, since it is associated with high risk of complications (infection, venous thrombosis, local bleeding), risk of failure, low cost-effectiveness and a relevant waste of time and resources. The twentieth century practice of 'blind' (or—euphemistically—'landmark-based') puncture of deep veins must be abandoned, too, since the introduction of ultrasound in clinical practice.

M. Pittiruti (✉)
Department of Surgery, Catholic University Hospital, Rome, Italy

D. G. Biasucci et al. (eds.), *Vascular Access in Neonates and Children*,
https://doi.org/10.1007/978-3-030-94709-5_15

Considering that ECC and UVC are appropriate only in neonates, all central VADs in infants and children should be currently placed by ultrasound-guided cannulation of deep veins (PICC, CICC or FICC). In the previous chapter, we have discussed PICCs (i.e., central VADs obtained by ultrasound guided cannulation of deep veins of the arm). Small infants do not usually have veins of the arm suitable for 3Fr catheters (which is the smallest size available for ultrasound guided PICCs), so that in this category of pediatric patients most central VADs are either CICCs or FICCs. On the other hand, PICC should be regarded as the first option for central venous access in children, because of their low invasiveness and the absence of potentially life-threatening complications at the time of insertion. Though, there are many clinical situations when a PICC cannot be inserted because of small caliber of the veins of the arm (both in the green zone and in the yellow zone) or because of other anatomical or pathological abnormalities of the upper limb. The presence of chronic renal failure likely to require an arterial-venous fistula is another important contraindication to PICC. In these situations, CICC or FICC insertion should be considered.

15.2 Indications

Central venous access is indicated when the child requires (a) infusion of solutions associated with potential endothelial damage (i.e., non-compatible with the peripheral route), (b) repeated daily blood sampling, (c) hemodynamic monitoring (central venous pressure, oxygen saturation in mixed venous blood, (d) hemodialysis, (e) prolonged intravenous access in the extra-hospital setting. In case of indication for hemodynamic monitoring, the tip of the central venous access must be located in SVC or RA. In case of indication for hemodialysis, a specific CICC or FICC with proper design (double lumen, stiff material, etc.) is necessary. In case of prolonged extra-hospital use, a tunneled-cuffed catheter (either PICC, CICC or FICC) should be used, or—preferably—a non-cuffed tunneled catheter secured by subcutaneous anchorage.

CICC insertion should be considered when contraindications to PICC insertion are present:

- small infants or children with arm veins of caliber <3 mm (and thus not suitable for 3Fr catheters)
- emergency central venous catheterization
- anatomical or pathological abnormalities of the arm, related to the vasculature (thrombosis), to the joints and bones (ankylosis, fractures, amputation), to the neuromuscular function (long standing paresis with muscle hypotrophy and consequent vascular hypoplasia), to the skin (burns, skin ulcers, infections)
- chronic renal failure stage 3B—4 or 5, probably requiring an arterial-venous fistula for hemodialysis

- central venous catheterization required for temporary hemodialysis (no PICC is appropriate for hemodialytic procedures)

On the other hand, FICC insertion may have specific indication in case of simultaneous contraindication to both CICCs and PICCs:

- emergency central venous catheterization in clinical situations when a supra/infra-clavicular puncture is considered at high risk (for example, in agitated patients) or logistically difficult (severe difficulty in the management of the airway or of the tracheotomy)
- surgical wounds or infections or burns of the chest area and of the arms
- mediastinal masses compressing the SVC
- agitated, non-collaborative child with previous accidental removal of PICCs and CICCs; an exit site in the lower limb may be part of a strategy of reducing the risk of removal, by placing the catheter out of reach of the hands of the child
- scheduled cardiac or head/neck surgery: in this case, the management of perioperative venous access will be easier if the exit site is at mid-thigh
- COVID patients, or other patients with severe respiratory distress, especially if treated by non-invasive ventilation using helmets or facial masks
- any child at high risk for accidental pleural injury in case of CICC insertion, if PICC insertion is simultaneously contraindicated.

Insertion of FICCs is increasingly used in pediatric clinical practice. Old-fashioned FICC insertion by placement of non-tunneled catheters after direct puncture of the common femoral vein (CFV) was inevitably associated with increased risk of infection, thrombosis, and dislodgement, because of the exit site at the groin. As direct puncture of the superficial femoral vein (SFV) and tunneling are being implemented in clinical practice, it is possible to insert FICCs placing the exit site at mid-thigh or even more caudally, either by accessing the SFV at mid-thigh or by accessing the CFV and then tunneling the catheter so to obtain an exit site at mid-thigh.

15.3 Materials

The traditional classification (short term—medium term—long term) is not appropriate anymore, since the same tunneled central VADs (especially if secured with subcutaneous anchorage) may be appropriate for short-, medium- and long-term use, both in Pediatric Intensive Care Unit and in the homecare setting. In fact, tunneling should not be regarded as an uncommon technique used exclusively for cuffed catheters, but as an option to be considered in any situation when the puncture site is not an ideal exit site (see Chap. 8).

In the intrahospital setting (both in intensive and non-intensive wards), tunneling is adopted on the basis of the clinical situation, according to the RAVESTO protocol (see Chap. 14), both for CICCs and FICCs; subcutaneous securement is recommended in all central venous access devices in children, with the only exception of devices which are expected to be removed within 48 hours (for example: FICCs inserted in emergency or CICCs inserted only for a short perioperative period).

In the extrahospital setting, if a CICC or a FICC is indicated, we recommend using non-cuffed tunneled catheters secured with subcutaneous anchorage or—as second option—cuffed-tunneled catheters. In very special conditions (long term intermittent use of the venous access, typically for antiblastic chemotherapy) venous access may be obtained by totally implantable venous access devices (PICC-ports, chest-ports, and femoral ports), that will be discussed in Chap. 16.

Based on the material, on specific design features, and on technique of insertion, the currently available CICCs and FICCs for pediatric use can be classified as follows:

1. polyurethane catheters (of different caliber, length, and number of lumens) to be inserted by simple Seldinger technique; these catheters are made of old-generation polyurethanes and often provided with non-optimal insertion kits (for example, kits including large bore needles, j-shaped guidewires, etc.). Since they are inserted by simple Seldinger technique ('catheter over guidewire') tunneling is often impossible. They cannot be trimmed, so that it is necessary to plan the expected length before insertion. Their use should be confined to emergency venous access, and—as any central or peripheral VAD inserted in emergency—they should be removed within 48 hours. Figure 15.1 shows a non-tunneled FICC placed in emergency.
2. Power injectable, non-cuffed, new-generation polyurethane catheters (of caliber 3-6Fr, single, double, or triple lumen), commonly marketed as PICCs but used 'off label' as CICCs and FICCs. They have many advantages: (a) they are made of new generation polyurethanes (Carbothane, Chronoflex, etc.), very resistant and very bio-compatible; (b) they are inserted by modified Seldinger technique ('catheter through introducer'), so that they can be easily tunneled, if needed; (c) the introducer kit is equipped with small bore echogenic needles (21G) and floppy straight tip 0.018″ nitinol guidewires, so to minimize trauma to the vein wall; (d) they are 40–60 cm long and they are supposed to be trimmed to the desire length, depending on the use (CICC vs. FICC), on the required intravascular tract, on the extent of the tunneling, and on the type of securement (standard sutureless securement vs. subcutaneous anchorage); the operator must choose the catheter just considering the caliber (based on the diameter of the available veins) and the number of lumens (based on the clinical indication). Figures 15.2 and 15.3 show tunneled power injectable polyurethane double-lumen CICCs in a child and in a small infant, respectively. Figure 15.4 shows a tunneled power injectable polyurethane single-lumen FICC in a small infant. Though silicon catheters and/or valved catheters are still available on the market, they should not be used; silicon catheters have no advantage over polyurethane catheters in terms of risk of infection or thrombosis, but they are more fragile, not appropriate for high flow and/or power injectable infusions, and prone to

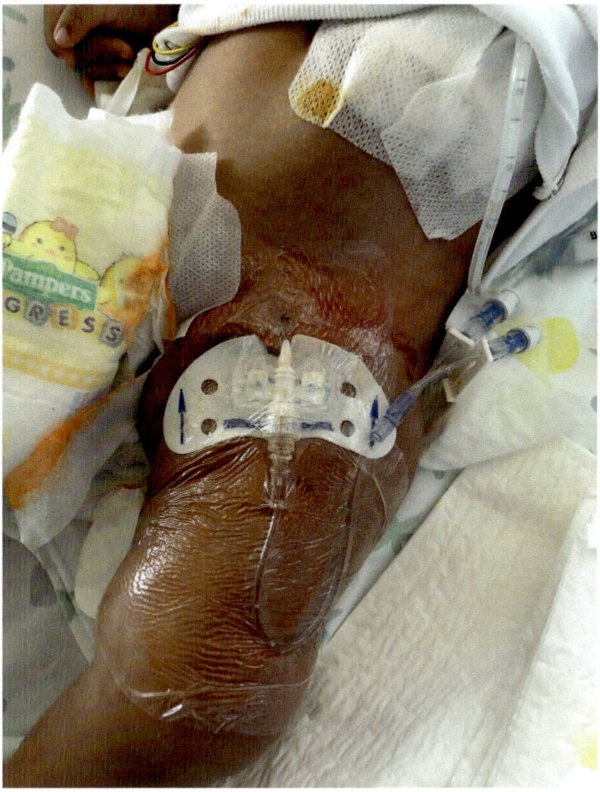

Fig. 15.1 FICC inserted in emergency in a small infant: puncture of the left common femoral vein; no tunneling; securement with skin-adhesive sutureless device

mechanical complications; valved catheters have an increased cost and no advantage in terms of prevention of lumen occlusion (catheter with distal valve are even characterized by high incidence of malfunction).

3. Power injectable, cuffed, new-generation polyurethane catheters, all of them to be inserted by modified Seldinger technique and necessarily tunneled. They are available in different sizes (5-7Fr), single or double lumen. They should be used exclusively in children requiring prolonged venous access in the extrahospital setting. The actual advantage of using a cuffed-tunnel catheter vs. a non-cuffed tunneled catheter secured with subcutaneous anchorage is still matter of debate. In the experience of many pediatric centers, subcutaneous anchorage seems to be associated with lower costs, more efficacy, and less complications if compared to the cuff. Also, non-cuffed tunneled catheters secured with subcutaneous anchorage are removed easily, while removal of a cuffed catheter requires a minor surgical procedure and some sedation and/or local anesthesia. Old fashioned silicon cuffed catheters, valved or non-valved (i.e., Broviac, Hickman, Groshong, Leonard), are still available on the market but they are not recommended, because of the high risk of rupture, mechanical complications, and malfunctions.

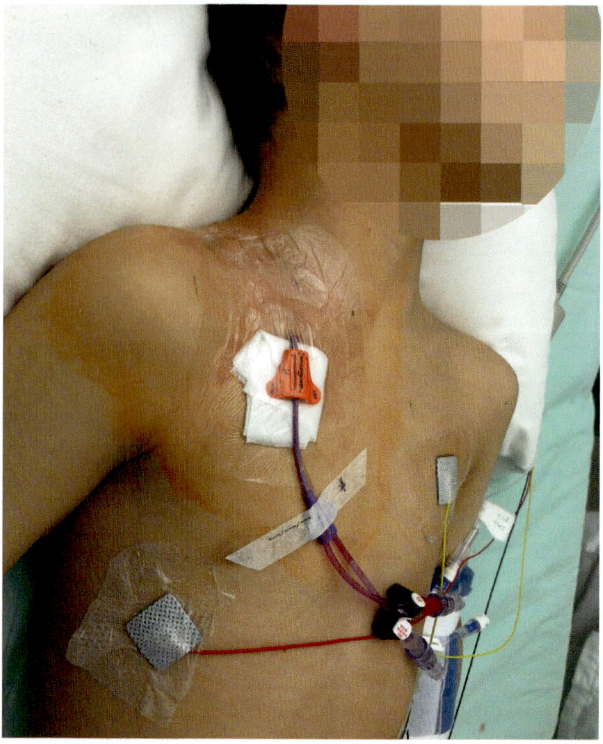

Fig. 15.2 Double lumen CICC inserted in a child: puncture of the right brachio-cephalic vein; tunneling to the infraclavicular area; securement by subcutaneous anchorage

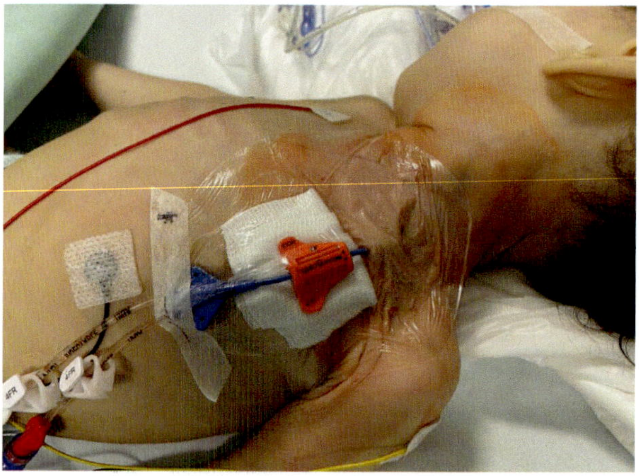

Fig. 15.3 Double lumen CICC inserted in a child: puncture of the left brachio-cephalic vein; tunneling to the infraclavicular area; securement by subcutaneous anchorage

4. Double lumen polyurethane catheters specifically designed for hemodialysis; they are available of different length, depending on the size of the child and whether they are meant to be used as CICCs (by right supraclavicular venous approach) or FICCs (by right or left femoral approach). Most of them are inserted by simple Seldinger technique.

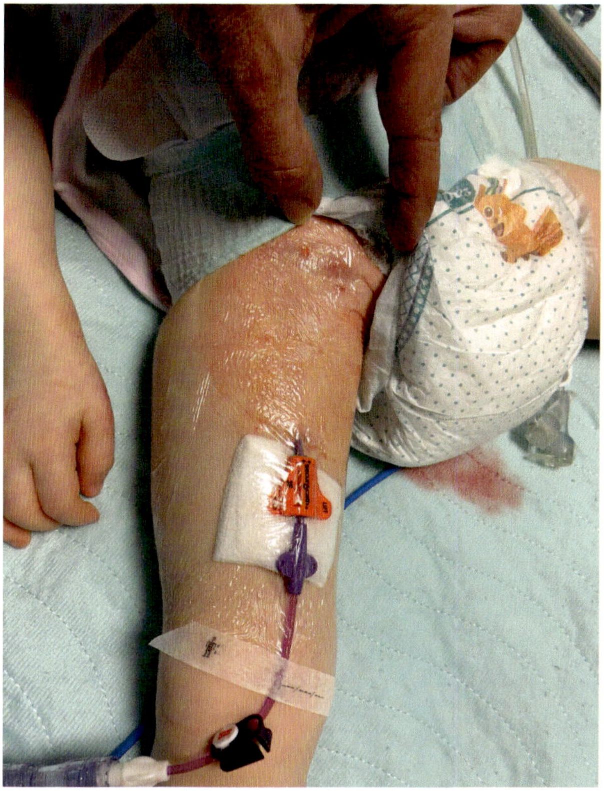

Fig. 15.4 Single lumen FICC inserted in a small infant: puncture of the right common femoral vein; tunneling to mid-thigh; securement by subcutaneous anchorage

15.4 Technique of CICC Insertion

The insertion of a CICC, as the insertion of any other VAD, should be performed following a well-defined 'bundle' that includes all current recommendations for optimizing the cost-effectiveness of the maneuver and avoiding complications. For CICCs, one insertion bundle already described in the literature is the SIC protocol (SIC = Safe Insertion of CICCs) (see Table 15.1). This protocol includes seven steps, which collect effectively and synthetically the most relevant phases of the procedure.

1. Preprocedural evaluation. The first step is an appropriate choice of the vein to be cannulated, adopting the RaCeVA protocol, i.e., a systematic ultrasound examination of the veins of the neck and of the supra/infraclavicular region (Fig. 15.5a). The ultrasound scan starts at mid-neck, with the linear transducer placed in a transversal position so to visualize the internal jugular vein (IJV) and the carotid artery in short axis; then, the probe slides downward along the neck, visualizing the area where the IJV (still visualized in short axis) crosses the subclavian artery (visualized in long axis, posteriorly to the IJV). Sliding even more caudally and tilting the probe, it is possible to visualize the brachio-cephalic vein

Table 15.1 The SIC protocol (SIC = Safe Insertion of CICC)

1.	Preprocedural evaluation—choice of the vein by systematic ultrasound examination of the veins of the neck and of the supra/infraclavicular region (RaCeVA protocol) and choice of the ideal exit site (Central ZIM)
2.	Appropriate aseptic technique—hand hygiene, skin antisepsis with 2% chlorhexidine in 70% alcohol, maximal barrier precautions
3.	Ultrasound-guided insertion—ultrasound-guided venipuncture, ultrasound verification of the correct direction of the guidewire (tip navigation) and of the absence of pneumothorax (pleural scan)
4.	Intra-procedural assessment of tip location—verification of the central position of the tip by intracavitary ECG and/or by transthoracic echocardiography, using the 'bubble test'
5.	Adequate protection of the exit site—reduction of the risk of bleeding and risk of contamination by sealing with cyanoacrylate glue
6.	Proper securement of the catheter—stabilization of the catheter using skin-adhesive sutureless devices, transparent dressing with integrated securement or subcutaneous anchorage
7.	Appropriate coverage of the exit site—use of semi-permeable transparent dressing, preferably with high breathability

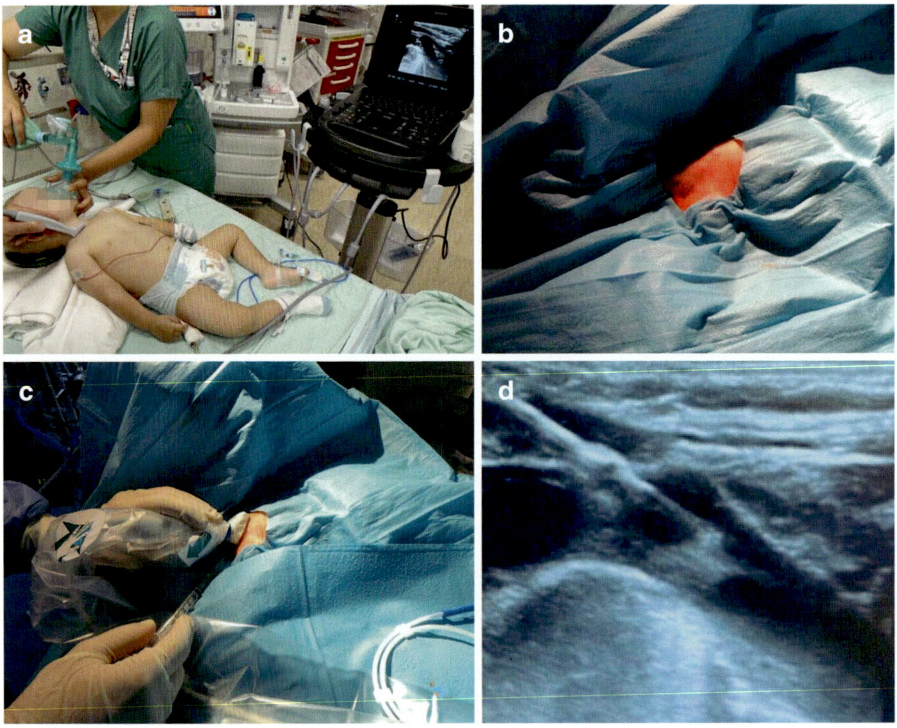

Fig. 15.5 Technique of CICC insertion in a small infant: preprocedural ultrasound evaluation (**a**); maximal barrier precautions (**b**); ultrasound guided cannulation of the brachio-cephalic vein (**c**), with real time visualization of the needle inside the vein (**d**)

(BCV) in long axis, in the anterior mediastinum. Sliding the transducer laterally along the clavicle, and further tilting it, the subclavian vein (SV) is seen in long axis; posterior, superior and parallel to the SV, the final tract of the external jugular vein (EJV) is visualized in long axis, too. Moving the probe to the infraclavicular area and placing it close to the lateral third of the clavicle, the axillary vein (AV) and the axillary artery can be visualized in short axis or—appropriately rotating the probe—also in oblique axis or in long axis. The final tract of the cephalic vein (CV) can also be visualized in the infra-clavicular area, at its merging into the AV. After this systematic evaluation of all major veins of the supra/infra-clavicular area, the most appropriate can be chosen, considering different factors: the size of the vein (which must be at least three times the external caliber of the catheter), its depth, its relationship with the surrounding structures, and so on. According to the Central ZIM (Zone Insertion Method), there are three zones in this area: the green zone corresponds to the infraclavicular area, the yellow zone to the supraclavicular fossa, and the red zone to the neck. The red zone should not be used as puncture site or exit site. The yellow zone is used as puncture site when a supraclavicular vein is chosen (IJV, SV, BCV, EJV), while the green zone is the puncture site when the AV or the CV are accessed. The yellow zone is acceptable as exit site, though in some situations (presence of tracheostomy, for example) the exit site should be moved elsewhere. The RAVESTO protocol (see Table 15.2) summarizes the different options for tunneling. The most frequent tunneling in the pediatric patient is the tunnel to the infraclavicular area after BCV puncture; especially in small infants, BCV is the largest and easiest vein to access, but its puncture site is not an ideal exit site because of the contamination of the skin and the instability of the dressing. Sometimes, when the catheter is cuffed, tunneling is mandatory. Tunneling is also recommended for pediatric patients in home care and/or receiving extra-hospital intravenous treatments, since tunneling is a very effective strategy against extraluminal bacterial contamination. In short, the preprocedural evaluation is focused on the choice of the vein (choice of the puncture site) and on the evaluation of the indication to tunneling (choice of the exit site). If a non-tunneled dialysis catheter is inserted, the best choice is the right BCV, with the exit site in the right supraclavicular area.

2. Appropriate aseptic technique (Fig. 15.5b). The three main strategies for infection prevention, that must be adopted in any central venous catheterization, are (a) proper hand hygiene, (b) skin antisepsis with 2% chlorhexidine in 70% isopropyl alcohol, and (c) maximal barrier precautions (mask, cap, sterile gloves, sterile gown, large sterile drapes over the child, long sterile cover for the probe). When CICC insertion is performed as an emergency, if these three precautions cannot be completely adopted, the VAD must be removed as soon as possible, within 48 hours.
3. Ultrasound-guided insertion. Ultrasound-guided venipuncture can be performed with different techniques in the pediatric patients, depending on the vein chosen for cannulation, always using a linear transducer. Supraclavicular veins should be preferably accessed by in-plane techniques (Fig. 15.5c, d), so to minimize the

Table 15.2 The RAVESTO protocol (RAVESTO = Rapid Assessment of Venous Exit Site and Tunneling Options)

Central venous access device	Type and path of tunnel	Indications for tunneling
PICC	Tunnel to Dawson's green area	Puncture site in Dawson's yellow area; non-hospitalized patients with expected long intravenous treatment
CICC (supraclavicular puncture)	Tunnel to infraclavicular area	Long term intravenous treatment in non-hospitalized patients (antibiotics, parenteral nutrition, chemotherapy); expected difficulties in management of the exit site in hospitalized patients (beard, humidity, tracheostomy, instability, etc.)
	Tunnel to arm	Compromised skin integrity of the chest area; oral or endotracheal secretions over chest; implanted device on ipsilateral chest; chest surgery; contracted shoulder; etc.
	Tunnel to back	Cognitive disorder resulting in device removal; contraindication to chest or arm exit site
CICC (infraclavicular puncture)	Tunnel to lower chest	Long term intravenous treatment in non-hospitalized patients (antibiotics, parenteral nutrition, chemotherapy); expected problems in management of the exit site in hospitalized patients (tracheostomy, etc.)
	Tunnel to arm	Compromised skin integrity of the chest area; oral or endotracheal secretions over chest; implanted device on ipsilateral chest; chest surgery; contracted shoulder; etc.
	Tunnel to back	Cognitive disorder resulting in device removal; contraindication to chest or arm exit site
FICC (puncture at the groin)	Tunnel to the abdomen	Non-emergency line in walking patients with contraindication to PICC/CICC
	Tunnel to mid-thigh	Non-emergency line in bedridden patients with contraindication to PICC/CICC
FICC (puncture at mid-thigh)	Tunnel to the abdomen	Non-emergency line in walking patients with contraindication to PICC/CICC
	Tunnel to distal thigh	Long term intravenous treatment in bedridden patients with contraindication to PICC/CICC

risk of accidental injury to the pleura or to the subclavian artery or to the carotid artery: IJV should be accessed by a short axis/in-plane or an oblique axis/in-plane approach, as the old-fashioned short axis/out-of-plane approach carries some risk of accidental arterial puncture; the BCV, SV and EJV are all accessed by a long axis/in-plane approach. The ideal approach to the AV is still not defined; short axis/out-of-plane, oblique axis/in-plane and long axis/in plane approaches have been described. Though, infra-clavicular veins (AV and CV) are usually quite small in all infants and in most children, so that they are not commonly selected for CICC insertion. A micro-introducer kit (21G needle, floppy straight tip 0.018″ nitinol guidewire, micro-introducer-dilator) is strongly recommended for any venipuncture (Fig. 15.6a). Soon after venipuncture, the linear transducer is used for verification of the correct direction of the guidewire (tip navigation according to the ECHOTIP-Ped protocol) (see Table 15.3)

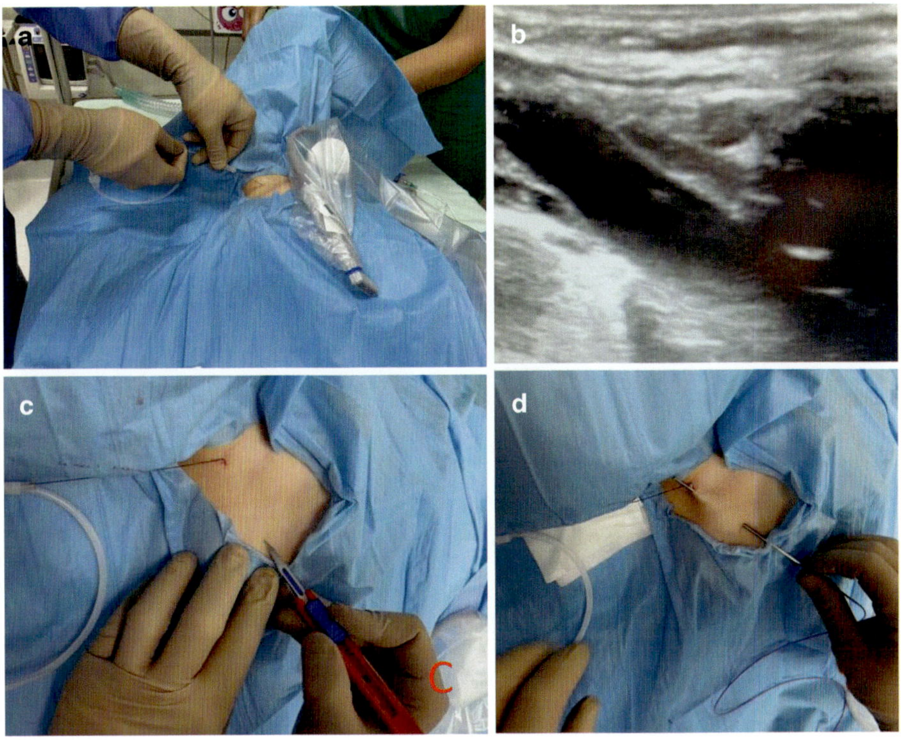

Fig. 15.6 Technique of CICC insertion in a small infant: insertion of the guidewire (**a**) and its real time visualization inside the vein (**b**); preparation of the tunnel (**c**) and (**d**)

Table 15.3 Summary of ECHOTIP-Ped for CICCs and FICCs

CVC	Protocol	Probe	Windows
CICC	Tip navigation	Linear probe 10–14 MHz	Same acoustic windows as RaCeVA
	Tip location	Small sectorial probe 3–7 MHz	Subcostal bi-caval or 4-chamber view
FICC	Tip navigation	Linear probe 10–14 MHz and micro-convex probe 4–8 MHz	Short/long axis of the femoral vein (linear probe) and of the inferior vena cava (micro-convex)
	Tip location	Micro-convex probe 4–8 MHz	Subcostal longitudinal view of the inferior vena cava

(Fig. 15.6b), and for ruling out pneumothorax (pleural scan: see Chap. 7). If a tunneling is required, it should be prepared after the insertion of the guidewire and before the insertion of the micro-introducer over the guidewire ('antero-grade tunneling': see Chap. 8), as shown in Figs. 15.6c, d, and 15.7a.

4. Intra-procedural assessment of tip location. According to all current guidelines, the verification of the central position of the tip should be done during the pro-

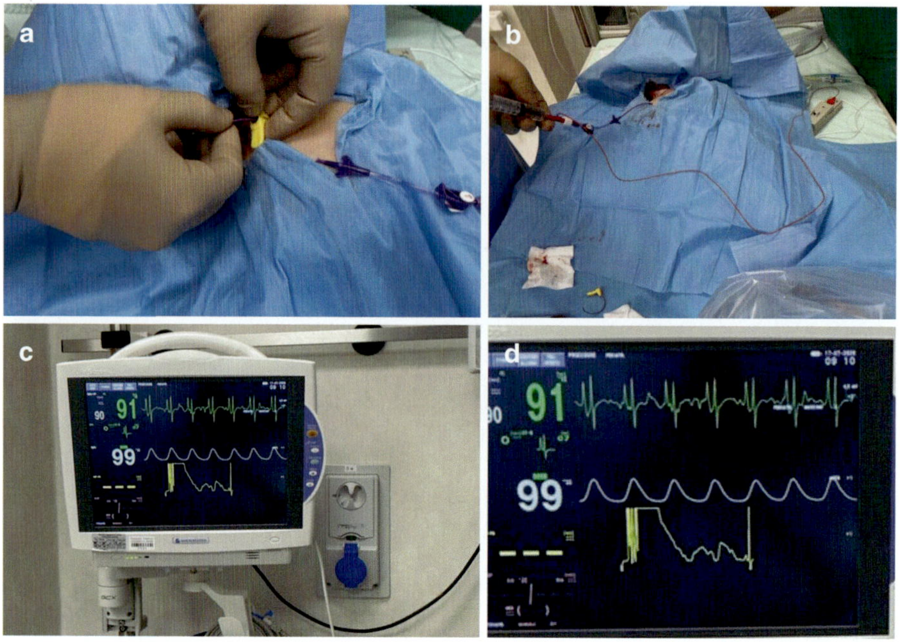

Fig. 15.7 Technique of CICC insertion in a small infant: insertion of the catheter through the micro-introducer (**a**); using a sterile cable (**b**), connection of the catheter to a standard ECG monitor (**c**); the appearance of the peak of the P wave (**d**) confirms the location of the tip at the junction between right atrium and superior vena cava

cedure; the old-fashioned strategy of approximate length estimation during the procedure and subsequent post-procedural chest x-ray is currently considered unacceptable in terms of safety, accuracy, and cost-effectiveness. Intraprocedural methods for tip location include intracavitary ECG (IC-ECG), fluoroscopy, trans-esophageal echocardiography (TEE), and trans-thoracic echocardiography (TTE) using the 'bubble test' (see Chap. 6). The most accurate methods are TEE and IC-ECG, the least accurate is fluoroscopy. However, both TEE and fluoroscopy are invasive, expensive, and logistically difficult to apply. For these reasons, tip location should be verified by IC-ECG and/or TTE. Interestingly, while IC-ECG have some limitations in adult patients (because of atrial fibrillation or complex cardiac arrhythmias), the applicability and feasibility of this method in children is 100%. Furthermore, TTE, if using the subcostal views, is very easy to perform in the pediatric patient. When a dialysis catheter is required, the IC-ECG method should be applied to both lumens: the correct tip position corresponds to a diphasic P wave on the distal lumen (intra-atrial location) and a high P wave on the proximal lumen (lower third of the superior vena cava). Figures 15.7 and 15.8 show how IC-ECG and TTE can be applied during the same procedure.

5. Adequate protection of the exit site. All exit sites of central venous access should be sealed with cyanoacrylate glue (see Chap. 8). Application of cyanoacrylate is

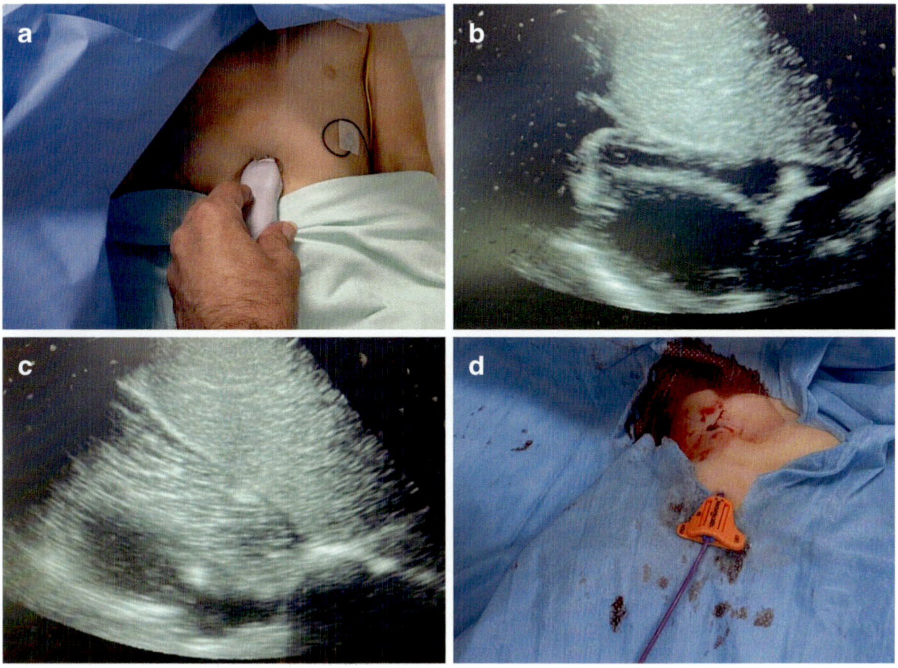

Fig. 15.8 Tip location by ultrasound: subcostal window (**a**), with visualization of the heart chambers (**b**) and appearance of the micro-bubbles soon after saline injection (**c**); securement with subcutaneous anchorage (**d**)

Fig. 15.9 Tunneled CICC: glue is used both for sealing the exit site and for closing the skin incision at the puncture site

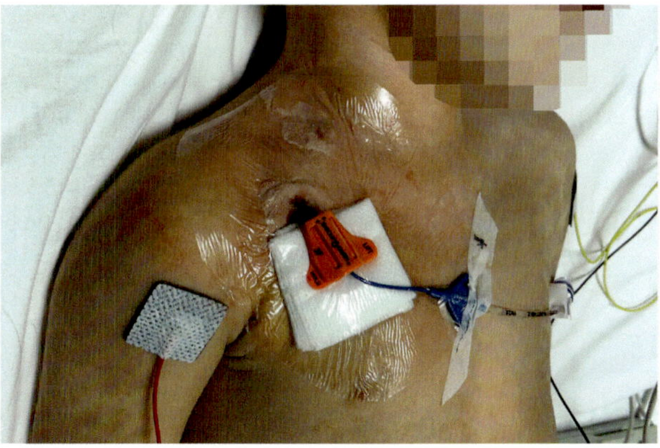

a safe and cost-effective strategy for reducing the risk of bleeding and the risk of bacterial contamination by the extraluminal route. If the catheter has been tunneled, cyanoacrylate is also used for closing the skin incision at the puncture site (Fig. 15.9). Clinical studies have proven that cyanoacrylate glue is completely safe, even in small neonates, and that its use is not associated with any chemical or physical damage of polyurethane catheters.

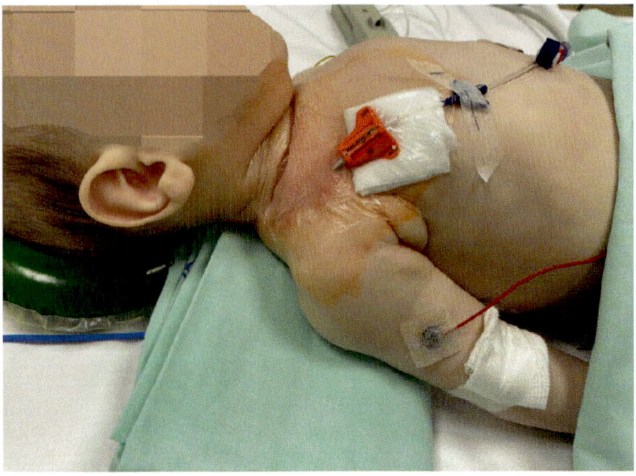

Fig. 15.10 Subcutaneous anchorage of a tunneled CICC in a small infant

6. Proper securement of the catheter. Stabilization of the CICC should be obtained with (a) skin-adhesive sutureless devices, or (b) transparent dressing with integrated securement or (c) subcutaneous anchorage. In most CICC inserted as elective procedure and expected to last for a prolonged period, either tunneled or non-tunneled, the best option is the subcutaneous anchorage, which has been proven to be safe and highly effective (Figs. 15.8d and 15.10). Subcutaneous anchorage should also be considered whenever there is a high risk of dislodgment (for example, in agitated and non-collaborative infants and children, or in case of skin abnormalities).
7. Appropriate coverage of the exit site. The exit site should be protected with a semi-permeable transparent membrane, placed directly over the catheter and the exit site (Fig. 15.11). Coverage with gauze dressing should be discouraged since it gives no protection against bacterial contamination. As bleeding and oozing are prevented by the glue, the transparent dressing is expected to stay in place for one week, in most cases, with no need of unscheduled dressing change. In all pediatric patients we recommend using membranes with high breathability (high MVTR = Moisture Vapor Transfer Rate) (see Chap. 8).

15.5 Technique of FICC Insertion

FICC insertion should be carried out using a proper 'insertion bundle', like the SIF protocol (Safe Insertion of FICCs) (see Table 15.4), in many aspects similar to the SIC protocol.

1. Preprocedural evaluation. The insertion of a femoral catheter should always start with a careful ultrasound scan of the femoral veins using the RaFeVA protocol (Rapid Femoral Vein Assessment). The RaFeVA has been designed to help the clinician in choosing the best puncture site, by a systematic ultrasound examina-

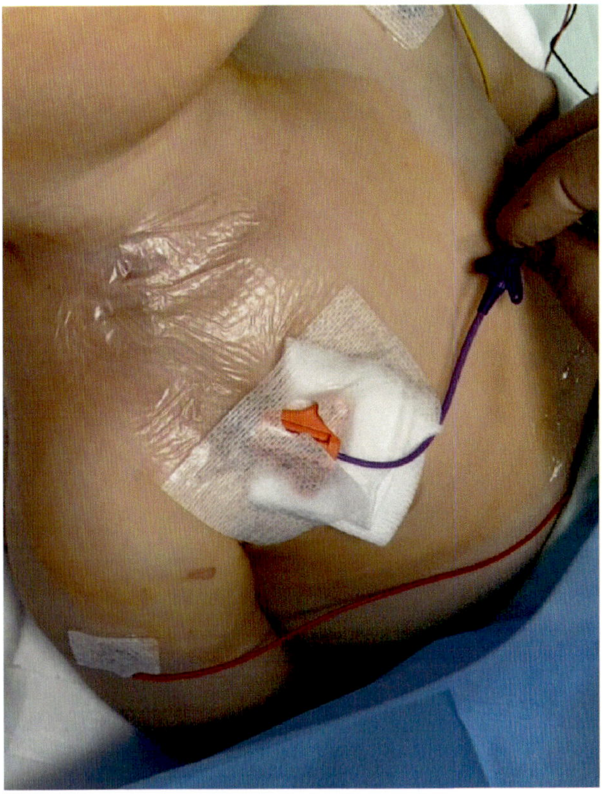

Fig. 15.11 Coverage of the exit site using a transparent membrane with high permeability

Table 15.4 The SIF protocol (SIF = Safe Insertion of FICC)

1. Preprocedural evaluation—choice of the vein by systematic ultrasound examination of the veins of the groin and the thigh (RaFeVA protocol) and choice of the ideal exit site (Femoral ZIM)
2. Appropriate aseptic technique—hand hygiene, skin antisepsis with 2% chlorhexidine in 70% alcohol, maximal barrier precautions
3. Ultrasound-guided insertion—ultrasound-guided venipuncture, ultrasound verification of the correct direction of the guidewire (tip navigation)
4. Intra-procedural assessment of tip location—if the tip must be in IVC, use length estimation by anthropometric measurement and consider post-procedural x-ray; if the tip must be in RA or at IVC/RAJ, use intracavitary ECG and/or by transthoracic echocardiography (in subcostal view, using the 'bubble test')
5. Adequate protection of the exit site—reduction of the risk of bleeding and risk of contamination by sealing with cyanoacrylate glue
6. Proper securement of the catheter—stabilization of the catheter using skin-adhesive sutureless devices, transparent dressing with integrated securement, or subcutaneous anchorage
7. Appropriate coverage of the exit site—semi-permeable transparent dressing, preferably with high breathability

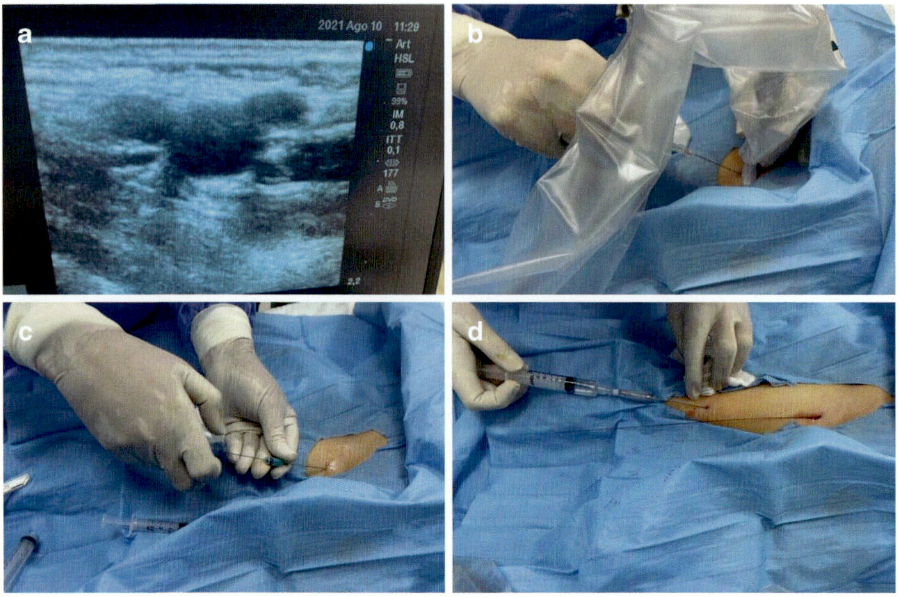

Fig. 15.12 Technique of FICC insertion in a child: visualization of the common femoral vein at the groin (**a**); ultrasound-guided venipuncture (**b**); insertion of the guidewire (**c**); preparation of the tunnel, planning the exit site at mid-thigh (**d**)

tion of all the major veins of the groin and the thigh. The scan starts at the inguinal groove, which corresponds to the transition between the common femoral vein (CFV) (in the groin area) and the external iliac vein (EIV) (visualized in the pelvic area, soon above the inguinal ligament); both veins can be visualized in short and long axis. The external iliac vein (EIV) may be an option for venous access in neonates and small infants; the CFV is usually the easiest target of the upper limb for FICC insertion at all ages (Fig. 15.12a). Sliding the probe downward, transverse to the axis of the main vessels, the great saphenous vein is visualized as it merges with the CFV; its size is very small, so it is rarely accessed by ultrasound in small infants. Sliding downward with the probe, the common femoral artery divides into deep and superficial femoral artery. Further downward, also the CFV divides into deep and superficial femoral vein. At mid-thigh, the superficial femoral vein (SFV) may be regarded as an interesting option for ultrasound cannulation in children. If the SFV is of appropriate size, it has the advantage of an exit site (at mid-thigh) much more aproppriate than the exit site obtained after CFV puncture (at the groin). Interestingly, the same exit site at mid-thigh can be achieved after CFV cannulation, it the FICC is tunneled downward. In neonates and infants, SFV is usually very small so that the ideal FICC is a tunneled FICC after CFV cannulation. In children, two options are feasible: tunneled FICC by CFV cannulation and tunneling to mid-thigh, or non-tunneled FICC by direct SFV cannulation without tunneling. Noteworthily, both CFV and

SFV cannulation may be difficult in the pediatric patient when the artery overlaps and hides the vein; such anatomic asset increases the risk for accidental arterial injury.
2. Appropriate aseptic technique. Same as for the SIC protocol (see above).
3. Ultrasound-guided insertion. Both the CFV and the SFV are commonly accessed by a short axis/out-of-plane approach, using a linear probe (Fig. 15.12b, c). A micro-introducer kit (21G needle, floppy straight tip 0.018″ nitinol guidewire, micro-introducer-dilator) is strongly recommended. Soon after the venipuncture, the same probe is used for visualizing the presence of the guidewire inside the vein (visualization in long axis). In small children, ultrasound can also be used for following the progression of the catheter through the iliac veins and the inferior vena cava (IVC), according to the tip navigation described in the ECHOTIP-Ped protocol (see Table 15.3). All dialysis catheters—if inserted as FICCs—should be placed by puncture/cannulation of the CFV. If a tunneling is required, it should be prepared after the insertion of the guidewire and before the insertion of the micro-introducer over the guidewire ('anterograde tunneling': see Chap. 8), as shown in Figs. 15.12d and 15.13a, b.
4. Intra-procedural assessment of tip location. The appropriate tip location depends on whether the FICC is meant to be used for hemodynamic monitoring or exclusively for infusion and blood sampling. In the first case, the tip must be in right atrium (RA) or at IVC/RA junction; the best intraprocedural methods are IC-

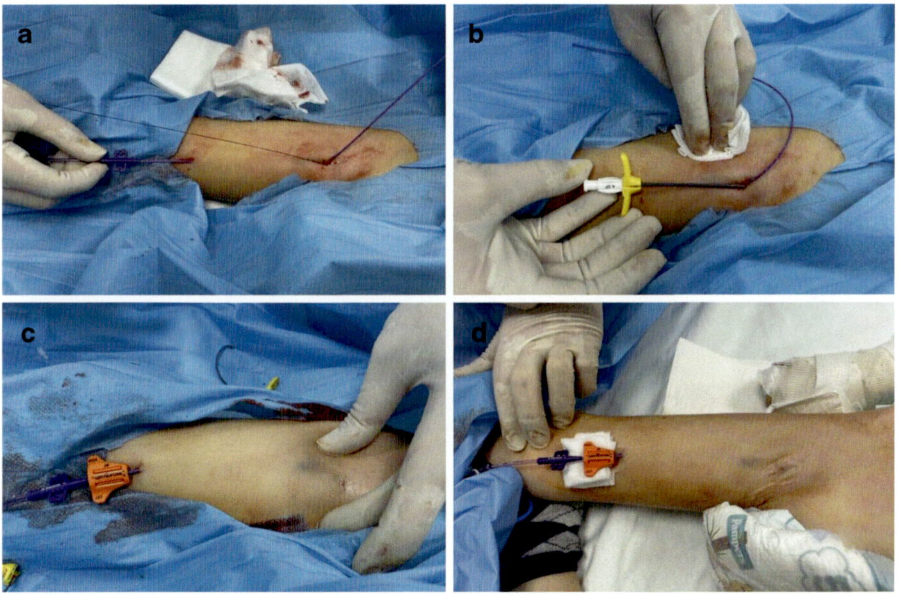

Fig. 15.13 Technique of FICC insertion in a child: the catheter is threaded through the tunnel (**a**); insertion of the micro-introducer (**b**); application of glue (**c**); and securement with subcutaneous anchorage (**d**)

ECG and TTE (in subcostal view, using the 'bubble test'). In the second situation (far more common), the tip is located in the middle portion of the IVC and TTE with bubble test is required; the correct position is confirmed by the appearance of the bubbles in the RA one second after injection (visualization by the subcostal view); if the bubbles appear immediately, the tip is very close to the IVC/RA junction; if the bubbles appear after two seconds or they do not appear, the catheter may be malpositioned in the iliac veins or in the lumbar veins. As an alternative option, when the tip must be in IVC, a post-procedural x-ray can be useful; though, x-ray is not accurate and does not discriminate between a catheter in IVC and a catheter in the right ascending lumbar vein. All dialysis catheters—if inserted as FICCs—must have the tip in the IVC.

5. Adequate protection of the exit site. Same as for the SIC protocol (see above). Glue is particularly important when the exit site is at the groin since this area is highly contaminated by bacteria.
6. Proper securement of the catheter. Same as for the SIC protocol (see above). We recommend using subcutaneous anchorage as often as possible, since FICCs are at high risk for dislodgment (Figs. 15.13c, d and 15.14).
7. Appropriate coverage of the exit site. Same as for the SIC protocol (see above).

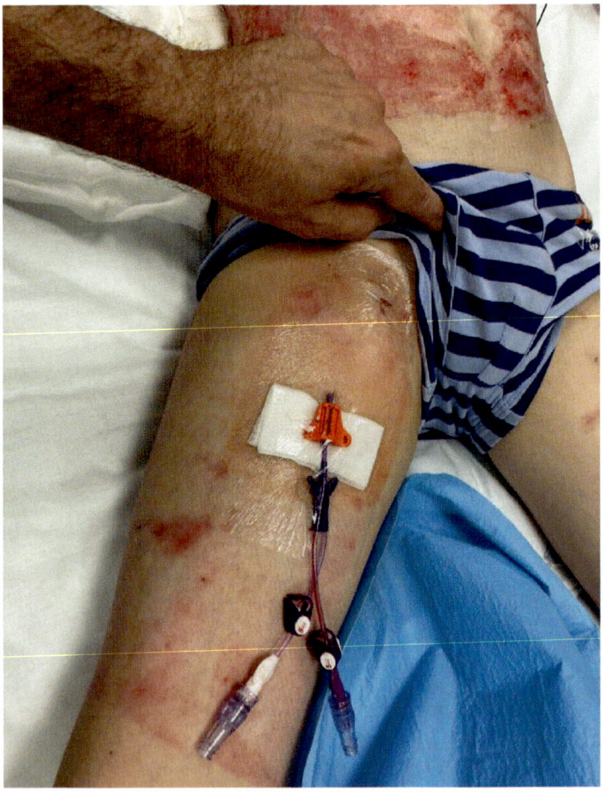

Fig. 15.14 Tunneled FICC in a burned child

15.6 Maintenance

As for any other central access device, the goal of maintenance is to protect the CICC and FICC from infective and non-infective complications.

The care of the exit site is focused on the prevention of dislodgment and of extraluminal bacterial contamination; for this purpose, the main recommended strategies are: (a) proper frequency of dressing change (every 7 days or more frequently, if the dressing is loose or wet or detached), (b) skin antisepsis with 2% chlorhexidine in alcohol, (c) weekly replacement of the skin-adhesive sutureless securement (if the catheter is not secured by subcutaneous anchorage), (d) weekly replacement of chlorhexidine-releasing sponge dressing (in non-tunneled catheters), and (e) weekly replacement of the semipermeable transparent dressing.

The care of the infusion lines is focused on the prevention of lumen occlusion and of intraluminal bacterial contamination, and the main recommended strategies for non-dialysis catheters are: (a) saline flushing with normal saline—using a push-stop technique—before and after each infusion, and at least every week if the catheter is not used; (b) adoption of neutral displacement needle free connectors, covered with disinfecting caps (so called 'port protectors'); (c) in specific cases at high risk for infection, periodic prophylactic lock of the catheter with 2% taurolidine. For dialysis catheters: (a) the lock solution must be 4% citrate (or—as a second option—heparin 500–1000 units/ml), since a local anticoagulant action is needed; (b) needle free connectors should be replaced by simple caps, since the presence of a needle free connector causes reduction of the flow; (c) in specific cases at high risk for infection, periodic prophylactic lock of the catheter with a taurolidine-citrate solution is recommended.

As far as the catheter is still indicated and there are no complications requiring removal, the device can be left in place for an unlimited period. The main limitation is related to the fact the child grows, so that a catheter with the tip properly located at the time insertion may become too short with the passing of time. Also, non-tunneled dialysis catheters should be left in place only for the acute treatment of the renal failure, and rapidly removed or replaced with an arterial-venous fistula depending on the clinical conditions.

15.7 Complications

As already mentioned, insertion-related complications are rare if adopting a proper insertion bundle as the SIC and SIF protocols. On the other hand, late complications may occur.

- *Infection*—Infection may occur as infection of the exit site, infection of the tunnel or catheter-related blood stream infection (CRBSI). The latter is a severe and possibly life-threatening complication, which may occur especially in immuno-

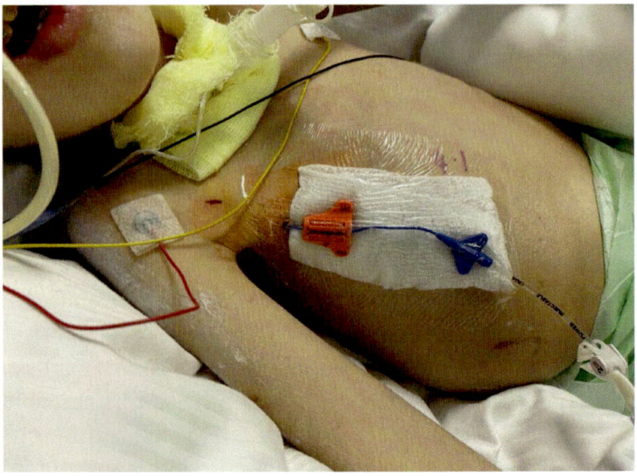

Fig. 15.15 Tunneled CICC in a small child with tracheostomy

compromised children and/or in central lines used for parenteral nutrition. The diagnosis is made by simultaneous blood cultures from peripheral vein and from the catheter, using the method of the Differential Time to Positivity (DTP). The standard treatment of CRBSI is removal of the catheter and antibiotic therapy. The prevention relies on proper policies of care of the exit site and of the infusion line. Figure 15.15 shows a CICC appropriately tunneled to the chest, so to move the exit site far from the tracheostomy. CRBSI should not be confused with catheter colonization (at DTP: catheter blood culture is positive, but peripheral blood culture is negative): the standard treatment of colonization is catheter removal, though in some situations (long term catheters in children with poor venous patrimony) a de-colonization using lock with 2% taurolidine should be considered.

- *Venous thrombosis*—Catheter-related thrombosis (CRT) may be symptomatic or asymptomatic and is usually caused by a mismatch between vein diameter and catheter caliber (a catheter that occupies >33% or >45% of the venous lumen), and/or by relevant damage of the vein during repeated attempts of venipuncture, and/or by an inappropriate location of the tip (i.e., far from the cavo-atrial junction), and/or by thrombophilia of the child. When adopting the SIC protocol, the occurrence of CICC-related thrombosis is minimized, both in adults and in children, and it may be expected to be 0–3% (slightly more frequent in children with leukemia). The expected rate of FICC-related thrombosis is higher, but some recent data suggest that when the exit site is at mid-thigh (CFV puncture + tunneling, or SFV puncture with/without tunneling) the incidence of CRT is less than when than the exit site is at the groin, probably because of the absence/presence of micro-movements of the catheter inside the vein. The expected incidence of CRT for dialysis catheters (either CICC or FICC) is higher, mainly because of the large caliber of these catheters; though, if a proper match between catheter caliber and vein diameter is assessed, the risk of CRT may be minimized. Diagnosis is based on ultrasound examination of the veins occupied by the catheter. The standard treatment is anticoagulation with low molecular weight hepa-

rin; the CICC/FICC is removed only if there is concomitant malfunction or infection. At the ultrasound examination, asymptomatic CRT should not be confused with fibroblastic sleeve (FS), a very common physiological phenomenon associated with vascular devices (much more frequent than CRT), which consists in a sleeve of connective tissue enwrapping the catheter in some segments. FS is a benign event that does not require treatment.
- *Lumen occlusion*—Malfunction due to lumen occlusion is a complication somehow more frequent in in children than in adults, because of the smaller caliber of the catheters, but completely preventable by a proper policy of flushing with saline (before starting the infusion, in between different infusions, at the closing of the line) and locking with the appropriate solution (saline, citrate, or taurolidine-citrate—depending on the clinical indication: see above). Occlusion may occur after blood sampling or after infusion of viscous solutions (blood, blood derivatives, lipids, contrast media, etc.), if the catheter is not properly flushed after being used. In non-dialysis catheters, heparinization of the catheter has no role in preventing lumen occlusion, and—as a matter of fact—may cause lumen occlusion by facilitating the precipitation of lipids and drugs with high pH. In dialysis catheters, heparin lock can be effectively replaced by 4% citrate lock.
- *Dislodgment*—Dislodgment used to be a very frequent cause of accidental CICC/FICC removal. Today, it can be successfully prevented by subcutaneous anchorage. We strongly recommend using subcutaneous anchorage in most central venous catheters used in children, with the possible exception of central lines inserted in emergency and/or scheduled to stay in place only for few days. The range of subcutaneous anchorage devices currently available (from 3Fr to 12Fr) covers most of the sizes of the CICCs and FICCs used in the pediatric patient.

15.8 Conclusion

Even if PICCs are the first option for any central venous access both in hospitalized and in non-hospitalized children, there are many situations when a CICC or a FICC is indicated: small caliber of the deep veins of the arm; chronic renal failure; emergency central venous access; need for hemodialysis; bilateral issues of the upper limb that contraindicate PICC insertion; and so on.

The basic principles of CICC and FICC insertion are:

- Power injectable, non-valved, polyurethane catheters should always be preferred, for both short- and long-term intravenous treatments
- For most CICC and FICC insertion, we recommend the ‘off label’ use of the catheters marketed as PICC, so to ensure the adoption of the best polyurethane available, of high-quality micro-introducer kits and of the modified Seldinger technique, which allows an easy tunneling (Fig. 15.16)
- A rapid ultrasound evaluation of the venous patrimony should always precede the procedure, according to the RaCeVA-RaFeVA protocols

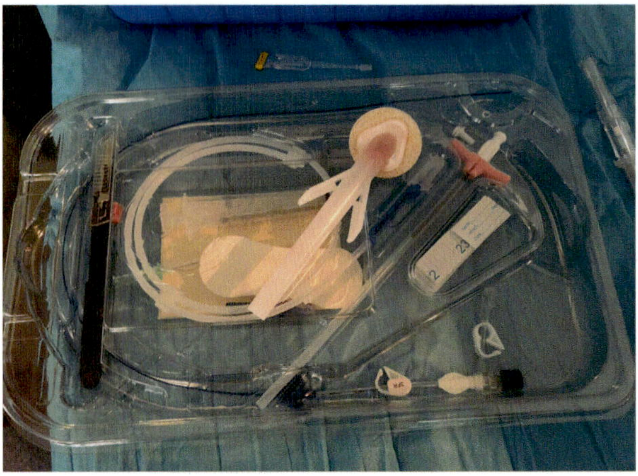

Fig. 15.16 Kit of a power injectable polyurethane PICC, used 'off label' as CICC or FICC in children

- All pediatric central lines should be inserted by ultrasound guided venipuncture, without any exception
- The proper location of the tip should always be assessed by an intraprocedural method (IC-ECG or TTE)
- The procedure should preferably be carried out adopting a systematic 'insertion bundle' such as the SIC or SIF protocol.

The key concept in the mind of the clinicians should be that most insertion-related complications (both immediate and late) are iatrogenic, and that they can avoided by adopting the appropriate evidence-based strategies.

Bibliography

1. Alexandrou E. Right assessment and vein selection. In: Moureau N, editor. Vessel health and preservation: the right approach for vascular access. Cham: Springer; 2019.
2. Biasucci DG, Pittiruti M, Taddei A, Picconi E, Pizza A, Celentano D, Piastra M, Scoppettuolo G, Conti G. Targeting zero catheter-related bloodstream infections in pediatric intensive care unit: a retrospective matched case-control study. J Vasc Access. 2018;19(2):119–24. https://doi.org/10.5301/jva.5000797.
3. Bodenham A, Lamperti M. Ultrasound guided infraclavicular axillary vein cannulation, coming of age. Br J Anaesth. 2016;116:325–7.
4. Brasher C, Malbezin S. Central venous catheters in small infants. Anesthesiology. 2018;128:4–5.
5. Brescia F, Pittiruti M, Ostroff M, Spencer TR, Dawson RB. The SIC protocol: a seven-step strategy to minimize complications potentially related to the insertion of centrally inserted central catheters. J Vasc Access. 2021;29:11297298211036002. https://doi.org/10.1177/11297298211036002.
6. Brescia F, Pittiruti M, Ostroff M, Biasucci DG. Rapid Femoral Vein Assessment (RaFeVA): a systematic protocol for ultrasound evaluation of the veins of the lower limb, so to optimize the insertion of femorally inserted central catheters. J Vasc Access. 2020;16:1129729820965063. https://doi.org/10.1177/1129729820965063.

7. Cellini M, Bergadano A, Crocoli A, Badino C, Carraro F, Sidro L, Botta D, Pancaldi A, Rossetti F, Pitta F, Cesaro S. Guidelines of the Italian Association of Pediatric Hematology and Oncology for the management of the central venous access devices in pediatric patients with onco-hematological disease. J Vasc Access. 2020;10:1129729820969309. https://doi.org/10.1177/1129729820969309.
8. Crocoli A, Cesaro S, Cellini M, Rossetti F, Sidro L, Pinelli F, Pittiruti M. In defense of the use of peripherally inserted central catheters in pediatric patients. J Vasc Access. 2021 May;22(3):333–6. https://doi.org/10.1177/1129729820936411.
9. Crocoli A, Martucci C, Sidro L, Delle Donne D, Menna G, Pittiruti M, De Pasquale MD, Strocchio L, Natali GL, Inserra A. Safety and effectiveness of subcutaneously anchored securement for tunneled central catheters in oncological pediatric patients: a retrospective study. J Vasc Access. 2021;4:11297298211009364. https://doi.org/10.1177/11297298211009364.
10. Crocoli A, Tornesello A, Pittiruti M, Barone A, Muggeo P, Inserra A, Molinari AC, Grillenzoni V, Durante V, Cicalese MP, Zanazzo GA, Cesaro S. Central venous access devices in pediatric malignancies: a position paper of Italian Association of Pediatric Hematology and Oncology. J Vasc Access. 2015;16(2):130–6. https://doi.org/10.5301/jva.5000314.
11. Doellman D, Buckner JK, Hudson Garrett J Jr, et al. Best practice guidelines in the care and maintenance of pediatric central venous catheters. 2nd ed. Herriman, UT: Association for Vascular Access; 2015.
12. Fraga MV, Stoller JZ, Glau CL, et al. Seeing is believing: ultrasound in pediatric procedural performance. Pediatrics. 2019;144:e20191401.
13. Gilbert RE, Mok Q, Dwan K, et al. Impregnated central venous catheters for prevention of bloodstream infection in children (the CATCH trial): a randomized controlled trial. Lancet. 2016;387:1732–42.
14. Gorski L, Hadaway L, Hagle M, et al. Infusion therapy standards of practice. J Infus Nurs. 2021;44(1S Suppl 1):S1–S224.
15. Habas F, Baleine J, Milési C, et al. Supraclavicular catheterization of the brachiocephalic vein: a way to prevent or reduce catheter maintenance-related complications in children. Eur J Pediatr. 2018;177:451–8.
16. Jijeh AM, Shaath G, Kabbani MS, et al. Ultrasound guided vascular access in pediatric cardiac critical care. J Saudi Heart Assoc. 2014;26:199–203.
17. Kim EH, Lee JH, Song IK, et al. Real-time ultrasound-guided axillary vein cannulation in children: a randomized controlled trial. Anaesthesia. 2017;72:1516–22.
18. Lai L, Yue X. Efficacy of antimicrobial-impregnated catheters for prevention of bloodstream infections in pediatric patients: a meta-analysis. Front Pediatr. 2021;9:632308.
19. Lamperti M, Caldiroli D, Cortellazzi P, et al. Safety and efficacy of ultrasound assistance during internal jugular vein cannulation in neurosurgical infants. Int Care Med. 2008;34:2100–5.
20. Lamperti M, Biasucci DG, Disma N, Pittiruti M, Breschan C, Vailati D, Subert M, Traškaitė V, Macas A, Estebe JP, Fuzier R, Boselli E, Hopkins P. European Society of Anaesthesiology guidelines on peri-operative use of ultrasound-guided for vascular access (PERSEUS vascular access). Eur J Anaesthesiol. 2020;37(5):344–76. https://doi.org/10.1097/EJA.0000000000001180. Erratum in: Eur J Anaesthesiol. 2020;37(7):623
21. Lau C, Chamberlain R. Ultrasound-guided central venous catheter placement increases success rates in pediatric patients: a meta-analysis. Pediatr Res. 2016;80:178–84.
22. Menéndez JJ, Verdú C, Calderón B, et al. Incidence and risk factors of superficial and deep vein thrombosis associated with peripherally inserted central catheters in children. J Thromb Haemost. 2016;14(11):2158–68.
23. Merchaoui Z, Lausten-Thomsen U, Pierre F, Ben Laiba M, Le Saché N, Tissieres P. Supraclavicular approach to ultrasound-guided brachiocephalic vein cannulation in children and neonates. Front Pediatr. 2017 Oct;5(5):211. https://doi.org/10.3389/fped.2017.00211.
24. Nakayama Y, Takeshita J, Nakajima Y, et al. Ultrasound-guided peripheral vascular catheterization in pediatric patients: a narrative review. Crit Care. 2020;24:592.

25. Nifong TP, McDevitt TJ. The effect of catheter to vein ratio on blood flow rates in a simulated model of peripherally inserted central venous catheters. Chest. 2011;140:48–53.
26. Ostroff MD, Moureau N, Pittiruti M. Rapid assessment of vascular exit site and tunneling options (RAVESTO): a new decision tool in the management of the complex vascular access patients. J Vasc Access. 2021;21:11297298211034306. https://doi.org/10.1177/11297298211034306.
27. Paterson RS, Chopra V, Brown E, et al. Selection and insertion of vascular access devices in pediatrics: a systematic review. Pediatrics. 2020;145:e20193474H.
28. Patil V, Jaggar S. Ultrasound guided internal jugular vein access in children and infant: a meta-analysis. Paediatr Anaesth. 2010;20:475.
29. Pinelli F, Pittiruti M, Van Boxtel T, Barone G, Biffi R, Capozzoli G, Crocoli A, Elli S, Elisei D, Fabiani A, Garrino C, Graziano U, Montagnani L, Prato AP, Scoppettuolo G, Zadra N, Zanaboni C, Zerla P, Konstantinou E, Jones M, Rosay H, Simcock L, Stas M, Pepe G. GAVeCeLT-WoCoVA Consensus on subcutaneously anchored securement devices for the securement of venous catheters: current evidence and recommendations for future research. J Vasc Access. 2020;2:1129729820924568. https://doi.org/10.1177/1129729820924568.
30. Pirotte T. Ultrasound-guided vascular access in adults and children: beyond the internal jugular vein puncture. Acta Anaesth Belg. 2008;59:157–66.
31. Pittiruti M, Hamilton H, Biffi R, et al. ESPEN guidelines on parenteral nutrition: central venous catheters (access, care, diagnosis and therapy of complications). Clin Nutr. 2009;28:365–77.
32. Pittiruti M, Scoppettuolo G, Dolcetti L, Celentano D, Emoli A, Marche B, Musarò A. Clinical experience of a subcutaneously anchored sutureless system for securing central venous catheters. Br J Nurs. 2019;28(2):S4–S14. https://doi.org/10.12968/bjon.2019.28.2.S4.
33. Pittiruti M. Ultrasound guided central vascular access in neonates, infants and children. Curr Drug Targets. 2012;13:961–9.
34. Pittiruti M, Van Boxtel T, Scoppettuolo G, Carr P, Konstantinou E, Ortiz Miluy G, Lamperti M, Goossens GA, Simcock L, Dupont C, Inwood S, Bertoglio S, Nicholson J, Pinelli F, Pepe G. European recommendations on the proper indication and use of peripheral venous access devices (the ERPIUP consensus): a WoCoVA project. J Vasc Access. 2021;4:11297298211023274. https://doi.org/10.1177/11297298211023274.
35. Rhondali O, Attof R, Combet S, et al. Ultrasound-guided subclavian vein cannulation in infants: supraclavicular approach. Paediatr Anaesth. 2011;21:1136–41.
36. Sayin M, Mercan A, Koner O, et al. Internal jugular vein diameter in pediatric patients: are the J-shaped guidewire diameters bigger than internal jugular vein? An evaluation with ultrasound. Paediatr Anaesth. 2008;18:745–51.
37. Sharp R, Cummings M, Fielder A, et al. The catheter to vein ratio and rates of symptomatic venous thromboembolism in patients with a peripherally inserted central catheter (PICC): a prospective cohort study. Int J Nurs Stud. 2015;52(3):677–85.
38. Singh Y, Tissot C, Fraga MV, et al. International evidence-based guidelines on point of care ultrasound (POCUS) for critically ill neonates and children issued by the POCUS Working Group of the European Society of Paediatric and Neonatal Intensive Care (ESPNIC). Crit Care. 2020;24:65.
39. Spencer TR, Pittiruti M. Rapid Central Vein Assessment (RaCeVA): a systematic, standardized approach for ultrasound assessment before central venous catheterization. J Vasc Access. 2019;20:239–49.
40. Takeshita J, Nakayama Y, Nakajima Y, et al. Optimal site for ultrasound-guided venous catheterisation in paediatric patients: an observational study to investigate predictors for catheterisation success and a randomised controlled study to determine the most successful site. Crit Care. 2019;19:15.
41. Timsit JF, Baleine J, Bernard L, et al. Expert consensus-based clinical practice guidelines management of intravascular catheters in the intensive care unit. Ann Intensive Care. 2020;10:118.
42. Tufegdzic B, Khozenko A, Lee St John T, et al. Dynamic variation of the axillary veins due to intrathoracic pressure changes: a prospective sonographic study. J Vasc Access. 2020;21:66–72.

43. Ullman AJ, Bernstein SJ, Brown E, Aiyagari R, Doellman D, Faustino EVS, Gore B, Jacobs JP, Jaffray J, Kleidon T, Mahajan PV, McBride CA, Morton K, Pitts S, Prentice E, Rivard DC, Shaughnessy E, Stranz M, Wolf J, Cooper DS, Cooke M, Rickard CM, Chopra V. The Michigan appropriateness guide for intravenous catheters in pediatrics: miniMAGIC. Pediatrics. 2020 Jun;145(Suppl 3):S269–84. https://doi.org/10.1542/peds.2019-3474I.
44. Zito Marinosci G, Biasucci DG, Barone G, D'Andrea V, Elisei D, Iacobone E, La Greca A, Pittiruti M. ECHOTIP-Ped: a structured protocol for ultrasound-based tip navigation and tip location during placement of central venous access devices in pediatric patients. J Vasc Access. 2021;13:11297298211031391. https://doi.org/10.1177/11297298211031391.

Chapter 16
Totally Implantable Venous Access Devices

Alessio Pini Prato, Elisa Cerchia, Claudio Carlini, and Mauro Pittiruti

16.1 Introduction

Since the early 80s, totally implantable venous access devices (ports) have been introduced in clinical practice for the administration of chemotherapy and for blood sampling in adult patients with cancer. Some years later, ports were introduced in pediatric clinical practice with enthusiasm and success. The first reports date back to 1985, when McGovern and colleagues described a series of 39 children who underwent successful port placement with acceptable complication rate, lower than 10%. Even since then, ports have been used world-wide in pediatrics and indications have included not only chemotherapy administration in malignancies, but also transfusions, parenteral nutrition, and long-term intravenous treatments in many clinical conditions (hematological disorders, cystic fibrosis, metabolic diseases, etc.). In 2007, Carausu and co-workers reported the first successful series of patients undergoing peripheral blood stem cell apheresis using ports and suggested that these devices may be effective and safe also for this purpose. This chapter will discuss the indications, the implantation technique and the complications associated to these devices.

A. P. Prato · E. Cerchia · C. Carlini
Alessandria Children Hospital, AON SS Antonio e Biagio e Cesare Arrigo, Alessandria, Italy
e-mail: apini@ospedale.al.it; ecerchia@ospedale.al.it; ccarlini@ospedale.al.it

M. Pittiruti (✉)
Department of Surgery, Catholic University Hospital, Rome, Italy

D. G. Biasucci et al. (eds.), *Vascular Access in Neonates and Children*,
https://doi.org/10.1007/978-3-030-94709-5_16

16.2 Indications and Contraindications to Port

According to current guidelines, the main indication to port insertion is the need for long term intermittent venous access in the extrahospital setting. Long term continuous venous access (daily or weekly access) is best obtained by tunneled catheters, either cuffed or non-cuffed but secured with subcutaneous anchorage. When venous access is intermittent and expected to be required for months or years, totally implantable VADs have many advantages: minimal requirement for maintenance, relative protection from the risk of infection, no risk of accidental dislodgment, optimal compliance of the patient since the port allows a near-normal quality of life. Drawbacks include low tolerance of the puncture necessary for accessing the port (which may be a relevant issue in younger children), more invasive insertion technique compared to other VADS, and need for surgical removal in case of complications or therapy cessation.

Therefore, the choice to insert a totally implantable venous device depends on the age and size of the patient, the expected duration and type of treatment, as well as the patient's or the family's choice, lifestyle, or preference.

At present, indications to port in children can be summarized as follows:

- Long term intermittent use (i.e., >3–4 months—infrequent use, less than once per week)
- Previous multiple episodes of accidental removal of external VADs
- Exhaustion of venous patrimony in children requiring frequent blood sampling or periodic intravenous treatments (cystic fibrosis, hemophilia, etc.)
- Strong preference of the patient, related to the conservation of a normal body-image
- Poor compliance to the basic practices necessary for the maintenance of an external VAD
- Skin abnormalities that impair the effectiveness of skin-adhesive sutureless securement have also been considered indication to port, though many of these problems are currently solved by subcutaneous anchorage

Contraindications to port are the same as in adults:

- severe, uncorrectable coagulopathy with low platelet count. Although a clear-cut limits do not exist, we suggest avoiding port placement in case platelets count is lower than 50–70.000/mm^3
- ongoing systemic infection, particularly in case of bloodstream infection due to Candida.
- severe cachexia due to malnutrition, as it may be associated with reservoir-related complications (skin decubitus and subsequent local infection).

16.3 Age Range for Port Insertion

Age and size of the patients neither limit the indication to the use of ports nor the feasibility of their insertion. In 2016, Kilic and co-workers published a retrospective study on 241 ports inserted in a 4-year period, showing that age is not related to the risk of complications. In small children, the only feasible port is usually the chest-port; in older children, PICC-port is also an option, if the veins of the arms are of appropriate diameter. Nevertheless, older children and adolescents represent the most frequent candidates for totally implantable venous system positioning given the poor tolerance of most infants and toddlers to port punctures.

16.4 Materials

Totally implantable VADs consists of a reservoir connected to a central venous catheter. The reservoirs are made of plastic, titanium, or both (hybrid); based on their height they are described as 'low profile' (approximately 10 mm) or 'very low profile' (approximately 8 mm); 'standard profile' reservoir have little or no indication in the pediatric patient; PICC-ports are preferably 'very low profile'. Although manufacturers offer reservoirs of different sizes, shapes and materials, there is no evidence-based criteria to prefer one from the others.

The catheter can be in silicone or polyurethane; silicon catheters with distal valve (Groshong) have been reported to be associated with catheter malfunction and should be avoided. For chest port, there is no clear preference between silicon or polyurethane, while PICC-ports should be preferably in polyurethane, so that the catheter may progress easily into the vasculature.

Most ports are single lumen, but double lumen ports do exist (double reservoir connected to a double lumen catheter) and they have some specific indications. Ports are usually power injectable, to allow the administration of contrast medium required for computed tomography or magnetic resonance; though, there is still a debate about the opportunity to administer contrast medium through a port: while the risk of structural damage due to high pressure is very low, the risk of irreversible occlusion of the system—because of the high viscosity of the contrast medium—is very high.

Insertion of a totally implantable VAD requires additional material, which may or may not be included in the insertion pack: micro-introducer kit with 21G needle, floppy straight tip 0.018″ nitinol guidewire and introducer-dilator of appropriate caliber; maximal barrier precautions (sterile gloves, gown and drapes, plus long sterile cover for the probe); applicator with 2% chlorhexidine in alcohol; non-coring needles for port access; sterile cable for the intracavitary ECG method of tip location (IC-ECG); scalpel; syringes and needles for the local anesthesia; disposable surgical tools (including a tunneling tool); centimetric tape; sterile gauzes; resorbable sutures; cyanoacrylate glue.

16.5 Choice of the Insertion Site

The puncture site may be a vein of the supra/infraclavicular area (chest-port), a vein of the upper arm (PICC-port) or a vein at the groin (FICC-port). Traditionally, most of the ports have been inserted as chest-ports for at least three decades, as the arm-ports had worse performance and worse compliance. Recently, a new type of arm port has been introduced into the clinical practice, the PICC-port: this can be defined as an arm port inserted according to the current advanced technology used for PICC insertion (ultrasound guided venipuncture at the upper arm, special consideration of the match between vein diameter and catheter caliber, ultrasound-based tip navigation, tip location using IC-ECG). The current literature suggests that there is no significant difference between PICC-ports and chest-ports in terms of performance, risk of infection and risk of thrombosis; though, PICC-ports are a less invasive procedure if compared to chest ports, and severe immediate insertion-related complications are unlikely. FICC-ports are an alternative option when venous access through veins of the arms or of the neck/chest region is contraindicated by an obstruction of the superior vena cava.

As regards the site of placement of the reservoir, the preferred locations are usually over the biceps muscle (for PICC-ports), over the pectoralis major muscle (for chest-ports) and over the quadriceps muscle (for FICC-ports), though many other options exist. For instance, it is possible (and sometimes advisable) to place the reservoir at the arm after cannulation of the brachio-cephalic vein (so-called 'chest-to-arm' tunneling). Also, the reservoir of a FICC-port can also be placed in the abdomen rather than at mid-thigh.

In infants and toddlers, the best veins usually available for cannulation are the supraclavicular veins, i.e., the brachio-cephalic vein (BCV), the internal jugular vein (IJV) and the subclavian vein (SV), so that most totally implantable VADs are chest-port with the reservoir placed in the infraclavicular region, over the pectoralis major muscle, with a short tunneling of the catheter over the clavicle. The best vein will be chosen after a RaCeVA assessment. In infants and toddlers, the BCV usually represents the best option. PICC-ports are unlikely to be inserted in these small patients given the insufficient size of the arm veins. In older children and adolescents, both PICC-ports and chest-ports may be considered. The choice of the puncture site and of the location of the reservoir depends on many factors: presence or absence of cervicothoracic issues contraindicating; previous scarring; patient's preference; and so on. Adolescents with cystic fibrosis are often the ideal candidates for PICC-ports (Figs. 16.1 and 16.2) as their arm veins are of appropriate size and their chest should be left untouched on the ground of the possibility for lung surgery (pneumothorax, transplantation, etc.).

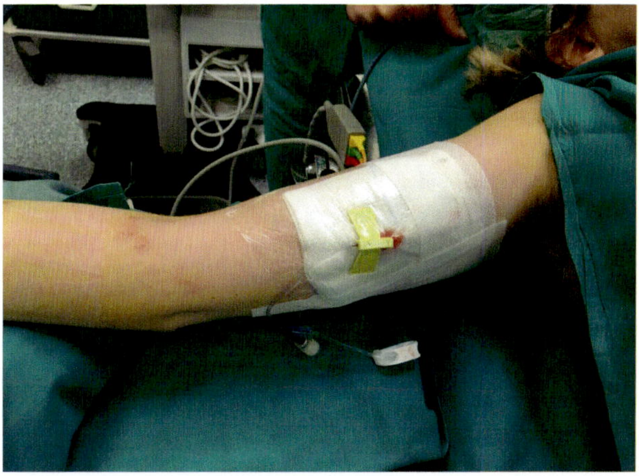

Fig. 16.1 PICC-port

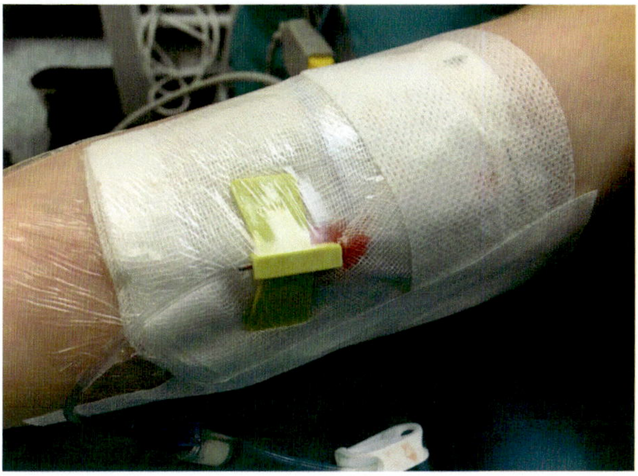

Fig. 16.2 Dressing over a PICC-port

16.6 Technique of Insertion

The implantation of a port should be preferably performed following a specific 'insertion bundle' including all the major recommended strategies for minimizing complications. An example of insertion bundle for chest-port and PICC-port are reported in Table 16.1 and 16.2, respectively.

Depending on the age, the clinical conditions, and the collaboration of the patient, the maneuver can be carried out in general anesthesia or in local anesthesia with or without sedation. In older children and in adolescent, especially if a PICC-port is planned, the whole maneuver can be performed with local anesthetic only (preferably ropivacaine 0.75%).

Table 16.1 Insertion bundle for chest-ports

1. Preprocedural ultrasound evaluation of the veins of the supra/infra-clavicular area according to the RaCeVA protocol.
2. Appropriate aseptic technique: hand hygiene, skin antisepsis with 2% chlorhexidine, maximal barrier precautions.
3. Ultrasound guided puncture and cannulation of the most appropriate vein.
4. Ultrasound scan of the pleura, for ruling out pneumothorax.
5. Ultrasound scan of the vasculature, for assessing the correct direction of the guidewire and of the catheter (tip navigation).
6. Intraprocedural assessment of tip location using intracavitary ECG and/or ultrasound-based tip location according to the ECHOTIP-Ped protocol
7. Placement of the reservoir over the pectoralis major muscle, at proper distance from the clavicle and from the humerus head.
8. Closure of the pocket with resorbable intradermic suture and cyanoacrylate glue

Table 16.2 Insertion bundle for PICC-ports

1. Preprocedural ultrasound evaluation of the veins of the upper arm and of the supra/infra-clavicular area according to the RaPeVA and RaCeVA protocols.
2. Appropriate aseptic technique: hand hygiene, skin antisepsis with 2% chlorhexidine, maximal barrier precautions.
3. Careful identification of the brachial artery and of the median nerve before the venipuncture.
4. Ultrasound guided puncture and cannulation of the most appropriate vein in terms of diameter, either in Dawson's green zone or yellow zone; if the vein is in the yellow zone and very close to the axilla, consider tunneling, so to place the reservoir in the green zone.
5. Ultrasound scan of the supraclavicular area, for assessing the correct direction of the catheter (tip navigation).
6. Intraprocedural assessment of tip location using intracavitary ECG and/or ultrasound-based tip location according to the ECHOTIP-Ped protocol.
7. Placement of the reservoir over the biceps muscle, preferably in Dawson's green zone.
8. Closure of the pocket with resorbable intradermic suture and cyanoacrylate glue.

After the preprocedural ultrasound examination of the vasculature, the first step of insertion regards infection prevention. An appropriate aseptic technique will include (a) hand hygiene, (b) skin antisepsis with 2% chlorhexidine in 70% isopropyl alcohol, and (c) maximal barrier precautions (MBP). MBP include cap, mask, sterile gloves, sterile gowns, a very wide sterile field all over the patient, and a long sterile cover for the ultrasound probe. All devices and clothes should be latex-free. Antibiotic prophylaxis is not recommended by current guidelines.

Ultrasound-guided puncture and cannulation of the vein represent the gold standard for any central venous catheterization in children and adults, and port insertion is no exception. A high frequency linear probe up to 15 MHz and a depth range of visualization of up to 5–6 cm is required. A hockey-stick linear probe is preferable in very small patients (Fig. 16.3) but even a conventional linear probe can work adequately. Depending on the chosen vein, a long or short axis visualization of the vein and "*in-plane*" or "*out-of-plane*" approach will be chosen. The veins of the

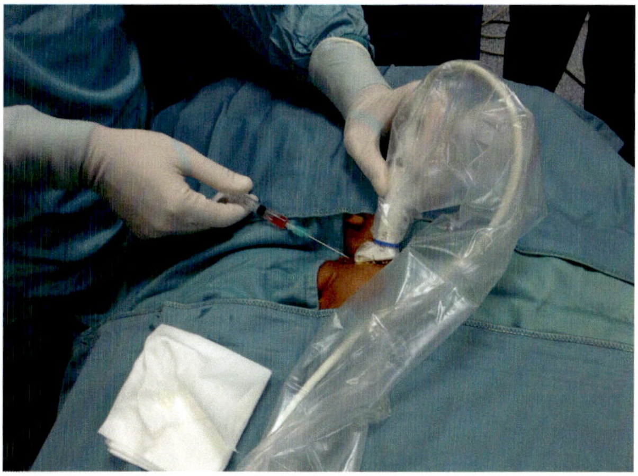

Fig. 16.3 Ultrasound guided venipuncture using 'hockey stick' linear probe

upper limb and lower limb should be punctured with a short axis/out-of-plane approach. All veins of the supraclavicular should be accessed by an in-plane approach, either in short/oblique axis (IJV) or in long axis (BCV, SV). The axillary vein in the infraclavicular area can be accessed with different techniques: short axis/out-of-plane, oblique axis/in-plane or long axis/in-plane. All venipunctures should be performed using small gauge echogenic needles (21G), floppy straight tip 0.018″ nitinol guidewires and micro-introducer-dilator.

Soon after the puncture, the proper trajectory of the guidewire can be assessed by using the linear probe (tip navigation). In case of chest-port insertion (particularly when the axillary vein or the SV has been accessed), the linear probe should also be used for ruling out a pneumothorax secondary to accidental pleural injury. As the catheter enters the vasculature, its correct direction can be assessed using again the linear probe: this is particularly useful during PICC-port insertion, when an ultrasound scan of the supraclavicular area can confirm that the catheter has entered the BCV (ultrasound-based tip navigation, according to the ECHOTIP-Ped protocol). Another option of tip navigation is fluoroscopy, but its use should be discouraged in the pediatric patient, since radiological methods are relatively inaccurate, expensive, and unsafe—since it implies x-ray exposure for the patient and for the operator (see Chap. 6).

The assessment of the final position of the tip (tip location), according to all current guidelines, should be performed using an intraprocedural method. The intraprocedural methods currently available for a real time verification of the proper position of the tip at the junction between right atrium and superior vena cava are (a) intracavitary ECG, (b) trans-thoracic echocardiography (TTE), (c) trans-esophageal echocardiography (TEE), and (d) fluoroscopy. The most accurate method is TEE, but it is invasive, expensive, and logistically difficult. Fluoroscopy is inaccurate (while the catheter tip is easily visualized, the location of the junction between superior vena cava and right atrium can be only inferred based on approximate radiological landmarks), expensive and unsafe. On the contrary, the IC-ECG method is accurate, non-invasive, inexpensive and safe; albeit this method may have some limitations in adult patients (for example, in the case of some arrhythmias), its applicability and feasibility are close to 100% in the pediatric patient. TTE is an alternative option, though less accurate than IC-ECG and less easy to perform; nonetheless, TTE is non-invasive, inexpensive, and its applicability and feasibility in the pediatric patient is 100%. TTE has a role particularly in the tip location of FICC-ports. IC-ECG is currently the standard for tip location during insertion of chest-ports and PICC-ports. It requires only a standard ECG monitor and a sterile cable for connecting the catheter to the electrode (such cable is often provided in the insertion pack). The maximal height of the P wave corresponds very precisely to the transition between superior vena cava and right atrium (Fig. 16.4a).

The next step is the preparation of the pocket for the placement of the reservoir. Depending on the puncture site, a tunneling might be required so to bring the catheter from the puncture site to the pocket. In PICC-ports with puncture site in Dawson's green zone and in chest-ports with puncture site in the infraclavicular area, tunneling is not required. When the puncture site is in the supraclavicular area (chest-port with BCV access, which is the most common occurrence), the catheter must be inevitably tunneled to the infraclavicular area since the reservoir must be placed over the major pectoral muscle.

If the procedure is performed in general anesthesia, the subcutaneous pocket is prepared by hydro-dissection with saline. If the child is awake or under slight sedation, the dissection of the subcutaneous tissue is made with local anesthetic. The pocket should be created deep enough so to place the reservoir above the muscle. Securement of the reservoir with sutures inside the pocket does not provide any advantages but increases the length of the procedure and its invasiveness.

The catheter is now connected to the reservoir and the reservoir inserted inside the pocket, paying attention to place it away from the skin incision. The correct functioning of the catheter (both in aspiration and infusion) must be checked before closing the pocket, using the non-coring needle included in the insertion pack

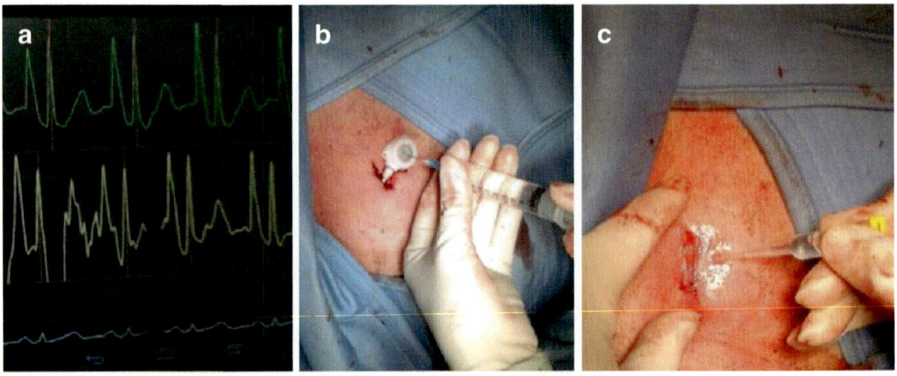

Fig. 16.4 Port insertion: tip location by IC-ECG (**a**); assessment of the possibility of infusion and withdrawal before closing the pocket (**b**); skin closure with cyanoacrylate glue (**c**)

(Fig. 16.4b). The wound is closed using intradermic absorbable stitches and cyanoacrylate glue (Fig. 16.4c). Transcutaneous suture is not recommended, as it leaves a route of bacterial contamination between the external surface and the subcutaneous tissue where the reservoir is located. All totally implantable VADs can be used immediately after the implantation, if needed. If this is the case, we recommend inserting the Huber needle immediately at the end of the procedure, so to avoid early painful punctures in children with lower likelihood of pain tolerance.

16.7 Maintenance

The basic principles of maintenance of ports include: (a) access the reservoir exclusively with Huber (non-coring) needles; (b) secure carefully the Huber on the reservoir using transparent membranes and additional securement (sterile strips) if needed; (c) do not leave the same Huber in place for more than one week; (d) flush and lock the port with saline only (there is no evidence that heparin lock may be more effective than saline in preventing occlusion; on the other hand, heparinization is associated with potential risks if not properly managed); (e) rinse the port with turbulent flush (using the push-pause technique) and leave a positive pressure when locking the system: this can be achieve by injecting saline during removal of the Huber or by using specific Huber needles that automatically inject saline, creating a positive pressure inside the reservoir, as they are removed; (f) In case the catheter is not in use, we recommend monthly flushing, though it has been suggested that flushing can be performed every two or three months, without increasing the risk of occlusion, at least in adulthood.

16.8 Complications

Complications of port insertion are not uncommon and should be divided into intraoperative and postoperative ones.

In the past, intraoperative complications were quite common (up to 18% of cases) and sometimes severe (pneumothorax, hemothorax, massive bleeding due to major vein laceration, air embolism, accidental arterial puncturing, cardiac arrhythmia, pericardial tamponade, heart injury, and brachial plexus injury). The introduction in clinical practice of ultrasound, micro-puncture kits, IC-ECG, and other new strategies (see Tables 16.1 and 16.2) has dramatically reduced the incidence of such complications. A retrospective study on more than 240 port catheters inserted in children showed that the current incidence of intraoperative complications is less than 3% and the most of them are minor complications.

As regards postoperative complications, infection is the most clinically relevant, being responsible of more than 50% of unscheduled removals of the port. Catheter related thrombosis (CRT) is a not to be considered a life-threatening complication and its incidence may be drastically reduced by a proper insertion technique (proper choice of the vein so that the vein diameter is at least 3 times the catheter caliber; ultrasound-guided venipuncture with micro-introducer kits; tip location by IC-ECG). Lumen occlusion is a completely preventable complication, essentially iatrogenic and caused by inadequate policies of flushing and locking (flushing and locking with saline only; exerting positive pressure inside the reservoir when removing the needle; flushing before and after each use). The use of port for parenteral nutrition or blood components increases the risk of infection or occlusion.

Infection is a severe complication and can lead to port removal. Although many Authors suggest that the prevalence of central line associated bloodstream infection (CLABSI) may be significantly lower for ports if compared to other central VADs, port-related infections have been reported with an incidence varying between 8 and 57% of cases. A study by Viana Taveira and colleagues reported a higher incidence of CLABSI within the first 2.5 months post-implantation, and a significant correlation between occurrence of CLABSI and the presence of risk factors such as malnutrition, immunodeficiency, or white blood cells count lower than 1000 mm^3 at implantation; *Klebsiella*, *Pseudomonas aeruginosa*, and *Coagulase-negative staphylococci* were the most frequently encountered microorganisms. On the other hand, Kilic and co-workers in 2016 reported a lower incidence of CLABSI (around 15%) with different pathogens (mainly *Staphylococcus aureus* and *Candida albicans*. Methodological issues, definition of CLABSI, type of patients addressed can explain these highly divergent results. Current guidelines recommend considering infection a 100% preventable complication; all efforts should be done to enforce the clinical strategies that are known to reduce the risk of bacterial contamination: strict aseptic technique during implantation; sterile gloves and appropriate skin antisepsis with 2% chlorhexidine while accessing the port with the Huber; proper aseptic technique in handling the infusion lines. In selected cases, lock with 2% taurolidine may be used for infection prevention in children at high risk for infection. Finally, in order to avoid unnecessary removal, it is of paramount importance to differentiate between CLABSI (which might be related to other sources of infection) and catheter-related blood stream infection (CRBSI) (which means that the colonization of the port is the actual source of the infection). The differential diagnosis between CRBSI and infection not related to the port can be done exclusively by the DTP method (Differential Time to Positivity), based on simultaneous blood cultures from a peripheral vein and from the port, comparing the time of positivity.

Not all infections are bloodstream infection. Local infection of the pocket of the reservoir may also occur (and they inevitably require port removal). Other non-infective complications of the reservoir include early complications (wound dehiscence, hematoma, seroma) and late complications (rotation of the reservoir inside the pocket with flipping and dislodgement, extravasation of drug or contrast medium, decubitus of the reservoir) (Fig. 16.5). Most of these local complications require port removal; though, most of them can be prevented by a proper technique of implantation (with special emphasis to the choice of the size of the reservoir and the choice of the site of the pocket).

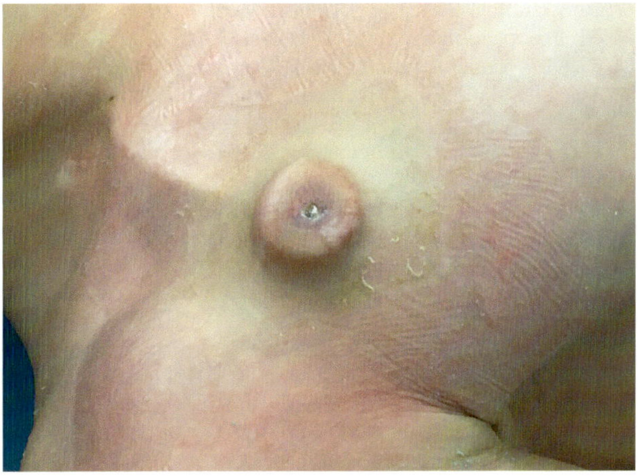

Fig. 16.5 Skin decubitus over the reservoir

16.9 Conclusions

As in adults, ports are the most appropriate device for children requiring long term intermittent venous access. While in the past this procedure has been regarded as invasive and has been associated with significant early and late complications, in the last decade new devices, new technologies and new strategies have changed the practice of port implantation and port maintenance, reducing dramatically the risks and suggesting a wider clinical application of this procedure.

Finally, even if totally implantable VADs are relatively protected by extraluminal contamination, infections still occur and they represent the most severe challenge for the clinicians, especially in malnourished and immunocompromised children.

Bibliography

1. Akahane A, Sone M, Ehara S, Kato K, Tanaka R, Nakasato T. Subclavian vein versus arm vein for totally implantable central venous port for patients with head and neck cancer: a retrospective comparative analysis. Cardiovasc Intervent Radiol. 2011;34(6):1222–9.
2. Al-Bassam A, Al-Rabeeah A, Fouda K, Al-Ashwal A, Ozand PT. Implantable central venous access devices in children with metabolic disease. Metabolism. 1998;47(8):900–2.
3. Ares G, Hunter CJ. Central venous access in children: indications, devices, and risks. Curr Opin Pediatr. 2017;29(3):340–6.
4. Bass J, Halton J, Drouet Y, Ni A, Barrowman N. Central venous catheter database: an important issue in quality assurance. J Pediatr Surg. 2011;46(5):942–5.
5. Biffi R, De Braud F, Orsi F, et al. A randomized prospective trial of central venous ports connected to standard open-ended or Groshong catheters in adult oncology patients. Cancer. 2001;92(5):1204–12.
6. Biffi R, Toro A, Pozzi S, Di Carlo I. Totally implantable vascular access devices 30 years after the first procedure. What has changed and what is still unsolved? Support Care Cancer. 2014;22:1705–14.

7. Bonciarelli G, Batacchi S, Biffi R, Buononato M, Damascelli B, Ghibaudo F, Orsi F, Pittiruti M, Scoppettuolo G, Verzè A, Borasi G, De Cicco M, Dosio R, Gazzo P, Maso R, Roman A, Ticha V, Venier G, Blackburn P, Goossens GA, Bowen Santolucito J, Stas M, Van Boxtel T, Vesely TM, de Lutio E. Gruppo Aperto di Studio Accessi Venosi Centrali a Lungo Termine (Study Group on Long-Term Central Venous Access). GAVeCeLT* consensus statement on the correct use of totally implantable venous access devices for diagnostic radiology procedures. J Vasc Access. 2011;12(4):292–305.
8. Carausu L, Clapisson G, Philip I, Sebban H, Marec-Bérard P. Use of totally implantable catheters for peripheral blood stem cell apheresis. Bone Marrow Transplant. 2007;40(5):417–22.
9. Cassey J, Ford WD, O'Brien L, Martin AJ. Totally implantable system for venous access in children with cystic fibrosis. Clin Pediatr (Phila). 1988;27(2):91–5.
10. Cellini M, Bergadano A, Crocoli A, Badino C, Carraro F, Sidro L, Botta D, Pancaldi A, Rossetti F, Pitta F, Cesaro S. Guidelines of the Italian Association of Pediatric Hematology and Oncology for the management of the central venous access devices in pediatric patients with onco-hematological disease. J Vasc Access. 2020;10:1129729820969309. https://doi.org/10.1177/1129729820969309.
11. Covey AM, Toro-Pape FW, Thornton RH, Son C, Erinjeri J, Sofocleous CT, Brody LA, Brown KT, Sepkowitz KA, Getrajdman GI. Totally implantable venous access device placement by interventional radiologists: are prophylactic antibiotics necessary? J Vasc Interv Radiol. 2012 Mar;23(3):358–62.
12. Crocoli A, Tornesello A, Pittiruti M, Barone A, Muggeo P, Inserra A, Molinari AC, Grillenzoni V, Durante V, Cicalese MP, Zanazzo GA, Cesaro S. Central venous access devices in pediatric malignancies: a position paper of Italian Association of Pediatric Hematology and Oncology. J Vasc Access. 2015;16(2):130–6.
13. Dal Molin A, Clerico M, Baccini M, Guerretta L, Sartorello B, Rasero L. Normal saline versus heparin solution to lock totally implanted venous access devices: results from a multicenter randomized trial. Eur J Oncol Nurs. 2015;19(6):638–43.
14. Doellman D, Buckner MA, Garrett JH, Catudal JP, Frey AM, Lamagna P, Runde D, Schears GJ, Whitehead M. Best Practice Guidelines in the care and maintenance of Pediatric Central Venous Catheters. 2nd ed. Association for Vascular Access; 2010.
15. Essex-Cater A, Gilbert J, Robinson T, Littlewood JM. Totally implantable venous access systems in paediatric practice. Arch Dis Child. 1989;64(1):119–23.
16. Geremia C, De Ioris MA, Crocoli A, Adorisio O, Scrocca R, Lombardi MH, Staccioli S, Stella P, Amendola P, Ciliento G, De Peppo F, Campana A. Totally implantable venous access devices in children with medical complexity: preliminary data from a tertiary care hospital. J Vasc Access. 2017;18(5):426–9.
17. Goossens GA, Stas M, Moons P. Management of functional complications of totally implantable venous access devices by an advanced practice nursing team: 5 years of clinical experience. Eur J Oncol Nurs. 2012;16(5):465–71.
18. Gorski L, Hadaway L, Hagle M, et al. Infusion therapy standards of practice. J Infus Nurs. 2021;44(1S Suppl 1):S1–S224.
19. Gyves JW, Ensminger WD, Niederhuber JE, et al. A totally implanted injection port system for blood sampling and chemotherapy administration. JAMA. 1984;25:2538–41.
20. Hsieh CC, Weng HH, Huang WS, et al. Analysis of risk factors for central venous port failure in cancer patients. World J Gastroenterol. 2009;15(37):4709–14.
21. Kılıç S, Soyer T, Karnak İ, Çiftçi AÖ, Tanyel FC, Şenocak ME. Evaluation of the removal reasons of totally implantable venous devices in children: a retrospective study. Turk J Pediatr. 2016;58(2):187–94.
22. Lamperti M, Biasucci DG, Disma N, Pittiruti M, Breschan C, Vailati D, Subert M, Traškaitė V, Macas A, Estebe JP, Fuzier R, Boselli E, Hopkins P. European Society of Anaesthesiology guidelines on peri-operative use of ultrasound-guided for vascular access

(PERSEUS vascular access). Eur J Anaesthesiol. 2020;37(5):344–76. https://doi.org/10.1097/EJA.0000000000001180. Erratum in: Eur J Anaesthesiol. 2020;37(7):623
23. McGovern B, Solenberger R, Reed K. A totally implantable venous access system for long-term chemotherapy in children. J Pediatr Surg. 1985;20(6):725–7.
24. Niederhuber JE, Ensminger W, Gyves JW, et al. Totally implanted venous and arterial access system to replace external catheters in cancer treatment. Surgery. 1982;92:706–12.
25. Palese A, Baldassar D, Rupil A, Bonanni G, Capellari Maria T, Contessi D, De Crignis L, Vidoni A, Piller Roner S, Zanini A. Maintaining patency in totally implantable venous access devices (TIVAD): a time-to-event analysis of different lock irrigation intervals. Eur J Oncol Nurs. 2014;18(1):66–71.
26. Pinelli F, Cecero E, Degl'Innocenti D, Selmi V, Giua R, Villa G, Chelazzi C, Romagnoli S, Pittiruti M. Infection of totally implantable venous access devices: a review of the literature. J Vasc Access. 2018;19(3):230–42. https://doi.org/10.1177/1129729818758999. Epub 2018 Mar 7
27. Pittiruti M, Bertollo D, Briglia E, Buononato M, Capozzoli G, De Simone L, La Greca A, Pelagatti C, Sette P. The intracavitary ECG method for positioning the tip of central venous catheters: results of an Italian multicenter study. J Vasc Access. 2012;13(3):357–65.
28. Rossetti F, Pittiruti M, Lamperti M, Graziano U, Celentano D, Capozzoli G. The intracavitary ECG method for positioning the tip of central venous access devices in pediatric patients: results of an Italian multicenter study. J Vasc Access. 2015;16(2):137–43. https://doi.org/10.5301/jva.5000281.
29. Royal College of Nurses. Standards for infusion therapy [internet document]. 2010. http://ivtherapyathome.heartofengland.nhs.uk/wp-content/uploads/2013/05/RCN-Guidlines-for-IV-therapy.pdf. Accessed 6 Oct 2014.
30. Schiffer CA, Mangu PB, Wade JC, et al. Central venous catheter care for the patient with cancer: American Society of Clinical Oncology clinical practice guideline. J Clin Oncol. 2013;31:1357–70.
31. Shiono M, Takahashi S, Kakudo Y, Takahashi M, Shimodaira H, Kato S, Ishioka C. Upper arm central venous port implantation: a 6-year single institutional retrospective analysis and pictorial essay of procedures for insertion. PLoS One. 2014 Mar 10;9(3):e91335.
32. Shulman RJ, Rahman S, Mahoney D, Pokorny WJ, Bloss R. A totally implanted venous access system used in pediatric patients with cancer. J Clin Oncol. 1987 Jan;5(1):137–40.
33. Spencer TR, Pittiruti M. Rapid Central Vein Assessment (RaCeVA): a systematic, standardized approach for ultrasound assessment before central venous catheterization. J Vasc Access. 2019;20:239–49.
34. Tabatabaie O, Kasumova GG, Eskander MF, Critchlow JF, Tawa NE, Tseng JF. Totally implantable venous access devices: a review of complications and management strategies. Am J Clin Oncol. 2017;40(1):94–105.
35. Ullman AJ, Bernstein SJ, Brown E, Aiyagari R, Doellman D, Faustino EVS, Gore B, Jacobs JP, Jaffray J, Kleidon T, Mahajan PV, McBride CA, Morton K, Pitts S, Prentice E, Rivard DC, Shaughnessy E, Stranz M, Wolf J, Cooper DS, Cooke M, Rickard CM, Chopra V. The Michigan appropriateness guide for intravenous catheters in pediatrics: miniMAGIC. Pediatrics. 2020;145(Suppl 3):S269–84. https://doi.org/10.1542/peds.2019-3474I.
36. van Gent MB, van der Made WJ, Marang-van de Mheen PJ, van der Bogt KE. Contemporary insertion of central venous access catheters in pediatric patients: a retrospective record review study of 538 catheters in a single center. Surg Infect. 2017;18(2):105–11.
37. Viana Taveira MR, Lima LS, de Araújo CC, de Mello MJ. Risk factors for central line-associated bloodstream infection in pediatric oncology patients with a totally implantable venous access port: a cohort study. Pediatr Blood Cancer. 2017;64(2):336–42.
38. Walser EM. Venous access ports: indications, implantation technique, follow-up, and complications. Cardiovasc Intervent Radiol. 2012;35(4):751–64.

39. Wesenberg F, Anker C, Sommerschild H, Flaatten H. Central venous catheter with subcutaneous injection port (Port-A-Cath): clinical experience with children. Pediatr Hematol Oncol. 1987;4(2):137–43.
40. Wiener ES, McGuire P, Stolar CJ, et al. The CCSG prospective study of venous access devices: an analysis of insertions and causes for removal. J Pediatr Surg. 1992;27:155–64.
41. Zito Marinosci G, Biasucci DG, Barone G, D'Andrea V, Elisei D, Iacobone E, La Greca A, Pittiruti M. ECHOTIP-Ped: a structured protocol for ultrasound-based tip navigation and tip location during placement of central venous access devices in pediatric patients. J Vasc Access. 2021;13:11297298211031391. https://doi.org/10.1177/11297298211031391.

Part IV
Arterial Access

Chapter 17
Umbilical Arterial Catheters

Roberta Centorrino, Valentina Dell'Orto, and Daniele De Luca

17.1 Background

Umbilical arterial catheters (UACs) are the most used form of arterial access in neonatal critical care irrespective of patients' size, given the immediate accessibility of the umbilical arteries and the relative simplicity of placement. UACs allow repeatable and painless blood drawing. They are the gold standard for blood gas analysis and for invasive monitoring of arterial blood pressure, as non-invasive monitoring blood pressure measurements are inaccurate and associated with both over- and under-estimation, especially in the sickest neonates.

Umbilical arteries are only accessible early after birth, although cases of successful UAC placement have been reported also in the first days after birth. The success of UAC placement depends on the condition of the umbilical artery (ability to identify it, patency of the lumen, wall tissue elasticity), on the patient's temperature, and on the status of oxygenation. UAC placement is easier in normothermic and hypoxic than in hypothermic and well oxygenated neonates, because low temperature and high partial pressure of oxygen cause vasoconstriction of the smooth muscle in the umbilical arterial wall. If UAC placement is anticipated, temperature control to achieve normothermia is advised and it might also be useful, at least transiently, to reduce inspired oxygen fraction to the minimum, but still compatible with an acceptable arterial saturation. Moisture over the umbilical cord may also theoretically increases the chance of a successful UAC insertion.

R. Centorrino · V. Dell'Orto · D. De Luca (✉)
Division of Pediatrics and Neonatal Critical Care, Medical Centre "A.Béclère", South Paris University Hospital, APHP and South Paris-Saclay University, Paris, France
e-mail: Valentina.dellorto@aphp.fr

D. G. Biasucci et al. (eds.), *Vascular Access in Neonates and Children*,
https://doi.org/10.1007/978-3-030-94709-5_17

Delayed separation of the umbilical cord may be associated with some forms of congenital immunodeficiency or local infection; in these cases, both arterial and venous umbilical lines have a high risk of infection.

UAC, since it consists of a long line placed in the aorta, represents the only form of 'central' arterial access that can be achieved at the bedside. UACs represent the first-line choice for arterial cannulation in critically ill neonates; however, placing a UAC may not always be technically possible and in such instances, a peripheral arterial line should be placed instead.

17.2 Indications

UACs share the same risks as other forms of arterial access, plus some additional risks due to their 'central' position. The risk-benefit balance should always be evaluated before UAC placement. Suggested indications for UAC placement are described in Table 17.1.

Table 17.1 Indication for UAC placement according to the clinical indication

Absolute indications
Early critical care of patients <750g[a]
Early critical care of extremely ill neonates (severe respiratory failure, hemodynamic instability, severe pulmonary hypertension; metabolic diseases, life-threatening congenital heart defects)
Need (or suspected need) for whole body hypothermia[b]
Need for arterio-venous exchange-transfusion[c]
Relative indications
Anticipated need for serial blood gas analysis or extremely difficult blood draws
Unavailability of other venous access in the setting of specific medical emergencies[d]

Note: In this table, "early" refers to the first 72 h of life

[a]This is not a fixed weight threshold, as the decision to place an UAC should be taken according to the clinical conditions

[b]During whole body hypothermia capillary blood gas analysis and transcutaneous blood gas monitoring may be significantly influenced, thus UAC placement is necessary. UAC placement should be performed before starting the hypothermic state

[c]This is rarely performed but it provides the highest efficiency amongst exchange-transfusion procedures and an UAC is needed to perform it

[d]Although rare, umbilical venous catheters may be impossible to place and, if other venous accesses are not immediately accessible or the intraosseous infusion is not feasible (lack of materials/experience, very preterm or very low birth weight neonates), UAC may be considered as a temporary emergency vascular access ONLY for some types of infusions (blood and its derivatives, 5–10% glucose solutions, normal saline). This relative indication clearly depends on the operator's experience, degree of emergency and availability of other accesses

17.3 Insertion Technique

UACs are placed by direct insertion as the umbilical arteries are immediately visible and accessible after cutting the umbilical cord. The catheter will advance through umbilical arteries of approximate intra-corporeal length of 2–5 cm. The final location of the catheter tip must be inside the aorta. The umbilical artery connects to the internal iliac artery at an acute angle, so that the catheter may pass via the internal iliac and common iliac arteries to the aorta, or it may proceed in the wrong direction to the femoral artery. UACs are usually placed simultaneously to the umbilical venous catheter, but the two procedures may also be performed at different times, depending on the clinical conditions. The insertion procedure for UACs is like that of umbilical venous catheters described in Chap. 10.

- *Clean the cord and the surrounding skin.*
- *Disinfect and prepare a sterile area* with 2% chlorhexidine in alcohol (see Chap. 10 and also 4.1).
- *Place a sterile umbilical tape at the base of the cord.* This is highly recommended if a UAC is to be placed.
- *Cut the umbilical cord.* It is advised to leave at least 1 cm if an UAC is to be inserted (see below).
- *Umbilical artery identification.* The cord usually has one vein and two arteries. Arteries are recognized by their smaller lumen and thicker wall. Either of the two arteries can be cannulated. Sometimes (especially in extremely low birth weight newborns) an additional cut of the entire cord, or a small cut performed diagonally on a small portion of the Wharton's jelly may be useful for a clearer visualization of the artery. A single umbilical artery is a common malformation and does not represent a contraindication for UAC placement. In some cases, a 4-vessel cord may be found because of the presence of a fully patent second umbilical vein, or other vascular malformations. These vascular anomalies do not represent a contraindication for UAC placement but may be associated with complex congenital malformations.
- *Remove visible thrombi.* Removal of thrombi is obtained with a small gauze and normal saline.
- *Arterial dilatation.* Dilatation is a step not needed for a UVC but necessary for UAC placement. The chosen umbilical artery should be gently opened with a stylet to make its surface more accessible. Then, a small, curved forceps is used to dilate the arterial lumen to a depth of about 0.5 cm. Dilatation should be repeated progressively while pulling the cord vertically with a second pair of forceps.

- *Choice of catheter*. The catheter diameter must be chosen according to the artery size and patient's gestational age. Two diameters are commonly available: 2.5 Fr and 3.5 Fr (rarely is a bigger one needed). The 3.5 Fr catheter is also stiffer than the smaller one. As full term and late preterm babies have higher blood pressure, the 3.5 Fr catheter is to be preferred in these cases. The smaller 2.5 Fr catheter may kink, or be displaced, or create intra-aortic loops due to its flexibility, under the effect of high blood pressure.
- *Catheter filling and insertion*. The catheter should be filled with saline. Contrary to umbilical vein catheterization, UACs must be inserted in the direction of the patient's feet and proper placement often requires two operators. While pushing the catheter, the umbilical tape is partially released, and the umbilical stump is retracted away from the body and tilted towards the head. While advancing the catheter, some resistance is felt at about 2–3 cm of depth, which should be easily overcome. The catheter can be easily visualized in the iliac arteries and in the aorta by real time ultrasound guidance. Once the catheter is in the aorta, blood should be easily aspirated and spontaneous reflux in the catheter should be detected. If blood return is not optimal, the possibility of catheter obstruction due to thrombi must be considered. Blood aspiration from a UAC must always be performed very slowly as it may affect cerebral hemodynamics in preterm patients. If the catheter does not advance beyond 2–4 cm, it is likely to be blocked by a vasospasm of the umbilical artery. In this case, successful placement is extremely unlikely and insertion in the other umbilical artery should be considered.

Difficult position of the UAC is the main intraprocedural complication of UACs. Sometimes the catheter does not advance towards the aorta but instead goes downwards into the femoral artery or may kink or loop inside the iliac arteries. If the catheter is left in such inappropriate location, the risk for thrombosis is high. Several measures have been suggested for facilitating the passage of the catheter from the iliac arteries to the aorta, such as the insertion of a second catheter or forcing the neonate to special positions, but none of these maneuvers have been studied in randomized trials and there are no clear evidence of their efficacy. Probably the best recommendation is to use ultrasound during the procedure, so to detect immediately, in real time, the wrong direction of the catheter (so-called 'tip navigation').

Ultrasound is also of paramount importance for assessing the final position of the tip (so called 'tip location'), and is superior to the traditional method of post-procedural X-ray. At x-ray, the proper position of the catheter (in the thoracic aorta) is assessed indirectly, using radiological landmarks (projection of the tip in the area between the vertebral bodies T6–T9); in the past, also 'low' positions of the tip in the sub-diaphragmatic aorta (at vertebral bodies L3–L5) have been considered acceptable (Fig. 17.1). Though, current guidelines (see 2021 Standards of the Infusion Nursing Society) recommend that UACs should have the tip in the thoracic portion of the descending aorta below the aortic arch, as this position is associated with decreased risk of complications. Ultrasound has several advantages over x-ray as method of tip location for UACs (Fig. 17.2): it is very accurate (since both the

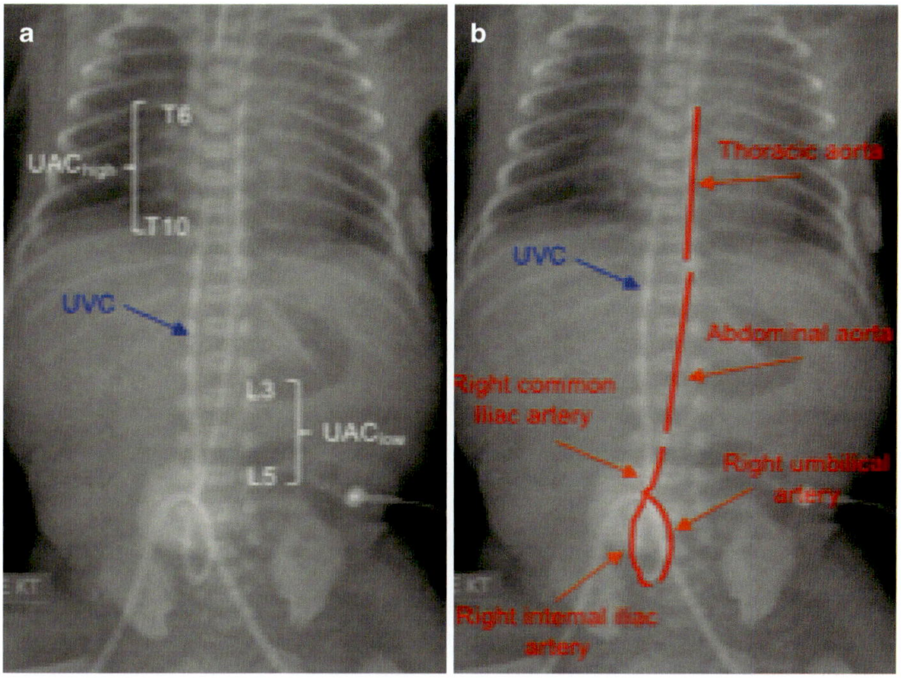

Fig. 17.1 Typical radiological imaging ("babygram") of a correctly placed UAC (Panel A) and the anatomical structures along the UAC course (Panel B). The characteristic acute angle between umbilical and iliac arteries is visible and the first part of the UAC is heading towards patient's feet. An umbilical venous catheter (UVC) is visible, as well. The preferred areas for correct placement (UAC_{high}) is between T6 and T10. The low position (UAC_{low}), between L3 and L5, is not currently recommended

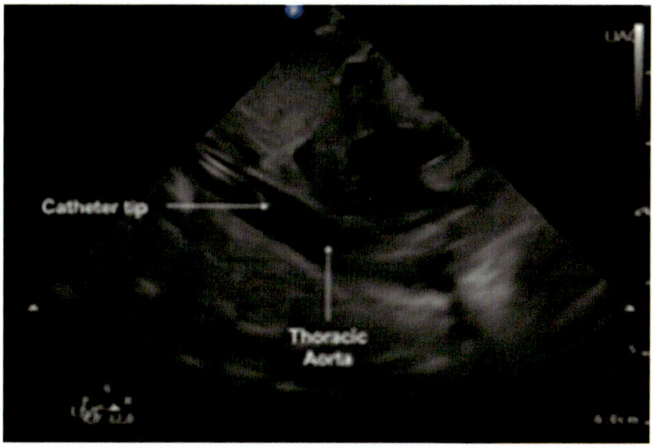

Fig. 17.2 Typical ultrasound imaging of a UAC. the UAC is visualized as a "double track" image in the thoracic aorta, above the diaphragm

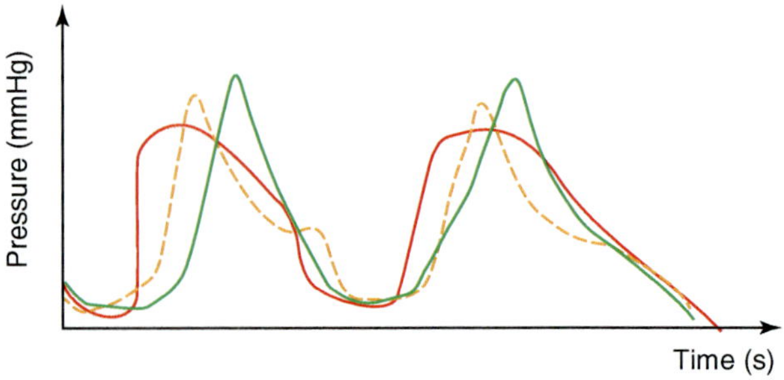

Fig. 17.3 Typical arterial pressure waveform obtained from a UAC (red curve), as compared to small peripheral arteries (orange and green curves). The waveform is less sharp and more rounded

catheter and the aorta are visualized directly and clearly); it is intraprocedural (so that it can be used also for tip navigation and it avoids the risk of secondary replacement of the catheter); it is non-invasive and safe (as it does not imply x-ray exposure); it is rapid and repeatable at any time in the following hours or days, so to detect possible secondary malpositions; it can detect vascular abnormalities; it is inexpensive; last but not least, ultrasound is widely available in any neonatal intensive care unit, since it is adopted for many other diagnostic and therapeutic procedures.

Once the catheter has been inserted, it is usually connected to a pressure transducer and a monitoring system. This will allow accurate, continuous, invasive, arterial pressure measurement. The arterial pressure waveform may also be evaluated. The waveform will be different from that obtained using arterial cannulas inserted in small peripheral arteries, since waveform from the aorta is less pointed and more rounded (Fig. 17.3).

Once the catheter position is checked (preferably by ultrasound), the catheter must be secured; as for the umbilical venous catheters, a combination of several strategies is used (surgical suture, plasters, glue, transparent dressing, etc.) and none of them is evidence-based. The most appropriate securement of umbilical catheters is still an unsolved issue (see Chap. 10).

At the time of removal, as opposed to umbilical venous catheters, UACs must be withdrawn very slowly, so to reduce the risk of bleeding. Once removed, if bleeding continues, plasters, cyanoacrylate glue, local pro-coagulants, or clamping of the umbilical stump may be necessary.

17.4 Materials

Catheters used for umbilical artery cannulation are the same as the ones used as UVC. They are usually made of polyurethane, 2.5 Fr or 3.5 Fr, and single lumen. Unlike other vascular accesses, UACs may require additional materials such as high-pressure valves, single or multiple stopcocks, and so on. Adequate pressure transducers and connectors to a monitoring system are needed for invasive arterial pressure monitoring.

17.5 Contraindications

Few conditions represent absolute contraindications to UAC placement: in these cases, a peripheral arterial catheter should be inserted.

UAC placement is usually impossible or unsuitable in abdominal wall malformations such as gastroschisis and omphalocele. In some cases of gastroschisis, the placement of UAC may be temporarily possible, although peripheral arterial access should be preferred. Complex vascular anomalies, genetic syndromes, or congenital abnormalities can make UAC placement difficult or even impossible even in the absence of a clearly defined vascular malformation. UACs are contraindicated in patients with of aortic coarctation as the catheter will reduce the aortic cross-sectional area available for blood flow. Neonates who had absent or reverse endo-diastolic flow in intrauterine life should not have an UAC, as the catheter may theoretically influence the restoration of normal hemodynamics.

UAC are relatively contraindicated in severe coagulopathy and when mesenteric or renal thrombosis is suspected. In some cases of thoraco-abdominal surgery, a UAC may be relatively contraindicated, depending on the surgical approach.

17.6 Complications

UACs do not seem to be more harmful than peripheral arterial catheters in terms of non-infective complications (Table 17.2). However, as central lines, UACs carry a higher infectious risk as compared to peripheral arterial lines. Insertion, care, and maintenance should be managed with strict sterile technique in the same manner as central venous lines, so to reduce the risk of infection. The most important intervention to reduce infection rates in neonates requiring central vascular access remains the introduction of a dedicated team and bundle to maintain and care for central lines.

Thrombotic events remain the most common and possibly scaring non-infective complication of UACs. The incidence of UAC-related thrombosis is unclear and may span from subclinical events that resolve spontaneously to catastrophic and life-threatening thrombosis. UACs share a similar thrombotic risk with peripheral artery cannulas but are associated with less thrombotic events than femoral arterial catheters (not commonly used in neonates). Risks factors for UAC-related thrombosis, both demonstrated and hypothesized, are listed in Table 17.3. When one or more of these risk factors are present, they should be considered in the risk-benefit ratio decision to place a UAC. The relationship between infection and thrombosis is not clear. Sepsis impacts the coagulation status but there no data proving a clear effect on UAC-related thrombosis. The catheter material does not seem to be important, since all catheters increase thrombogenicity; however, polyvinyl-chloride catheters carry a higher risk of thrombosis and they have been replaced by polyurethane catheters.

Table 17.2 Non-infectious complications of UAC

Decreased urine output
Retrograde embolization
Visceral infarction
Hemoperitoneum
Vasospasms
Skin/limb/gluteal necrosis
Refractory hypoglycemia[a]
Spinal cord injury/paraplegia[b]
Peripheral neural injury
Aneurysm and pseudoaneurysm[c]
Thrombosis
Catheter retention or rupture

Note: The list should not be considered exhaustive, and conditions are listed just on the basis of their literature description. Some of these complications may be associated and some may be related to pre-existing underlying conditions or to others that may be superimposed (e.g.: thrombo-embolic predisposition, infections). A direct cause-effect relationship cannot be clearly proven in some cases

[a]Hypoglycemia has been described when an UAC has been incorrectly used for parenteral nutrition

[b]This type of injury has been related to UAC malposition into the Adamkiewicz artery or local thrombo-embolic events

[c]Aneurysms have been described (both in the aorta and in the iliac arteries) years after UAC placement

Table 17.3 Risk factors for UAC-related thrombotic events

UAC of smaller diameter
Absence if heparin in the infusate
Presence of calcium or some drugs in the infusate[a]
Polyvinyl-chloride catheters
UAC misplaced in iliac arteries or creating loops
UAC with the tip in the abdominal aorta
Low cardiac output
High hematocrit
Inherited or acquired thrombophilia
Duration of UAC *in situ*

[a]ONLY blood and its derivatives, 5–10% glucose solutions or normal saline may be infused through UAC in case of medical emergencies and in absence of other accesses. All other drugs must be avoided

17.7 Conclusions

UACs are extremely useful in the management of the critically ill neonate. Though, they are potentially associated with severe infective and thrombotic complications. The safe insertion and maintenance of UACs is based on the following important strategies:

1. *UAC placement should be performed exclusively by specifically and properly trained operator, familiar with the techniques of ultrasound.* The most important thing is to develop an adequate bundle with a formal protocol to insert and maintain UACs. UAC should be placed only when the benefits overcome the risks and this evaluation must be done by an expert attending neonatologist or pediatric intensivist. Healthcare professionals must be well informed and trained for UAC insertion and maintenance.
2. *The desired final position of the tip must be in the thoracic aorta.* Tip positions below the diaphragm are associated with higher risk of thrombotic events and lower limb complications due to the lower diameter of the iliac arteries and the pro-thrombotic effect of the catheter itself. A Cochrane meta-analysis of six studies showed that UACs with tip in the thoracic aorta are associated with a lower incidence of clinical vascular complications, without an increase in any adverse sequelae. The occurrence of intraventricular hemorrhage, necrotizing enterocolitis and death is not affected by the position of the tip below or above the diaphragm.
3. *The final position of the tip should be assessed during the procedure, using ultrasound.* The old-fashioned method of pre-procedural length estimation + post-procedural x-ray assessment is not recommended anymore. Length estimation is highly approximative: though many methods have been described (see Table 17.4), none of them has been proven to be consistently accurate. Also, as

Table 17.4 Advantages and disadvantages of the different methods to estimate or measure the insertion depth for UAC

Name	Technique/Formula	Pro's	Con's
Shukla-Ferrara formula	(BW × 3 + 9)	Accurate. Easy and similar to UVC formula	May be wrong in SGA and VLBW patients
Wright formula	(BW × 4 + 7)	Easy and similar to UVC formula. Slightly more accurate	None
Dunn Nomogram	Determined by shoulder-umbilical length on the Dunn nomogram	Accurate	Cumbersome (require unusual measurements)

(conitnued)

Table 17.4 (continued)

Name	Technique/Formula	Pro's	Con's
Surface anatomy method	Umbilicus to nipple distance—1 cm plus twice the distance from umbilicus to symphysis pubis	Accurate	Cumbersome (require unusual measurements)
Lateral look method	1.1 × (xiphoid-ASIS + umbilicus-ASIS) + 1.6, where ASIS is the anterior superior iliac spine	Accurate	Cumbersome (require unusual measurements)
Thai method	Suprasternal notch to superior iliac spine length (SSSL)	Accurate	Cumbersome (require unusual measurements)
Length method	Heel-to-crown length × 0.33 (cm)	Accurate	Very old. Not proven on very preterm neonates

Note: Birth weight and length are to be considered in kilograms and centimeters, respectively
Abbreviations: BW: birth weight; SGA: small for gestational age; UAC: Umbilical artery catheters; UAC: Umbilical artery catheters placed in the thoracic aorta; UVC: Umbilical venous catheter; VLBW: Very low birth weight

noted above, x-ray assessment is less accurate than ultrasound, since it visualizes only the catheter, while the vascular structures are located on the basis of indirect radiological landmarks.

4. *The UAC should be maintained under continuous heparinization.* The use of heparin is especially important in situations that are at highest risk of thrombosis such as critically ill babies, polycythemia, narrow catheters, or presence of calcium in the infusate. A Cochrane meta-analysis of five randomized controlled trials showed that heparinization of the fluid infused through the UAC decreases the likelihood of catheter occlusion; though, it has no effect on the occurrence of aortic thrombosis or other thrombotic and ischemic events, including intraventricular hemorrhage. Heparinization is also associated with a reduction in arterial hypertension. Very low concentrations (0.25 units/mL) have been shown to be effective but doses up to 1 unit/mL have been used with no adverse effects. It seems prudent to use heparin starting at the lowest effective concentration (0.25–0.5 units/mL) in isotonic saline (the use of isotonic saline seems to reduce the risk of hemolysis during blood sampling. Heparinization of flushes without heparinizing the infusate resulted ineffective in preventing catheter occlusions or other complications: furthermore, flushes may be harmful, being associated with retrograde embolization. UAC may be maintained using electronically controlled infusion pumps or pressurized bag pumps. Electronic pumps should probably be preferred for a better volume control in the smallest patients.
5. *UAC should be used only for blood sampling and infusion of heparinized isotonic saline.* Infusions of normal saline, glucose solutions, or blood and blood derivatives are acceptable only in case of emergencies and in absence of other forms of access.

6. *Remove the catheter within 5 days after its insertion*. The duration of UACs *in situ* seem to affect the occurrence of clinically evident thrombosis, even if neo-intimal proliferation and increased thrombogenicity have been demonstrated even after a short application of a UAC. Neonates with UAC-related thrombotic events have a mean duration of 8.3 ± 3.9 days versus 4.8 ± 3.5 days of those not experiencing this complication. Thus, we advise to keep UACs for 5 days and to place a peripheral arterial line later, should arterial monitoring still be needed.
7. *UAC functionality should be tested regularly, and UACs should be removed as soon as possible if a complication is suspected*. Signs of possible complications are: (1) transient blanching, erythema, or reduced pulse at the affected extremity, (2) decreased urine output, (3) decreased regional saturation (by near infrared spectroscopy) or altered perfusion index on the affected extremity, (4) reduced temperature at the affected extremity, (5) low platelet count. In all these cases, an ultrasound examination should be performed, and the UAC should be removed if a thrombosis is demonstrated or suspected. An established UAC-related thrombosis should be promptly treated with thrombolytic therapy, heparin and heparin-derivatives, or caudal blockade. In the absence of evidence-based data, there are no clear recommendations on the best strategy to be applied. Conversely, enteral feeding can be continued in babies with (or at risk for) UAC-related thrombotic events. In fact, stable preterm neonates in stable condition receiving enteral feedings do not have an increased incidence of feeding problems, as compared to those who stopped the enteral feeding.

Bibliography

1. Barrington KJ. Umbilical artery catheters in the newborn: effects of position of the catheter tip. Cochrane Database Syst Rev. 2000;(2):CD000505.
2. Barrington KJ. Umbilical artery catheters in the newborn: effects of heparin. Cochrane Database Syst Rev. 2000;(2):CD000507.
3. Bhatt MD, Paes BA, Chan AK. How to use unfractionated heparin to treat neonatal thrombosis in clinical practice. Blood Coagul Fibrinolysis. 2016;27:605–14.
4. Blondiaux E, Miquel J, Thomas P, Laloum D, Watelet J, Dacher JN. Calcified aneurysm of the abdominal aorta 12 years after umbilical artery catheterization. Pediatr Radiol. 2008;38:233–6.
5. Blood withdrawal and infusion via umbilical catheters: effect on cerebral perfusion and influence of ibuprofen. Biol Neonate. 2003;84:187–93.
6. Brotschi B, Hug MI, Latal B, Neuhaus D, Buerki C, Kroiss S, Spoerri C, Albisetti M. Incidence and predictors of indwelling arterial catheter-related thrombosis in children. J Thromb Haemost. 2011;9:1157–62.
7. Cornelius A, Fischer J, Frey B, Baenziger O, Gerber A, Weiss M. Pressurized bag pump and syringe pump arterial flushing systems: an unrecognized hazard in neonates? Intensive Care Med. 2002;28:1638–43.
8. Dannevig I, Dale HC, Liestøl K, Lindemann R. Blood pressure in the neonate: three non-invasive oscillometric pressure monitors compared with invasively measured blood pressure. Acta Paediatr. 2005;94:191–6.

9. De Carolis MP, Romagnoli C, Gasbarrini A, de Francisci G, Piersigilli F, Cremonini F, Cittadino M, Pola P, Tortorolo G. Caudal blockade as alternative therapeutic approach in neonatal arterial thrombosis. Eur J Pediatr. 2001;160:61–2.
10. Deliège R, Cneude F, Barbier C, Rakza T, Bourlet A, Vaillant C, Bonnevale M, Storme L. Ruptured mycotic aneurysm with hemoperitoneum: an unusual septic complication of umbilical arterial catheter. Arch Pediatr. 2003;10:716–8. [Article in French]
11. Ergaz Z, Simanovsky N, Rozovsky K, Leil SA, Ofek-Shlomai N, Revel-Vilk S, Bar-Oz B. Clinical outcome of umbilical artery catheter-related thrombosis—a cohort study. J Perinatol. 2012;32:933–40.
12. Escourrou G, De Luca D. Lung ultrasound decreased radiation exposure in preterm infants in a neonatal intensive care unit. Acta Paediatr. 2016;105:e237–9.
13. Fleming SE, Kim JH. Ultrasound-guided umbilical catheter insertion in neonates. J Perinatol. 2011;31:344–9.
14. Fluss J, Dinomais M, Kossorotoff M, Vuillerot C, Darteyre S, Chabrier S. Perspectives in neonatal and childhood arterial ischemic stroke. Expert Rev Neurother. 2017;17:135–42.
15. Franta J, Harabor A, Soraisham AS. Ultrasound assessment of umbilical venous catheter migration in preterm infants: a prospective study. Arch Dis Child Fetal Neonatal Ed. 2017;102:F251–5.
16. Gazula S. Umbilical venous catheter insertion in gastroschisis. Indian J Pediatr. 2014;81:1261–2.
17. Gorski L, Hadaway L, Hagle M, et al. Infusion therapy standards of practice. J Infus Nurs. 2021 Jan–Feb 01;44(1S Suppl 1):S1–S224.
18. Gupta AO, Peesay MR, Ramasethu J. Simple measurements to place umbilical catheters using surface anatomy. J Perinatol. 2015;35:476–80.
19. Jackson JK, Biondo DJ, Jones JM, Moor PJ, Simon SD, Hall RT, Kilbride HW. Can an alternative umbilical arterial catheter solution and flush regimen decrease iatrogenic hemolysis while enhancing nutrition? A double-blind, randomized, clinical trial comparing an isotonic amino acid with a hypotonic salt infusion. Pediatrics. 2004;114:377–83.
20. Kieran EA, Laffan EE, O'Donnell CP. Estimating umbilical catheter insertion depth in newborns using weight or body measurement: a randomised trial. Arch Dis Child Fetal Neonatal Ed. 2016;101:F10–5.
21. Klaassen IL, van Ommen CH, Middeldorp S. Manifestations and clinical impact of pediatric inherited thrombophilia. Blood. 2015;125:1073–7.
22. König K, Casalaz DM, Burke EJ, Watkins A. Accuracy of non-invasive blood pressure monitoring in very preterm infants. Intensive Care Med. 2012;38:670–6.
23. Kotnis R, Salloum A, Hitchcock R. Retained umbilical artery catheter presenting as an umbilical abscess. Arch Dis Child Fetal Neonatal Ed. 2000;83(1):F77.
24. Kumar N, Uhing MR, Powell M. Congenital absence of ductus venosus: an umbilical catheter with an abnormal path. J Perinatol. 2009;29:646–8.
25. Kumar PP, Kumar CD, Nayak M, Shaikh FA, Dusa S, Venkatalakshmi A. Umbilical arterial catheter insertion length: in quest of a universal formula. J Perinatol. 2012;32:604–7.
26. Lean WL, Dawson JA, Davis PG, Theda C, Thio M. Accuracy of 11 formulae to guide umbilical arterial catheter tip placement in newborn infants. Arch Dis Child Fetal Neonatal Ed. 2018;103(4):F364–9. https://doi.org/10.1136/archdischild-2017-313039. Epub 2017 Aug 17
27. Lei T, Xie HN, Feng JL. Prenatal diagnosis of four-vessel umbilical cord with supernumerary vein varix: a case report and literature review. J Obstet Gynaecol Res. 2017;43:1200–4.
28. Li J, Kong JY, James TE, Chandran S. Umbilical lines in a sick, extremely low birth weight infant: clinical quandary of X-ray images. BMJ Case Rep. 2016 Jun 22;2016
29. Limperopoulos C, Gauvreau KK, O'Leary H, Moore M, Bassan H, Eichenwald EC, Soul JS, Ringer SA, Di Salvo DN, du Plessis AJ. Cerebral hemodynamic changes during intensive care of preterm infants. Pediatrics. 2008;122:e1006–13.
30. McAdams RM, Winter VT, McCurnin DC, Coalson JJ. Complications of umbilical artery catheterization in a model of extreme prematurity. J Perinatol. 2009;29:685–92.

31. Mehler K, Nowak M, Oberthuer A, Hahn M, Roth B, Kribs A. Blood sampling via a peripheral artery catheter decreases cerebral oxygenation index in very low-birthweight infants. Acta Paediatr. 2014;103:1227–32.
32. Mendeloff J, Stallion A, Hutton M, Goldstone J. Aortic aneurysm resulting from umbilical artery catheterization: case report, literature review, and management algorithm. J Vasc Surg. 2001;33:419–24.
33. Michel F, Brevaut-Malaty V, Pasquali R, Thomachot L, Vialet R, Hassid S, Nicaise C, Martin C, Panuel M. Comparison of ultrasound and X-ray in determining the position of umbilical venous catheters. Resuscitation. 2012;83:705–9.
34. Piersigilli F, Bersani I, Giliberti P, Ronchetti MP, Mancinelli RL, Cavadenti I, Dotta A. Neonatal limb ischemia: caudal blockade and NIRS monitoring. Eur J Pediatr. 2014;173:1599–601.
35. Roll C, Hüning B, Käunicke M, Krug J, Horsch S. Umbilical artery catheter blood sampling decreases cerebral blood volume and oxygenation in very low birthweight infants. Acta Paediatr. 2000;89:862–6.
36. Roll C, Hüning B, Käunicke M, Krug J, Horsch S. Umbilical artery catheter blood sampling volume and velocity: impact on cerebral blood volume and oxygenation in very-low-birthweight infants. Acta Paediatr. 2006;95:68–73.
37. Romantsik O, Bruschettini M, Zappettini S, Ramenghi LA, Calevo MG. Heparin for the treatment of thrombosis in neonates. Cochrane Database Syst Rev. 2016;11:CD012185.
38. Schlesinger AE, Braverman RM, DiPietro MA, Pictorial essay. Neonates and umbilical venous catheters: normal appearance, anomalous positions, complications, and potential aid to diagnosis. AJR Am J Roentgenol. 2003;180:1147–53.
39. Shahid S, Dutta S, Symington A, Shivananda S; McMaster University NICU. Standardizing umbilical catheter usage in preterm infants. Pediatrics. 2014;133:e1742–52.
40. Shibata M, Kanehiro H, Shinkawa T, Fujita Y, Yada K, Kamamoto T, Arai I, Nishikubo T, Sakata M, Kobayashi H, Takeda M, Nonomura A, Takahashi Y. A neonate with umbilical arteriovenous malformation showing hemorrhagic shock from massive umbilical hemorrhage. Am J Perinatol. 2009;26:583–6.
41. Simanovsky N, Ofek-Shlomai N, Rozovsky K, Ergaz-Shaltiel Z, Hiller N, Bar-Oz B. Umbilical venous catheter position: evaluation by ultrasound. Eur Radiol. 2011;21:1882–6.
42. Slow blood sampling from an umbilical artery catheter prevents a decrease in cerebral oxygenation in the preterm newborn. Pediatrics. 2003;111:e73–6.
43. So MJ, Kobayashi D, Anthony E, Singh J. Pseudoaneurysm formation after umbilical arterial catheterization: an uncommon but potentially life-threatening complication. J Perinatol. 2012;32:147–9.
44. Sritipsukho P, Sritipsukho S, Wattanaruangkowit P. Accuracy of the distance between suprasternal notch and superior iliac spine to determine umbilical arterial catheter length. J Med Assoc Thail. 2010;93:183–6.
45. Sritipsukho S, Sritipsukho P. Simple and accurate formula to estimate umbilical arterial catheter length of high placement. J Med Assoc Thail. 2007;90:1793–7.
46. Takada H, Yoshikawa H, Imaizumi M, Kitamura T, Takeyama J, Kumaki S, Nomura A, Hara T. Delayed separation of the umbilical cord in two siblings with Interleukin-1 receptor-associated kinase 4 deficiency: rapid screening by flow cytometer. J Pediatr. 2006;148:546–8.
47. Takci S, Esenboga S, Gonc N, Yigit S. Persistent hypoglycemia caused by umbilical arterial catheterization. J Pediatr Endocrinol Metab. 2011;24:1081–3.
48. Vali P, Fleming SE, Kim JH. Determination of umbilical catheter placement using anatomic landmarks. Neonatology. 2010;98:381–6.
49. van de Vijver E, van den Berg TK, Kuijpers TW. Leukocyte adhesion deficiencies. Hematol Oncol Clin North Am. 2013;27:101–16.
50. Weiss M, Balmer C, Cornelius A, Frey B, Bauersfeld U, Baenziger O. Arterial fast bolus flush systems used routinely in neonates and infants cause retrograde embolization of flush solution into the central arterial and cerebral circulation. Can J Anaesth. 2003;50:386–91.

51. Wellenstein MB, Stevenson DK. New technique for umbilical artery catheter placement in the neonate. J Pediatr. 2015;166:501.
52. Wieland I, Jack T, Seidemann K, Boehne M, Schmidt F, Happel CM, Koeditz H, Bertram H, Sasse M. Neonatal aortic arch thrombosis: analysis of thrombophilic risk factors and prognosis. Cardiol Young. 2014;24:33–9.
53. Wright IM, Owers M, Wagner M. The umbilical arterial catheter: a formula for improved positioning in the very low birth weight infant. Pediatr Crit Care Med. 2008;9:498–501.
54. Wyers MR, McAlister WH. Umbilical artery catheter use complicated by pseudoaneurysm of the aorta. Pediatr Radiol. 2002;32:199–201.
55. Zhou J, Elkhateeb O, Lee KS. Comparison of non-invasive vs invasive blood pressure measurement in neonates undergoing therapeutic hypothermia for hypoxic ischemic encephalopathy. J Perinatol. 2016;36:381–5.

Chapter 18
Peripheral Arterial Lines

Daniele G. Biasucci

18.1 Introduction

Arterial catheter placement is a common and essential procedure performed in many clinical settings like medical and surgical emergencies, major elective and emergency surgeries, and intensive care unit stay, mainly for hemodynamic monitoring and repeated arterial blood sampling.

The site most used for arterial cannulation is the radial artery (Fig. 18.1). Further sites include the femoral, axillary, brachial and dorsalis pedis arteries. The radial artery is the first choice for invasive blood pressure monitoring primarily because of the superficial nature of the vessel, the low rate of complications and the optimal nursing and dressing. The second most common site for arterial cannulation after radial artery is the femoral artery (Fig. 18.2). One advantage of femoral artery cannulation is that the vessel is larger than the radial artery, however, it is associated with a higher risk of infections, especially in critically ill children. Axillary artery is associated with high risks of hematoma, pneumothorax, and infections. The brachial artery is usually not recommended for cannulation since it is an 'end' artery, and its damage would endanger the circulation of the whole upper limb.

Contraindications for arterial line placement include absent pulse, burned skin over the cannulation site, inadequate circulation to the extremity with inadequate collateral flow, infection at the cannulation site, and presence of synthetic vascular grafts.

The traditional approach for arterial catheter placement is the pulse palpation method in which the pulse of the artery is the landmark for puncture site and needle

D. G. Biasucci (✉)
Intensive Care Unit, Department of Emergency, Anesthesiology and Intensive Care,
Fondazione Policlinico Universitario "A. Gemelli" IRCCS, Rome, Italy
e-mail: danieleguerino.biasucci@policlinicogemelli.it

D. G. Biasucci et al. (eds.), *Vascular Access in Neonates and Children*,
https://doi.org/10.1007/978-3-030-94709-5_18

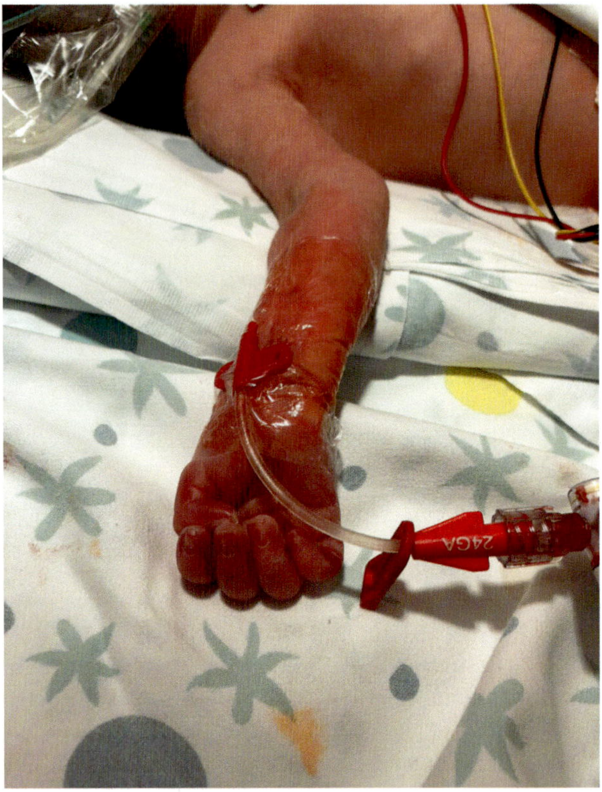

Fig. 18.1 Arterial catheter in brachial artery

direction. However, due to the small caliber of the arteries, arterial cannulation can be challenging in pediatric patients, especially in neonates, small infants and small children. In these patients, the traditional pulse palpation method is technically difficult since it does not allow accurate localization of such small arteries. Multiple cannulation attempts are common and may account for serious complications. In the emergency settings, dehydration or hemodynamic instability—making the pulse weak and difficult to find—can further complicate this situation.

The most frequent complications are represented by arterial occlusion, hematoma formation and nerve injury. Although rare, other serious complications, such as permanent ischemic damage, sepsis and pseudoaneurysm formation, may occur.

For this reason, the use of doppler assistance and ultrasound guidance has been recently proposed for those developmental age patients particularly at risk for severe complications, given the well-known difficulties in achieving an arterial access.

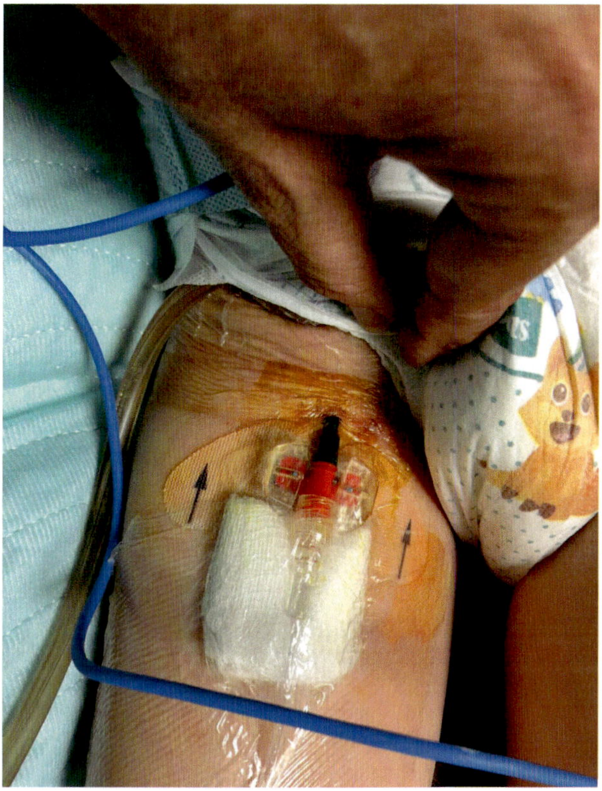

Fig. 18.2 Arterial catheter in femoral artery

18.2 Pulse Palpation Technique

For radial artery cannulation, the patient is in the supine position. The arm is placed in neutral position, with the palm up and the wrist dorsiflexed to 30–45 ° with a gauze under its dorsal surface. Excessive dorsiflexion must be avoided because it may compress the radial artery.

For femoral artery cannulation, the patient is also in the supine position, with the hip in mild external rotation. The artery is palpated at the midpoint between the anterior superior iliac spine and the pubic tubercle. The puncture site should be 2.5 cm below the inguinal ligament to allow control of bleeding and prevention of bleeding into the pelvis.

The non-dominant hand palpates the artery, while the dominant hand manipulates the intravascular needle or catheter, which is inserted at a 30-to-45-degree angle and is advanced slowly until pulsatile blood flow returns.

As already discussed above, pulse palpation technique is inaccurate for localization of small arteries in neonates, small infants, and small children, especially in emergency conditions in which hypotension and dehydration further complicate the procedure making the pulse weak and difficult to find. These special categories of patients often require multiple attempts which may account for complications.

18.3 Doppler Assistance

Doppler auditory assistance has been described as an alternative to the traditional pulse palpation method. This method allows to locate vascular flow and differentiate between veins and arteries whose flows have different patterns and tones. Thin pencil-like probes 9–10 MHz are used. Doppler assistance allows to locate the exact position of the artery where the area of the maximum tone of a pulsatile flow can be heard. The Doppler probe is maintained over the artery throughout the puncture. The right direction of the needle tip is identified by increased pitch or loss of Doppler tones when compressing tissues above the artery or the artery itself with the needle tip. The needle is then advanced until Doppler tones return to baseline, indicating re-expansion of the artery, or pulsatile blood flow appears from the needle hub. Unfortunately, this technique has been reported to have a success rate only at 46%, which is low, and a first-time success rate at 15%, which is very low [5].

18.4 Ultrasound Guidance

The use of ultrasound guidance for arterial catheters insertion has been proposed recently and most authors advocate for its use. Randomized controlled trials and a couple of systematic reviews and meta-analyses have been published on this topic. Current guidelines (2020 guidelines of the European Society of Anesthesia; 2021 Standards of the Infusion Nursing Society) recommend the use of ultrasound guidance for all arterial cannulations in pediatric patients.

Published evidence proves that ultrasound guidance significantly decreases the number of attempts improving the first attempt success rate and the success rate after only two attempts, as compared with traditional pulse palpation or Doppler assistance, both for radial artery—which is the first choice—and for femoral artery. Furthermore, complications like hematoma formation can be significantly reduced using ultrasound compared with any other methods.

Particularly, studies show that ultrasound guidance gains its maximum effectiveness and the greatest value in neonates, small infants, and small children. In fact, as previously commented, these are developmental ages in which a high risk for difficult arterial cannulation exists, since palpation for location of such small arteries may be inaccurate, especially when hemodynamic instability and hypovolemia make the pulse weak and much more difficult to find. Kantor and coworkers have found that factors most likely to interfere with peripheral arterial catheterization are patient age, patient systolic blood pressure, patient body mass index, degree of fluid status. In older children there is not a clear advantage of ultrasound guidance compared with pulse palpation technique, however, it is always undoubtedly useful in emergency and critical conditions like hypotension and hypovolemia.

Ultrasound has been shown to offer further advantages. Particularly, ultrasound allows an accurate sonographic-based pre-procedural assessment of all possible arterial options. The easiest and safest artery to be punctured, in terms of early and late complications, can be chosen using ultrasound. Particularly, pre-procedural sonographic assessment allows to perform a catheter/artery ratio to choose the most appropriate outer diameter of the arterial catheter for a given inner diameter of the artery. This kind of assessment allows to avoid arterial damage and thrombotic occlusion. In a study on adults, authors showed that if more than 20% of the radial artery lumen is occupied by catheter there is a significantly greater risk of thrombosis. Varga and coworkers have found that, usually, in children there are discrepancies between the measured real inner diameter of a radial artery and the catheter size proposed on the base of anthropometric characteristics. These discrepancies not only make the placement difficult but also have the potential for arterial injury. For all these reasons, it is important to measure the internal diameter of arteries in neonates, small infants, and small children prior to insertion of an intra-arterial catheter.

Regarding training and experience, studies have found that ultrasound guidance significantly increases first attempt success rate as compared with the pulse palpation technique when an expert operator, proficient in ultrasound-guided vascular cannulation, performs the procedure. No significant advantages have been found when the procedure had been performed by operators with an experience of less than 10 ultrasound guided vessel catheterizations. Other authors have found that the level of operators training and experience is one of the factors most likely affecting success rate of ultrasound guided arterial cannulation. An expert operator should perform no less than 10 supervised procedures to become proficient.

18.5 Insertion Technique

Disregarding the puncture technique (pulse palpation method, doppler assistance or ultrasound guidance), arterial catheterization can be performed using multiple methods.

The most commonly used methods are the following:

- Catheter over-the-needle
- Catheter over-the-wire, which includes:
  - direct Seldinger technique
  - modified Seldinger technique.

The choice of the appropriate method is determined by location. For radial artery cannulation, either the '*catheter over-the-needle*' technique or the '*catheter over-the-wire*' technique may be used. The latter is more common in adults and older children, whilst the former is more common in small infants and neonates. For femoral artery cannulation, the '*catheter over-the-wire*' technique is preferred.

Arterial cutdown for arterial access is not recommended and should be discouraged since it is associated with a high risk of arterial damage and infections.

Catheter over-the-needle technique. This technique is performed puncturing the skin over the artery and advancing the needle towards the pulsation with its bevel up and various angle's degrees, depending on the depth of the artery. Once the needle is in the arterial lumen, a flash of bright red blood can be seen in the hub. Once this flash has been obtained, the needle-catheter must be lower to an angle of 10–20° from the skin and inserted about 1–2 mm further, so to advance the catheter into the lumen of the artery. During ultrasound guided cannulation, the operator can follow, in real time, both the entry of the needle tip and that of the tip of the cannula. Only when the needle tip and the cannula are both in the lumen of the artery the outer cannula can be advanced into the artery over the needle which, at the end, must be retracted.

Catheter over-the-wire technique. The catheter over-the-wire method is a further option for arterial catheterization. This technique includes the Seldinger and modified Seldinger techniques which are very similar since both involve entering the artery with a needle, then advancing a wire into the artery through the needle, and finally threading the catheter over the wire into the artery. However, whereas the Seldinger technique uses separate components, the modified Seldinger technique uses an integrated needle-catheter-wire system. Catheter over-the-wire techniques can be used for superficial arteries like radial artery and are the recommended method for femoral arteries cannulation. This method should not be used routinely for radial artery cannulation in neonates and small infants, since inner diameter of the vessel is too small to allow an easy advancement of the guide wire.

18.6 Ultrasound-guided Puncture

Ultrasound guidance allows to follow, in real time, the advancement of the needle tip through the soft tissues into the lumen of the artery. When using catheter over-the-needle technique, ultrasound allows to visualize when also the cannula has entered the vessel so that only the cannula is advanced over the needle which, in turns, can be removed. On the other hand, when using a catheter over-the-wire technique, ultrasound allows real time visualization and control of wire advancement into the artery first, and then the catheter entry over the wire.

Ultrasound guided arterial puncture can be performed with any ultrasound device equipped with a linear probe dedicated to ultrasound guided vascular access

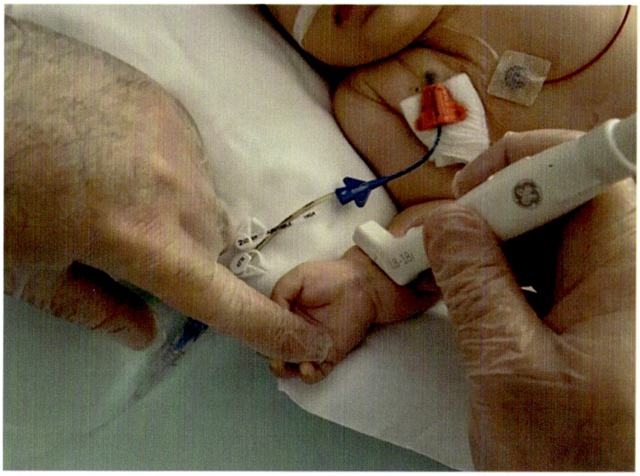

Fig. 18.3 Ultrasound scan of the brachial artery using a linear 'hockey stick' probe

procedures for neonates and children. In fact, in neonates and small infants, radial and femoral ones are superficial and have small diameters. For this reason, an ultrasound probe allowing maximum resolution of very superficial tissues—even if penalized by a low penetration in depth—is required. Currently, most of the ultrasound transducers used for this purpose have a frequency range of 7–15 MHz, which may imply a lack of resolution to allow accurate ultrasound guided cannulation of very shallow and small vessels like in neonates or small infants (Fig. 18.3). In these cases, Latham and coworkers have proposed the use of high-frequency micro-ultrasound transducers with a frequency range of 15–50 MHz which allows much higher resolution as compared with conventional ultrasound.

Currently, there are two techniques for ultrasound guided arterial cannulation: the short axis + out-of-plane technique (SA + OP) and the long axis + in-plane technique (LA + IP). Each of these techniques has advantages and disadvantages and both require appropriate training. However, despite obtaining LA requires longer time, there is no significant difference in the total time to successful cannulation between the two techniques.

Arteries can be visualized in short axis (SA) placing the probe perpendicular to the course and the long axis of the vessel. On the other hand, long axis (LA) can be obtained placing the probe parallel to the course of the vessel. SA and LA are imaging techniques and refer to the mutual position of the probe in respect to the vessel course.

The terms 'out-of-plane' (OP) and 'in-plane' (IP) refer to the direction of the needle in respect to the probe plane. OP and IP techniques are puncture techniques. In the OP puncture technique, the needle is directed perpendicular to the probe plane and the ultrasound beam, and it is visualized, in its short axis, as a hyperechogenic dot. Performing the IP technique, the needle is directed in a plane aligned with the major axis of the probe plane and the ultrasound beam. During the IP puncture, the entire needle tip and shaft can be visualized in its long axis.

18.6.1 Out-of-plane Puncture in Short Axis (SA + OP)

Arteries can be punctured OP using a SA view (Fig. 18.4). As discussed above, this technique is performed visualizing the artery in its SA in the middle of the screen so that he midpoint of the probe footprint becomes the reference point for puncture. The needle is then directed perpendicular to the midpoint of the probe with an angle greater than 45 ° and depending on the depth of the vessel. Using this technique, the needle appears as a hyper-echogenic dot. The operator can use or not the probe '*tilting*' technique to follow the needle tip during the procedure which consists in moving only the tail of the probe towards the needle hub so that the needle tip may be always included in the ultrasound beam. Using this '*tilting*' technique is possible to visualize the needle in the subcutaneous tissues and then, moving the tail of the probe so to have the needle tip always inside the ultrasound beam, to follow it until it entries the arterial lumen. The tilting technique requires some additional abilities especially when puncturing very superficial and small arteries. However, an adequate training may overcome any difficulties. If the tilting technique is not performed, the operator can hold the probe perpendicular to the artery inserting the needle with the above-described direction so that indirect soft tissues movement can be seen and then, if the right angle has been maintained, the needle tip as a hyper-echogenic dot entering the arterial lumen can be visualized. The SA + OP technique

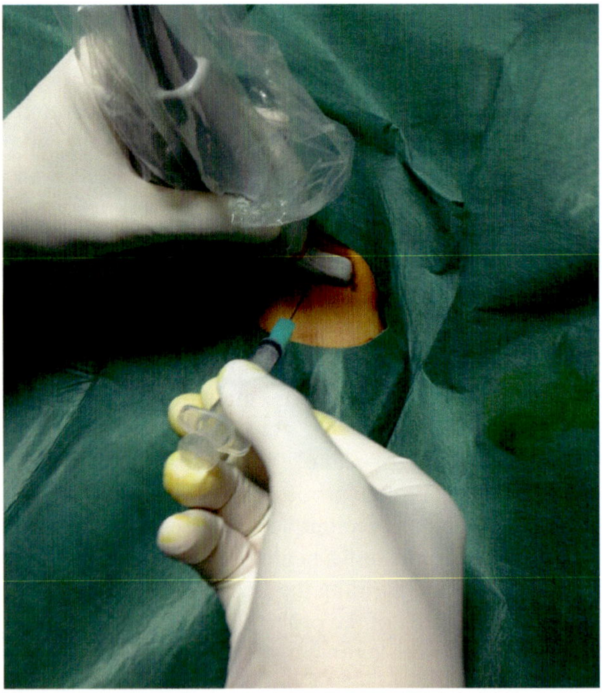

Fig. 18.4 Short axis/out of plane puncture

combines the advantages of the SA view, which gives us the appropriate panoramic view of the artery, and, eventually, of the accompanying nerves and veins (as in case of the femoral artery approach), with the disadvantage of the OP puncture technique which mainly consists in the difficulty to follow the needle tip appearing as a hyper-echogenic dot. Using this technique, the operator may inadvertently visualize a part of the needle shaft misinterpreting it as the tip of the needle. SA + OP technique may appear to be more comfortable when very small arteries are approached, and LA is difficult to obtain. However, posterior wall puncture rate has been found to be higher using this technique, as compared with LA + IP, due to the known difficulties to follow the tip of the needle.

18.6.2 In-plane Puncture in Long Axis (LA + IP)

On the other hand, the LA-IP technique combines the advantages of the IP puncture which allows better visualization of the needle tip and shaft trajectory, with the disadvantages of LA view of the vessel which does not allow a panoramic view of the nerve-vascular bundle. Using this technique, the operator may inadvertently visualize and/or puncture the accompanying veins. In fact, once the vessel has been visualized in its LA, the needle must be directed in a plane aligned and parallel with the probe plane exactly in the middle of the transducer footprint so to have the entire needle tip and shaft always included in the ultrasound beam not getting out of it. Even if LA requires longer time as compared with SA, the LA + IP technique has been found to have a lower rate of posterior wall penetration since it allows easier real time control of the needle tip and shaft trajectory.

During catheter over-the-needle cannulation technique, disregarding the puncture technique, LA view can be performed to accurately verify when also the outer cannula has entered the artery so to decide when it can be safely advanced visualizing real time advancement into the lumen. LA can be also used to be sure of the correct placements of wires and catheters into the arterial lumen even when catheter over-the-wire technique is performed.

18.7 Conclusions

- Radial artery is the first choice since it is associated with fewer complications and offers a nice reliability of hemodynamic parameters. Femoral artery is not considered the first choice since it is associated with a higher risk of infection complications.
- Compared to pulse palpation and doppler assisted methods, ultrasound guidance has been shown to be effective in reducing the number of attempts, increasing first attempt success rate and reducing complications.

- Ultrasound guidance is strongly recommended in small infants and small children and in all cases of emergency conditions when hypotension or dehydration and hypovolemia may further complicate the procedure.
- Proper ultrasound equipment must be used. Probes should have a high range of frequency so to obtain the highest resolution of superficial tissues.
- Ultrasound must be used for pre-procedural evaluation of all possible arterial options to choose the safest and easiest artery to be punctured in that specific patient in that specific clinical situation.
- Particularly, ultrasound must be used for pre-procedural evaluation of internal diameters of the artery so to choose an artery and a catheter caliber with optimal catheter/artery ratio to prevent early mechanical arterial damage and late thrombotic complication.
- There are two techniques for ultrasound-guided arterial cannulation: SA + OP and LA + IP. Each of these techniques has advantages and disadvantages and both require appropriate training.
- Ultrasound must be used also after puncture, to guide and verify correct advancement of wires and catheters.
- Ultrasound can also be used to diagnose eventual late complications like thrombotic occlusion of an artery with a catheter inside.
- Ultrasound guidance reaches its maximum effectiveness when performed by operators who had already fulfilled no less than 10 supervised ultrasound guided vascular access procedures.

Bibliography

1. Anantasit N, Cheeptinnakorntaworn P, Khositseth A, Lertbunrian R, Chantra M. Ultrasound versus traditional palpation to guide radial artery cannulation in critically ill children: a randomized trial. J Ultrasound Med. 2017 Dec;36(12):2495–501. https://doi.org/10.1002/jum.14291.
2. Aouad MT, Kanazi GE, Abdallah FW, Moukaddem FH, Turbay MJ, Obeid MY, Siddik-Sayyid SM. Femoral vein cannulation performed by residents: a comparison between ultrasound-guided and landmark technique in infants and children undergoing cardiac surgery. Anesth Analg. 2010 Sep;111(3):724–8. https://doi.org/10.1213/ANE.0b013e3181e9c475.
3. Aouad-Maroun M, Raphael CK, Sayyid SK, Farah F, Akl EA. Ultrasound-guided arterial cannulation for paediatrics. Cochrane Database Syst Rev. 2016 Sep 14;9:CD011364. https://doi.org/10.1002/14651858.CD011364.pub2.
4. Bedford RF. Radial arterial function following percutaneous cannulation with 18- and 20-gauge catheters. Anesthesiology. 1977;47:37–9.
5. Biasucci DG, La Greca A, Scoppettuolo G, Pittiruti M. Ultrasound-guided central venous catheterization: it is high time to use a correct terminology. Crit Care Med. 2015 Sep;43(9):e394–6. https://doi.org/10.1097/CCM.0000000000001069.
6. Ganesh A, Kaye R, Cahill AM, Stern W, Pachikara R, Gallagher P, et al. Evaluation of ultrasound-guided radial artery cannulation in children. Pediatr Crit Care Med. 2009;10(1):45–8.
7. Gorski L, Hadaway L, Hagle M, et al. Infusion therapy standards of practice. J Infus Nurs. 2021 Jan–Feb 01;44(1S Suppl 1):S1–S224.

8. Gu WJ, Tie HT, Liu JC, Zeng XT. Efficacy of ultrasound-guided radial artery catheterization: a systematic review and meta-analysis of randomized controlled trials. Crit Care. 2014 May 8;18(3):R93. https://doi.org/10.1186/cc13862.
9. Hansen MA, Juhl-Olsen P, Thorn S, Frederiksen CA, Sloth E. Ultrasonography-guided radial artery catheterization is superior compared with the traditional palpation technique: a prospective, randomized, blinded, crossover study. Acta Anaesthesiol Scand. 2014 Apr;58(4):446–52.
10. Ishii S, Shime N, Shibasaki M, Sawa T. Ultrasound-guided radial artery catheterization in infants and small children. Pediatr Crit Care Med. 2013;14(5):471–3.
11. Kantor DB, Su E, Milliren CE, Conlon TW. Ultrasound guidance and other determinants of successful peripheral artery catheterization in critically ill children. Pediatr Crit Care Med. 2016 Dec;17(12):1124–30.
12. King MA, Garrison MM, Vavilala MS, Zimmerman JJ, Rivara FP. Complications associated with arterial catheterization in children. Pediatr Crit Care Med. 2008;9(4):367–71.
13. Lamperti M, Biasucci DG, Disma N, Pittiruti M, Breschan C, Vailati D, Subert M, Traškaitė V, Macas A, Estebe JP, Fuzier R, Boselli E, Hopkins P. European Society of Anaesthesiology guidelines on peri-operative use of ultrasound-guided for vascular access (PERSEUS vascular access). Eur J Anaesthesiol. 2020;37(5):344–76. https://doi.org/10.1097/EJA.0000000000001180. Erratum in: Eur J Anaesthesiol 2020 Jul;37(7):623
14. Latham GJ, Veneracion ML, Joffe DC, Bosenberg AT, Flack SH. Low DK High-frequency micro-ultrasound for vascular access in young children—a feasibility study by the High-frequency UltraSound in Kids studY (HUSKY) group. Paediatr Anaesth. 2013 Jun;23(6):529–35. https://doi.org/10.1111/pan.12131.
15. Liu L, Tan Y, Li S, Tian J. "Modified dynamic needle tip positioning" short-axis, out-of-plane, ultrasound-guided radial artery cannulation in neonates: a randomized controlled trial. Anesth Analg. 2018 May 21—Volume Publish Ahead of Print—Issue—https://doi.org/10.1213/ANE.0000000000003445.
16. Mitchell JD, Welsby IJ. Techniques of arterial access. Surgery. 2004;22(1):3–4.
17. Scheer BV, Perel A, Pfeiffer UJ. Clinical review: complications and risk factors of peripheral arterial catheters used for haemodynamic monitoring in anaesthesia and intensive care medicine. Crit Care. 2002;6(3):198–204.
18. Schindler E, Kowald B, Swess H, Niehaus-Borquez B, Tausch B, Brecher A. Catheterization of the radial or brachial artery in neonates and infants. Paediatr Anaesth. 2005;15(8):677–82.
19. Schwemmer U, Arzet HA, Trautner H, Rauch S, Roewer N, Greim CA. Ultrasound-guided arterial cannulation in infants improves success rate. Eur J Anaesthesiol. 2006;23(6):476–80.
20. Siddik-Sayyid SM, Aouad MT, Ibrahim MH, Taha SK, Nawfal MF, Tfaili YJ, Kaddoum RN. Femoral arterial cannulation performed by residents: a comparison between ultrasound-guided and palpation technique in infants and children undergoing cardiac surgery. Paediatr Anaesth. 2016 Aug;26(8):823–30. https://doi.org/10.1111/pan.12935.
21. Song IK, Choi JY, Lee JH, Kim EH, Kim HJ, Kim HS, Kim JT. Short-axis/out-of-plane or long-axis/in-plane ultrasound-guided arterial cannulation in children: a randomised controlled trial. Eur J Anaesthesiol. 2016 Jul;33(7):522–7. https://doi.org/10.1097/EJA.0000000000000453.
22. Ueda K, Puangsuvan S, Hove MA, Bayman EO. Ultrasound visual image-guided vs Doppler auditory-assisted radial artery cannulation in infants and small children by non-expert anaesthesiologists: a randomized prospective study. Br J Anaesth. 2013;110(2):281–6.
23. Varga EQ, Candiotti KA, Saltzman B, Gayer S, Giquel J, Castillo-Pedraza C, et al. Evaluation of distal radial artery cross-sectional internal diameter in pediatric patients using ultrasound. Paediatr Anaesth. 2013;23(5):460–2.

Part V
Special Considerations in Pediatric Vascular Access

Chapter 19
Access for Dialysis and Apheresis

Xavier Torterüe and Pierre Tissières

19.1 Introduction

Success of dialysis or apheresis is due to a large part to the good choice of vascular access. Indeed, for both dialysis and apheresis, the blood flow in the catheter should remain as laminar as possible so to maintain correct suction and reinjection pressures and reduce hemolysis. Optimal blood flow is directly related to the site of insertion, length, and diameter of the catheter. This chapter will summarize current recommendations for vascular access in children with renal failure requiring dialysis or affected by clinical conditions requiring apheresis.

19.2 Material

The type of the catheter must be chosen according to the therapeutic objectives. Blood flow rate of 3 to 5 ml/kg min (in adult patient: 200–300 ml/min) should be targeted to allow a good efficacy of hemofiltration or dialysis, while lower flows (0.5–1 ml/kg min, 30–60 ml/min) may be sufficient for most apheretic procedures. Considering that blood flow is also dependent on the location of the tip, dialysis catheters are invariably central venous devices (i.e., tip in the right atrium, superior vena cava or inferior vena cava), while apheresis may be performed also with peripheral venous access devices.

X. Torterüe · P. Tissières (✉)
Pediatric Intensive Care and Neonatal Medicine, Le Kremlin-Bicêtre, France
e-mail: pierre.tissieres@aphp.fr

D. G. Biasucci et al. (eds.), *Vascular Access in Neonates and Children*,
https://doi.org/10.1007/978-3-030-94709-5_19

Another major difference is that while dialysis requires a specific double lumen central catheter, apheresis can be carried out either with a double lumen central catheter or with two different catheters (both peripheral, both central, or even one central and one peripheral).

As for double lumen dialysis catheters, manufacturers indicate the maximum blood flow allowed by the device depending on the diameter and length. Most catheters are in polyurethane, since the wall must be rigid enough to tolerate high pressures. The selection of the most adequate catheter is based on the adequacy of the catheter to the size and weight of the patient. As a rule, a large diameter must be preferred to decrease the risk of blood flow limitation. Though, the main limitation is the inner diameter of the vein chosen for cannulation. Catheters that occupy more than 33–45% of the diameter of the vein are prone to a high risk of catheter- related thrombosis. Examples of catheter size according to patient size are indicated in Table 19.1; it is understood that the final size of the catheter will also consider the size of the vein. If the double lumen catheter is needed for apheresis, catheters smaller than 6.5 Fr may be enough; in this case, it is recommended to use—'off label'—double lumen power injectable 5Fr and 6Fr catheters marketed as PICCs (Fig. 19.1).

Non-tunneled double lumen dialysis catheters are appropriate for renal replacement therapy for acute kidney injury. On the other hand, cuffed-tunneled dialysis catheters have a role only for periodic dialysis in children with chronic renal failure.

Table 19.1 Double lumen catheters for dialysis and apheresis

Patient size	Catheter size	Maximal blood flow
Neonate	6,5Fr	30–60 ml/min
3–6 kg	7Fr	30–60 ml/min
6–15 kg	8Fr	60–100 ml/min
15–30 kg	9Fr	75–150 ml/min
>30 kg	10–12Fr	150–200 ml/min
Adult	>12Fr	200–300 ml/min

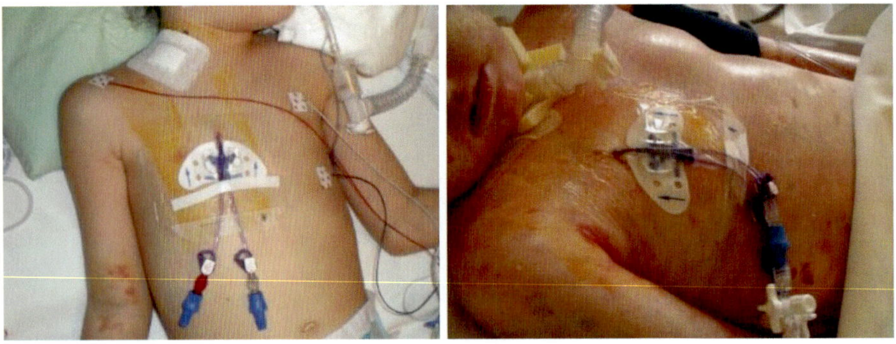

Fig. 19.1 Double lumen 5Fr power injectable PICCs inserted as CICC and used 'off-label' as tunneled, non-cuffed catheters for apheresis

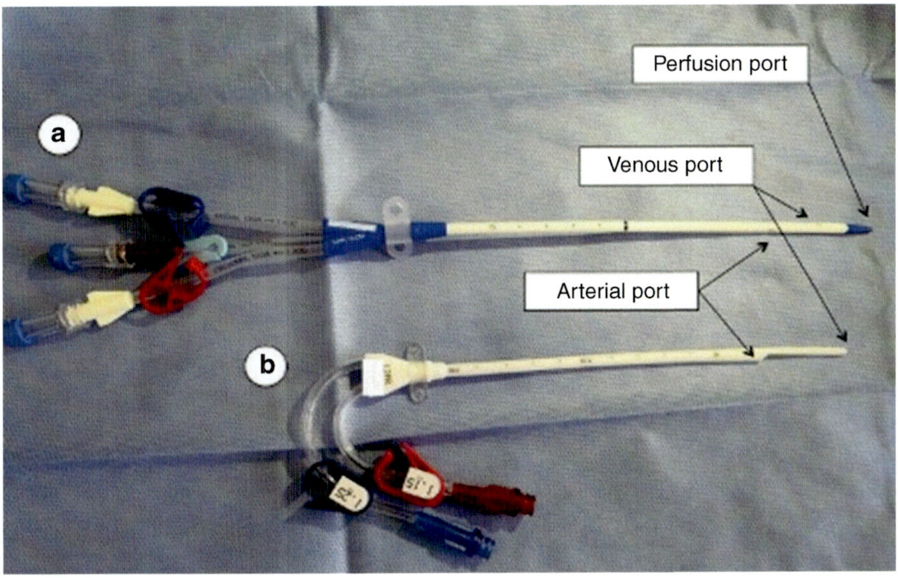

Fig. 19.2 Two different types of non-tunneled dialysis catheter (**a**) Multi-lumen dialysis catheter with perfusion line and straight extensions. (**b**) Step tip dual lumen dialysis catheter and J-curved extensions

Despite the demonstrated reduction in catheter related bloodstream infection and local skin infection as well as a better function, the indication to cuffed-tunneled catheters in the acutely ill patient is quite limited. Nonetheless, cuffed-tunneled dialysis catheters could be used also in Pediatric Intensive Care Units if an extended period of treatment is expected. A significant variability exist in the type of lumen and tip configuration (Fig. 19.2), but no significant blood flow and recirculation rate difference exist between the different catheter tip designs. Currently no recommendation exists on the type of configuration of dialysis catheter lumen and tip.

19.3 Insertion of Dialysis Catheters

Treatment efficacy and specific complications are associated with different insertion sites. The right supraclavicular area is the first choice as insertion site for dialysis catheters. In this area, ultrasound guidance allows a safe puncture either of the internal jugular vein (IJV) or of the brachiocephalic vein (BCV). Venipuncture of the BCV is easy in infants and children and it should be preferred since the diameter of the BCV is consistently larger than the IJV (thus reducing the risk of thrombosis). Recent studies suggest that in the pediatric population BCV puncture is safer than IJV puncture. Access to the subclavian vein or to the axillary vein should be avoided when placing a dialysis catheter, because of the high incidence of catheter

Table 19.2 Catheter insertion site choice

	Insertion site
1st choice	Right supraclavicular area
2nd choice	Left or right inguinal area
3rd choice	Left supraclavicular area

dysfunction, venous thrombosis and of late venous stenosis. Thrombosis or stenosis of subclavian/axillary vein may jeopardize the creation of future arteriovenous fistula in patients requiring chronic hemodialysis. Access to veins in the left supraclavicular area is not recommended since it is associated with risk of catheter dysfunction.

Non-tunneled dialysis catheters can also be inserted at the groin, accessing—by ultrasound guidance—either the right or the left common femoral vein (CFV). The insertion site in the groin area is nonetheless associated with a higher rate of infective complications compared to the supraclavicular area. Dialysis catheter dysfunction rate is similar between the supraclavicular and the femoral approach. Both femoral veins allow a direct insertion of the catheter inside the inferior vena cava, provided that the catheter is long enough (Table 19.2).

Regardless of the vein chosen (right BCF, right IJV, left or right CFV), the use of ultrasound guidance is mandatory. Access to the vein should also be obtained preferably using micro-puncture kits, so to reduce the local trauma and the risk of puncture-related complications.

As for all catheter insertions, a proper infection prevention strategy is of paramount importance, and it is based on proper hand hygiene, skin antisepsis with 2% chlorhexidine in 70% isopropyl alcohol, and maximal barrier precautions.

Cuffed-tunneled dialysis catheters are usually inserted only in the right supraclavicular area and the exit site is moved to the right infraclavicular area. The technique of insertion is the same that for non-tunneled catheter, except for the necessity to create a tunnel (see Chap. 8). The tunnel must be planned so that the Dacron cuff surrounding the catheter is placed inside the tunnel, at least 2.5 cm far from the exit site. Cuffs placed too close to the exit site are often associated with local infection, extrusion of the cuff and loss of the device.

19.4 Tip Position of Dialysis Catheters

To reduce catheter dysfunction and recirculation, the tip of catheter must be in a large vein. After access to the right BCV or IJV, the tip of the dialysis catheter must be located in the upper portion of the right atrium, just below the cavo—atrial junction. As tip location is of great importance for the proper performance of the dialysis, it should be assessed with the most accurate methodology, i.e., using the intracavitary ECG method and/or echocardiography (see Chap. 6), rather than radiological methods. With femoral access, the extremity of the dialysis catheter must be located in the inferior vena cava: catheters with tip in the iliac veins are inevitably associated with catheter dysfunction. This implies that the length of the catheters must be selected so to to ensure proper position of the catheter tip.

19.5 Removal of Dialysis Catheters

The dialysis catheter, due to its diameter and position, is at high risk of complications: local infection and sepsis, thrombosis, and vascular stenosis. The actual need for the non-tunneled dialysis catheter should be reassessed on a daily basis and the device should be removed as soon as possible, with a maximum dwelling time of 1–3 weeks. In children with acute renal failure, incidence of dialysis dependence significantly decreases at 6 and 12 months following initiation. Therefore, use of a cuffed-tunneled catheter should be considered in patients for whom prolonged hemodialysis is expected.

19.6 Access for Apheresis

If apheresis is performed using a non-tunneled dialysis catheter, the same recommendations above reported are valid. If the apheresis is planned only for few days, a femoral approach may be as good as a right supraclavicular approach, considering that the risk of infection or of thrombosis is quite low if the catheter is removed within 48–72 h.

On the other hand, apheresis—due to the low flow required for withdrawal/reinfusion of blood—can also be performed with a variety of techniques that depend on the venous patrimony of the child and on the presence of pre-existing central lines. For example, blood withdrawal can be done through a single lumen central or peripheral catheter and the reinfusion through a pre-existing central venous catheter (PICC, or CICC, or FICC) or through a large bore peripheral cannula. If a pre-existing central line is used for reinfusion, it should be vigorously flushed with saline (3–4 times the priming volume) after the apheresis.

19.7 Maintenance

Dialysis and apheresis catheters do not differ from the other central lines in terms of maintenance strategies: proper securement, surveillance of the exit site, skin antisepsis with 2% chlorhexidine, dressing change on a weekly basis, and so on. The only difference is that—in order to maintain an optimal functionality—dialysis and apheresis catheters should be flushed with saline but locked with an anticoagulant solution (either heparin or citrate). Lock with 4% citrate seems to have the same effectiveness of heparin lock, but a wider margin of safety.

19.8 Arteriovenous Fistula

Arterio-venous fistulas are reserved as vascular access for chronic hemodialysis in selected children with end stage renal disease. Due to high risk of complication (infection, thrombosis, bleeding, aneurysm, hematoma), the creation and the maintenance of the fistula should be assigned to specifically trained operators. Arterio-venous fistulas have been proposed also for children with chronic need for apheresis, though they are seldom used for this purpose.

Bibliography

1. Klouche K, Amigues L, Deleuze S, Beraud J-J, Canaud B. Complications, effects on dialysis dose, and survival of tunneled femoral dialysis catheters in acute renal failure. Am J Kidney Dis Off J Natl Kidney Found. 2007;49(1):99–108.
2. Mendu ML, May MF, Kaze AD, Graham DA, Cui S, Chen ME, et al. Non-tunneled versus tunneled dialysis catheters for acute kidney injury requiring renal replacement therapy: a prospective cohort study. BMC Nephrol. 2017;1z8(1):351.
3. Parienti J-J, Mégarbane B, Fischer M-O, Lautrette A, Gazui N, Marin N, et al. Catheter dysfunction and dialysis performance according to vascular access among 736 critically ill adults requiring renal replacement therapy: a randomized controlled study. Crit Care Med. 2010;38(4):1118–25.
4. Rewa O, Bagshaw SM. Acute kidney injury—epidemiology, outcomes and economics. Nat Rev Nephrol. 2014;10(4):193–207.
5. Schillinger F, Schillinger D, Montagnac R, Milcent T. Post catheterisation vein stenosis in haemodialysis: comparative angiographic study of 50 subclavian and 50 internal jugular accesses. Nephrol Dial Transplant Off Publ Eur Dial Transpl Assoc—Eur Ren Assoc. 1991;6(10):722–4.
6. Van Vong L, Osman D, Vinsonneau C. Groupe d'experts. Épuration extrarénale en réanimation adulte et pédiatrique. Recommandations formalisées d'experts sous l'égide de la Société de réanimation de langue française (SRLF), avec la participation de la Société française d'anesthésie-réanimation (SFAR), du Groupe francophone de réanimation et urgences pédiatriques (GFRUP) et de la Société francophone de dialyse (SFD). Réanimation. 2014;23(6):714–37.
7. Vazquez MA. Vascular access for dialysis: recent lessons and new insights. Curr Opin Nephrol Hypertens. 2009;18(2):116–21.
8. Vesely TM, Ravenscroft A. Hemodialysis catheter tip design: observations on fluid flow and recirculation. J Vasc Access. 2016;17(1):29–39.

Chapter 20
Intraosseous Access

Diego Neuhaus and Thomas Engelhardt

20.1 Introduction

The intraosseous infusion technique is a well-established alternative access in situations with difficult venous access or otherwise time-critical need for acute parenteral therapy. It usually represents a "life-line" that is meant to function as a bridge to a more durable and stable venous access, such as a central venous line.

Timely establishment of intravenous access in pediatric patients can be very demanding not only in emergency but also in pediatric anesthesia. Alternative techniques for difficult venous access such as ultrasound guided central or peripheral venous catheterization may not be feasible for lack of properly trained operators or lack of specific equipment, while there may be urgency to establish the parenteral access.

The technique of intraosseous infusion is generally considered easy to learn with a high first attempt success rate even in less experienced providers. A low risk profile and high reliability results in an extensive preclinical use and increasingly in clinical emergencies.

The correct technique is of utmost importance especially in infants where the most common puncture site, the proximal tibia, can be very difficult to palpate.

D. Neuhaus (✉)
Department of Anesthesia, University Children's Hospital, Zurich, Switzerland
e-mail: Diego.Neuhaus@kispi.uzh.ch

T. Engelhardt
Department of Anesthesia, Royal Aberdeen Children's Hospital, Aberdeen, UK

D. G. Biasucci et al. (eds.), *Vascular Access in Neonates and Children*,
https://doi.org/10.1007/978-3-030-94709-5_20

20.2 Access Sites

The most common puncture site in pediatric patients is the proximal antero-medial tibia. Other options are the distal femur, the distal tibia, or very rarely, the proximal humerus. The sternum is contraindicated due to possible mediastinal extravasation, which is unlikely in adults.

The tibia remains the preferred location for intraosseous infusion in pediatric emergency care. In school-aged children, this area for puncture is relatively easy to identify, palpate, and large, guaranteeing effective administration of fluids and drugs. It is important to realize, however, that in infants and toddlers subcutaneous tissue may sometimes impair the proper identification of the tibial puncture site. The relatively small tibial bone is covered by a substantial layer of subcutaneous tissue making complications such as dislocation, extravasation, and compartment syndrome more difficult to recognize. A practical and reliable 'step by step' approach to effective puncturing of the proximal tibia for these patients is offered below.

The medial malleolus is the distal part of the tibia. It is easy to find but the small external anatomical dimensions also indicate a small metaphysis for absorption. This area is, therefore, rarely a reliable alternative to the proximal tibia in infants and toddlers. The EZ-IO intraosseous infusion system has received an expanded CE mark approval for insertion in pediatric patients in the distal femur in 2011. The distal femur insertion target area is described as relatively large (measuring approximately 3 cm in length and 2 cm width for a newborn infant) and the anatomical landmarks (superior patella and distal femur) can easily be identified. There are currently only very few clinical reports of its use in pediatric patients, possibly due to a lack of information for clinical daily routine. Though, according to our personal experience, the distal femur is easy to identify and offers stable needle positioning with a very effective resorption time.

The proximal humerus is rarely used in pediatric patients. While it is a common puncture site in adult patients (for example, in car crash victims trapped in a car), the pediatric patient probably offers other more easily accessible puncture sites on the lower limbs.

20.3 Intraosseous Equipment

Several manufacturers offer a variety of different specialized systems to establish intraosseous access. These are either manual needles or assisted devices. Manual needles, such as the Cook Intraosseous Infusion Needle, have advantages of being inexpensive. However, they have some disadvantages: With the manual needles, it takes longer until the infusion to get started (30–60s); also, manual drilling is rarely straight, and therefore it produces a less stable and beveled drill hole; the needles

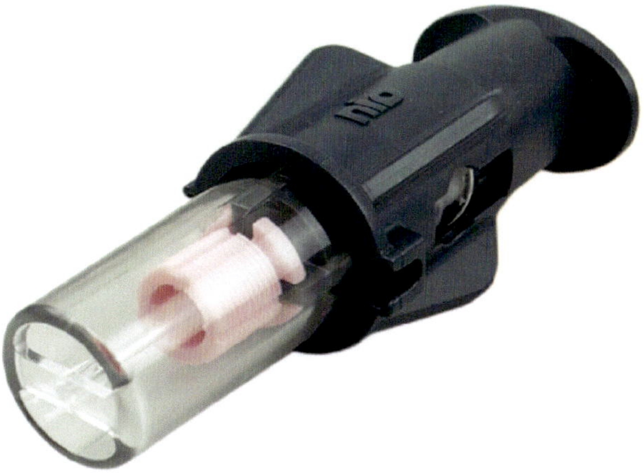

Fig. 20.1 Assisted device for intraosseous access (NIO)

might bend or break under effort and are reported to be more painful; last, fractures at the puncture site have also been described.

The EZ-IO and the NIO are assisted devices, very effective in pediatric patients.

- they remove the stress of manual drilling
- they offer better control over the needle
- they create effortlessly a stable cylindrical drill hole.

NIO (Fig. 20.1) has the additional advantage of not being dependent on an energy supply. While general principles of intraosseous insertion apply to all situations, the method that one ultimately adopts will depend on individual resources and experience.

20.4 Technique

Several general principles apply regardless of the technique used. These include aseptic precautions, use of local anesthetics at the puncture site in the awake patient, stable and firm fixation of the needle, and continuous monitoring during administration to prevent extravasation and swelling.

The process of intraosseous puncture at the proximal tibia in pediatric patients, for both the assisted devices or the manual needle, can be described as follows:

1. Identify anatomical landmarks (tuberosity of the tibia: from the lower edge of the patella, two fingers caudal and one finger medial). If this is not evident due to subcutaneous tissue, start palpation proximally with thumb and index finger on the tibial condyles, and proceed downwards where the bone is still clearly cone-shaped (Fig. 20.2). The puncture site is then in the middle of the still cone-shaped antero-medial edge, before reaching the cylindrical diaphysis, strictly between thumb and index finger (Fig. 20.3).

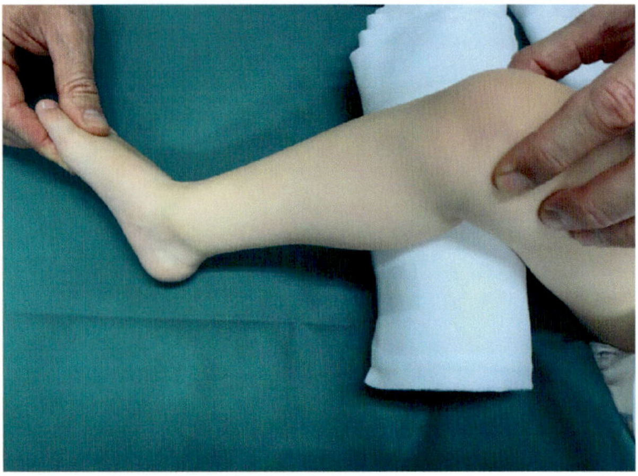

Fig. 20.2 Identification of bone landmarks

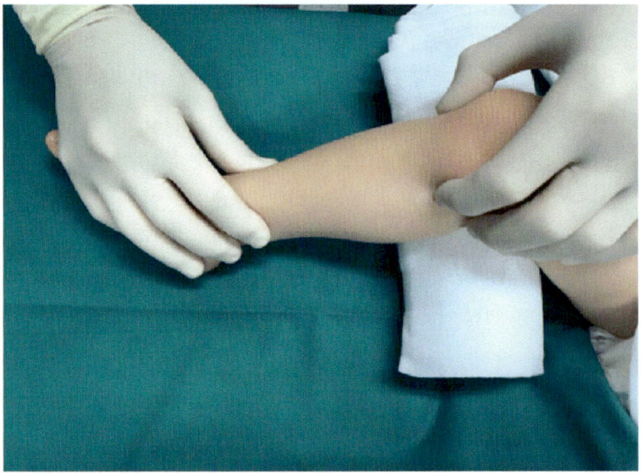

Fig. 20.3 Fixation of the bone between thumb and index of the non-dominant hand

2. Disinfect skin with 2% chlorhexidine in alcohol and take aseptic precautions (hand hygiene).
3. Consider periosteal local anesthesia in the awake patient.
4. Intraosseous puncture:

   (a) Always handle the tibia firmly between thumb and index finger of the non-dominant hand to ensure so that the target on the bone is as central as possible (Fig. 20.4)
   (b) Insert needle through skin without rotation (Fig. 20.5)
   (c) Verify the contact with the bone surface by "palpating" with the needle tip and ensure that at least 5 mm of the needle shaft is left over to advance the needle (Fig. 20.6)
   (d) Drill until loss of resistance is felt after penetrating the cortex (Fig. 20.7)
   (e) Check that needle is firmly inserted inside the bone (it must not move) (Fig. 20.8)

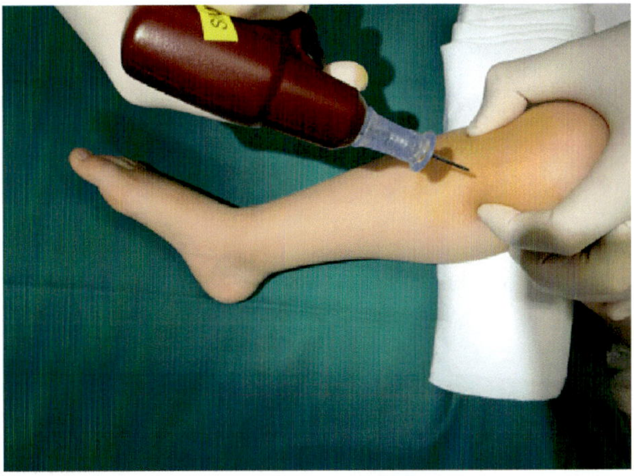

Fig. 20.4 Identification of the puncture site (the assisted device in the figure is EZ-IO)

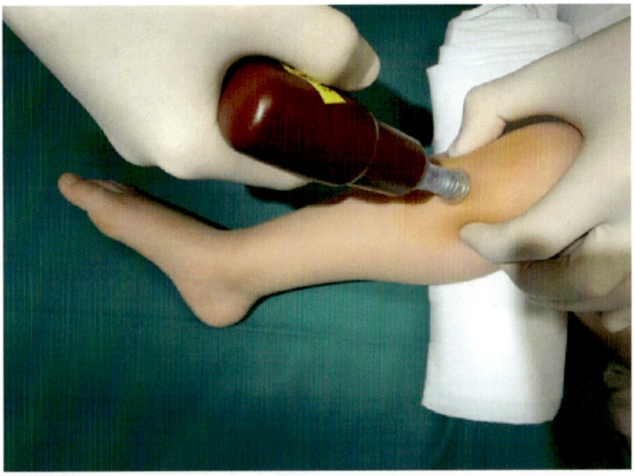

Fig. 20.5 Insertion of the needle through the skin

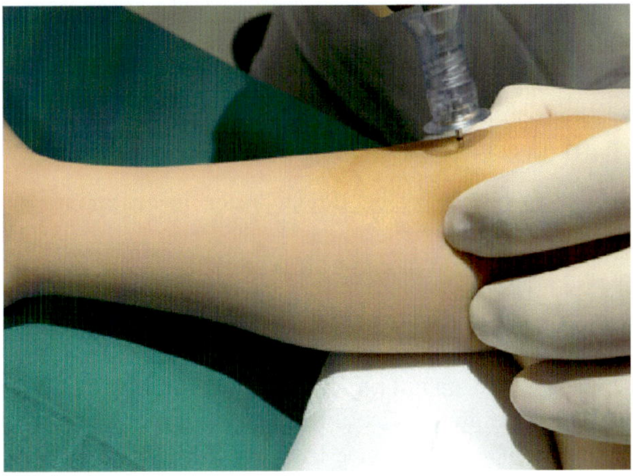

Fig. 20.6 Verification of the contact of the needle with the bone, with 5 mm left outside

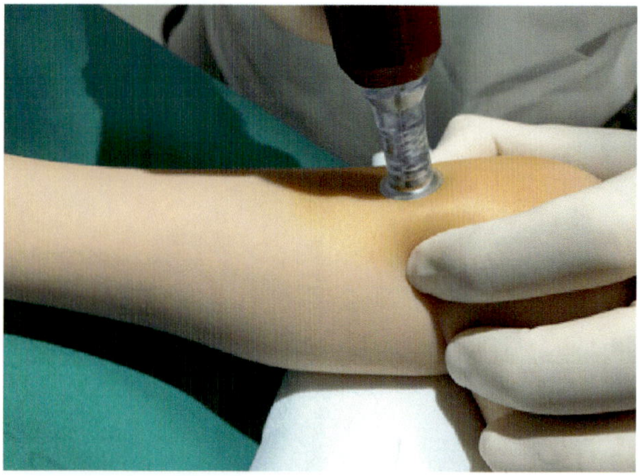

Fig. 20.7 Complete penetration of the needle inside the cortex of the bone

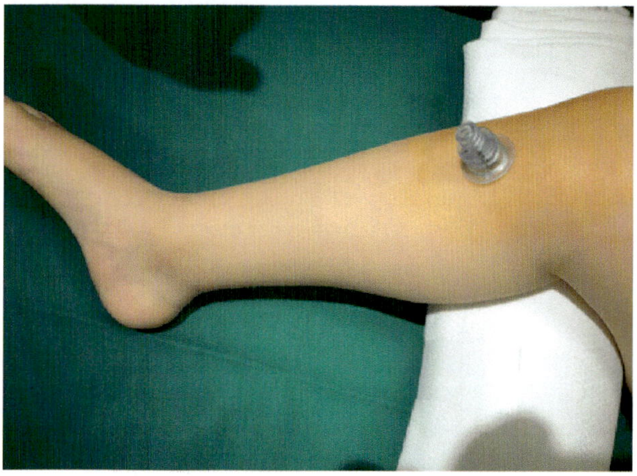

Fig. 20.8 Check the stability of the needle

(f) Aspiration of bone marrow is reassuring but not essential
(g) Consider the infusion of local anesthetic in the intramedullary spaces (if appropriate/necessary) in awake patient
(h) Secure the needle with a stabilizer (Figs. 20.9 and 20.10)
(i) Inject a 5–10 ml bolus of saline, to rule out extravasation (Fig. 20.11)

5. Check regularly the device after insertion, to detect secondary dislocation, extravasation, and compartment syndrome.

Please note that the puncture and the penetration of cortex and periosteum are often significantly less painful than the intramedullary injection. In unconscious patients, analgesia concerns are not an issue. In somnolent patients, placement of the intraosseous needle does not typically cause arousal, however, the patient might respond to the intramedullary injection. It is important to recognize that this is an expected response and not evidence that something went wrong. Pain upon injection can be

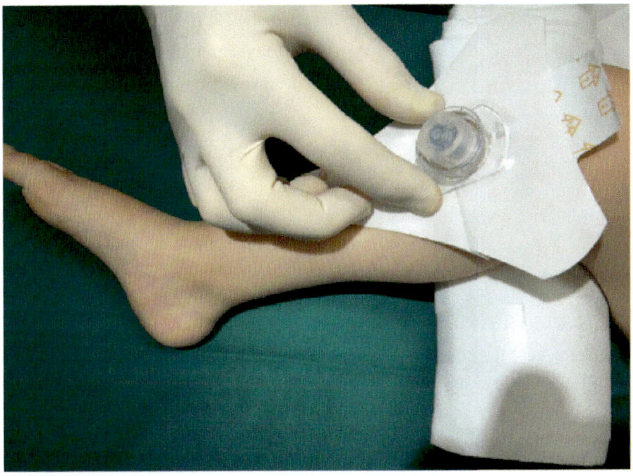

Fig. 20.9 Application of the securement

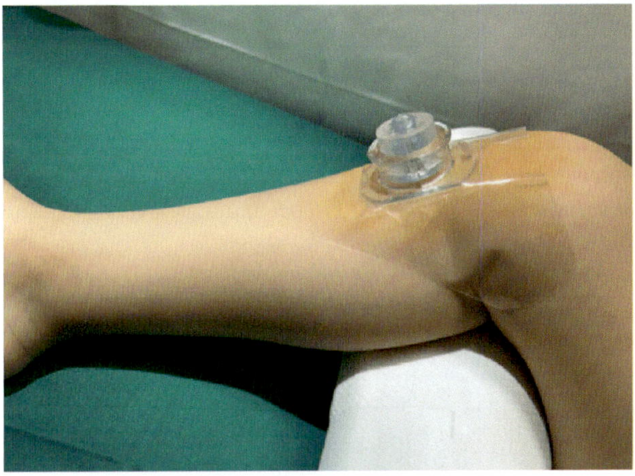

Fig. 20.10 The securement is applied, and the stability is verified again

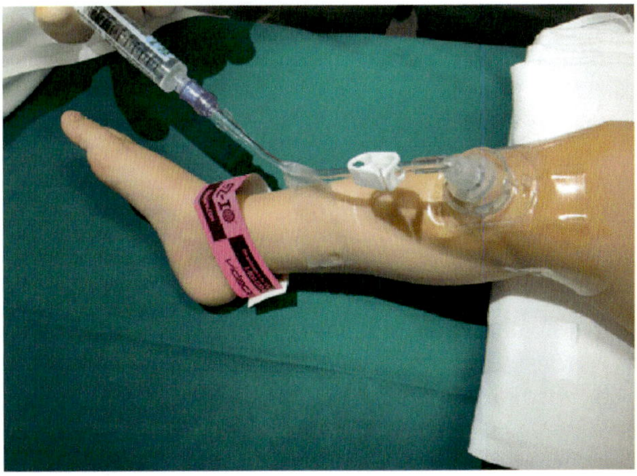

Fig. 20.11 Injection of a first bolus of 5–10 ml of saline

reduced by warning the awake patient, by slow injection (sensitivity diminishes rapidly after a few seconds) or by administering intramedullary local anesthetics (i.e. lidocaine). Subcutaneous and periosteal infiltration with local anesthetic is rarely required.

20.5 Complications

Once the intraosseous infusion is correctly established, the operator has the responsibility for checking periodically the limb for any signs of extravasation, swelling, or discoloration (pale or livid). While the intraosseous infusion is a safe and reliable procedure, it is only designed to provide a short-term access, as a bridge to a secure intravenous access: it should never be left in place for convenience.

Intraosseous infusions can result in complications that every provider must be aware of. Needle dislocation and extravasation are the most common complications. These complications occur either due to initial misplacement or due to forceful manipulation during transport or positioning of the child, and they are often associated with improvised securement techniques. Dislocation can lead to compartment syndrome or drug-induced tissue necrosis, and implies loss of the access. Therefore, correct securement and local monitoring are of paramount importance. There are several reports of severe tissue damage, even amputation, after dislocation of the needle tip.

Osteomyelitis can be a severe and significant complication of intraosseous access. To reduce the risk of osteomyelitis, aseptic technique during insertion and maintenance of the access plays a critical role. Some authors support a single dose administration of a first-generation broad spectrum cephalosporin antibiotic, though this practice is not based on scientific evidence. Osteomyelitis might also result from blood-borne contamination from other sources, regardless of aseptic precautions. Overall, osteomyelitis following intraosseous insertion is rare and should not prevent the practitioner from using the intraosseous technique when required.

Injury of the growth-plate and consecutive growth deviation has not been reported in humans. The operator must adhere to the recommended landmarks in order to minimize this theoretical risk.

20.6 Contraindications

There are very few contraindications for insertion of an intraosseous needle, if a patient really requires an urgent access. Nevertheless, some special situations need to be considered. Absolute contraindications include local fractures, or recent orthopedic manipulation at the site of needle insertion, or prior unsuccessful intraosseous access. A previously penetrated cortex will cause extravasation of the administered medication, with local tissue damage. There are also descriptions of extravasation through a bore hole of a freshly lost intraosseous needle at the proximal tibia after injecting through an intraosseous infusion at the distal tibia. An alternative insertion site should be considered.

Relative contraindications include local infection at the site of the planned needle insertion, osteogenesis imperfecta, osteopetrosis, and thermal injury at the puncture site. Again, an alternative insertion site should be considered.

20.7 Conclusions

The establishment of an access in patients with difficult venous access requires a contingency plan, regular training, and good preparation. Easy and quick access to appropriate equipment that requires little or no preparation time is essential in emergency situations. Therefore, we recommend that the intraosseous kits should be readily available in all areas where pediatric patients are cared for, especially in the operating room, emergency room, and trauma wards. Training in intraosseous infusion techniques should be tailored to the specific needs of small children with a special regard to the anatomical landmarks, the correct securement methods, and the necessity to monitor periodically the device. To maintain competency, intraosseous infusion training should be accessible to all team members on a regular basis, at least twice a year. Task fixation and/or the anesthetist's pride in situations where venous access is difficult should no longer delay the onset of parenteral therapy by way of intraosseous access.

The intraosseous infusion technique is a quick, reliable, and safe alternative especially in pediatric patients. Following general and insertion technique-specific safety principles, it is one of the best alternative option for patients with challenging venous access and an urgent need for parenteral treatment.

Bibliography

1. Burgert JM. A primer on intraosseous access: history, clinical considerations, and current devices. Am J Disaster Med. 2016;11(3):167–73.
2. Hallas P, Brabrand M, Folkestad L. Complication with intraosseous access: scandinavian users' experience. West J Emerg Med. 2013;14(5):440–3.
3. Hallas P, Folkestad L, Brabrand M. How many training modalities are needed to obtain procedural confidence in intraosseous access? A questionnaire study. Eur J Emerg Med. 2011;18(6):360–2.
4. Hansen M, Meckler G, Spiro D, Newgard C. Intraosseous line use, complications, and outcomes among a population-based cohort of children presenting to California hospitals. Pediatr Emerg Care. 2011;27(10):928–32.
5. Kwon OY, Park SY, Yoon TY. Educational effect of intraosseous access for medical students. Korean J Med Educ. 2014;26(2):117–24.
6. Maurin O, de Regoix S, Legonidec E, Tourtier JP, Kaiser E. Leg ischemia complicating the intraosseous infusion of epinephrine for a Djiboutian child. Med Sante Trop. 2014;24(2):214–6.

7. Neuhaus D. Intraosseous infusion in elective and emergency pediatric anesthesia: when should we use it? Curr Opin Anaesthesiol. 2014;27(3):282–7.
8. Oesterlie GE, Petersen KK, Knudsen L, Henriksen TB. Crural amputation of a newborn as a consequence of intraosseous needle insertion and calcium infusion. Pediatr Emerg Care. 2014;30(6):413–4.
9. Petitpas F, Guenezan J, Vendeuvre T, Scepi M, Oriot D, Mimoz O. Use of intraosseous access in adults: a systematic review. Crit Care. 2016;20:102.
10. Reuter-Rice K, Patrick D, Kantor E, Nolin C, Foley J. Characteristics of children who undergo intraosseous needle placement. Adv Emerg Nurs J. 2015;37(4):301–7.
11. Schwindt JC. Intraosseous access-of no value in neonatal resuscitation? Resuscitation. 2016:103–5.
12. Suominen PK, Nurmi E, Lauerma K. Intraosseous access in neonates and infants: risk of severe complications—a case report. Acta Anaesthesiol Scand. 2015;59(10):1389–93.
13. Tobias JD, Ross AK. Intraosseous infusions: a review for the anesthesiologist with a focus on pediatric use. Anesth Analg. 2010;110(2):391–401.
14. Yamamoto T, Schindler E. Anasthesiol Intensivmed Notfallmed Schmerzther. Vascular access in pediatric patients in emergency situations. 2017;52(1):55–64.

Chapter 21
Prevention and Treatment of Catheter-Related Complications

Mauro Pittiruti, Giancarlo Scoppettuolo, and Davide Celentano

21.1 Infection

Infections represent the most severe and most dangerous complication potentially related to venous access devices (VADs), in the pediatric patient (neonate, infant, child) as much as in adults. Any VAD implies a breakthrough of the defense barriers of the body, with the possibility of invasion of bacteria inside the tissues and into the bloodstream. Such invasion may happen through different routes, the most important being the so-called 'extraluminal route' (i.e., bacteria entering in the breech between the catheter and the surrounding skin, colonizing the external wall of the catheter and/or entering the bloodstream) and the so-called 'intraluminal route' (i.e., bacteria colonizing the internal walls of the catheter after entering through the infusion line, sometimes originating from contaminated solutions but more frequently through hubs and stopcocks). There is no such thing as a 'sterile' catheter: few hours after insertion any venous access device is already colonized. Bacteria and yeasts stick to the internal walls of the catheter producing a special glyco protein medium (also containing lipids and nucleic acids), called 'biofilm', which acts as a matrix that includes and protects the micro-organisms. The degree of colonization

M. Pittiruti (✉)
Department of Surgery, Catholic University Hospital, Rome, Italy

G. Scoppettuolo
Department of Infective Diseases, Fondazione Policlinico Universitario "A. Gemelli" IRCCS, Rome, Italy
e-mail: giancarlo.scoppettuolo@policlinicogemelli.it

D. Celentano
Pediatric Intensive Care Unit, Fondazione Policlinico Universitario "A. Gemelli" IRCCS, Rome, Italy
e-mail: Davide.celentano@policlinicogemelli.it

D. G. Biasucci et al. (eds.), *Vascular Access in Neonates and Children*,
https://doi.org/10.1007/978-3-030-94709-5_21

may be low enough to be detected only by electronic microscopy; heavier colonization (or more massive mobilization of the bacteria from the biofilm) may be detected by microbiological methods, either direct (culture of the catheter after removal) or indirect (culture of blood drawn from the catheter). A massive colonization will be potentially associated with inoculation of a relevant number of micro-organisms from the device into the blood, eventually causing clinically detectable bacteremia and catheter-related bloodstream infection (CRBSI). Though central VADs are traditionally considered more prone to CRBSI, this life-threatening complication may occur also with peripheral VADs.

Not all catheter-related infections are necessarily associated with bacteremia. Local infection may occur, such as exit site infection, tunnel infection or (in the case of totally implantable venous access devices) pocket infection. These 'local' infections are nonetheless clinically relevant: an exit site infection of a non-tunneled VAD is likely to become a catheter-related bloodstream infection, so that the suspicion of a bacterial infection of the exit site (except for tunneled catheters) is an indication to remove the device. Tunnel infection and pocket infection are almost inevitably associated with the need of device removal.

As explained below, diagnosis, treatment and prevention of catheter-related infection does not differ significantly in neonates and children vs. adult patients.

21.1.1 Infection of the Exit Site

It is the most common type of infection for peripheral VADs, but it may occur also in central VADs. Diagnosis is usually made by inspection and palpation: the simultaneous presence of redness and tenderness of the exit site is considered highly suspicious for a local infection, and the presence of infection is certain if other local signs are detected, such as purulent secretions (Fig. 21.1). In some cases, culture of local secretions may be indicated. For short peripheral cannulas, an exit site infection may appear as a local phlebitis (tenderness, redness, swelling, loss of function of the device), though the differential diagnosis between mechanical phlebitis and chemical phlebitis may be difficult. In fact, inflammation of a small superficial vein—regardless of the cause—is invariably associated with venous thrombosis and edema/infiltrate of the vein wall.

The treatment of an exit site infection—for both peripheral and central VADs—is always the removal of the device, except for the case of a tunneled central VAD: in this case, the exit site infection (if it has not evolved into an infection of the tunnel) may be initially treated with systemic antibiotics (preferably after culture of the local secretions) and daily antisepsis of the exit site.

The prevention of exit site infections (which are usually the results of an uncontrolled bacterial contamination of the skin around the VAD) is based on evidence-based strategies directed to minimize extraluminal contamination:

- Proper choice of the exit site. Short peripheral cannulas placed in flexion areas (back of the hand and antecubital fossa) are more prone to phlebitis than cannulas

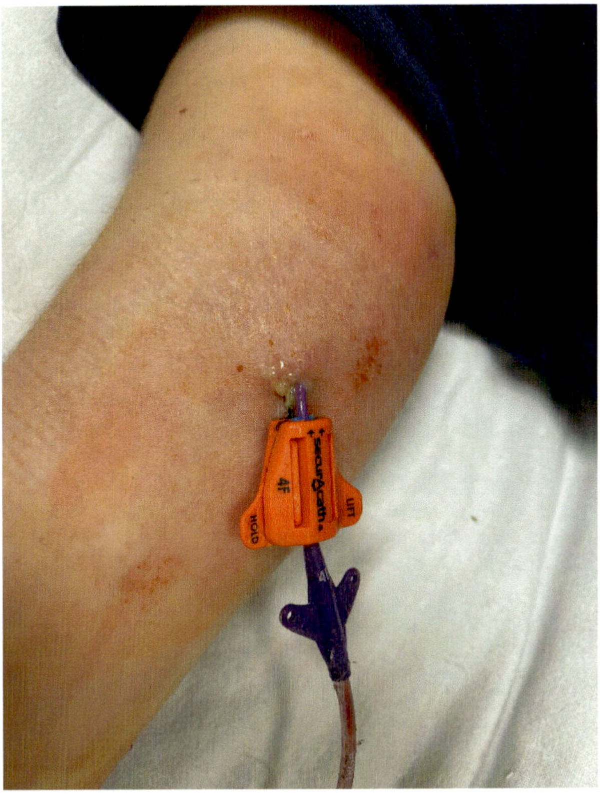

Fig. 21.1 Exit site infection

placed at the forearm. If the peripheral cannula is placed as an elective maneuver and is expected to last for several days, flexion areas must be avoided. The exit site of a central VAD should be far from contaminated areas and from areas associated with instability of the dressing. Bacterial contamination of the skin is secondary to three factors: (a) the proximity to natural or iatrogenic communications with the internal cavity of the body (nose, mouth, urethra, vagina, anus; tracheostomy, gastrostomy, jejunostomy, ileostomy, colostomy, chest drainage, biliary drainage, nephrostomy, etc. etc.); (b) the degree of humidity of the skin (maximal at skin folds); (c) the presence and quantity of hairs. Also, the instability of the catheter and of the dressing, causing micro-movements of the device, increases the risk of extraluminal contamination. In short, the worst areas for the exit site of a central VADs are the neck, the groin, and any area too close to a stoma. The areas to be preferred are the mid-portion of the upper arm, the infraclavicular area (unless a tracheostomy is present) and the mid-thigh. The supraclavicular area may be acceptable in older children, but not in neonates or in infants. The strongest tool for modulating the exit site of a central venous access is the technique of tunneling (see Chap. 8). Exit sites at the neck or at the groin are acceptable only as emergency central lines: as such, they should be removed as soon as possible (within 24–48 h) and replaced with an elective central

VAD. The only central VADs that do not consent tunneling are the epicutaneo-cava catheters (ECC) and the umbilical venous catheters (UVC) in the neonate. All the other central lines in neonates, infants and children can be easily tunneled, especially if adopting catheters that are meant to be inserted by modified Seldinger technique. Peripherally inserted central catheters (PICC) should have the exit site in Dawson's green zone; if there is no vein of proper caliber in the green zone, venipuncture can be done in the yellow zone and the catheter tunneled so to get the exit site in the green zone. Centrally inserted central catheters (CICC) are usually inserted in the supraclavicular area (by ultrasound-guided cannulation of the internal jugular vein or of the brachio-cephalic vein) and they should be tunneled to the infraclavicular area (Fig. 21.2); in older children, CICC placed by ultrasound-guided cannulation of the axillary vein may be left non-tunneled or tunneled downward (if a tracheostomy is present) (Fig. 21.3). Femorally inserted central catheters (FICC) should have the exit site—prefera-

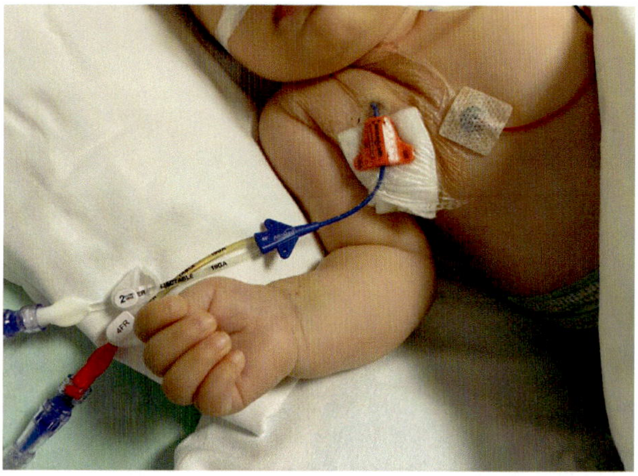

Fig. 21.2 CICC tunneled to the infraclavicular area after supraclavicular venipuncture

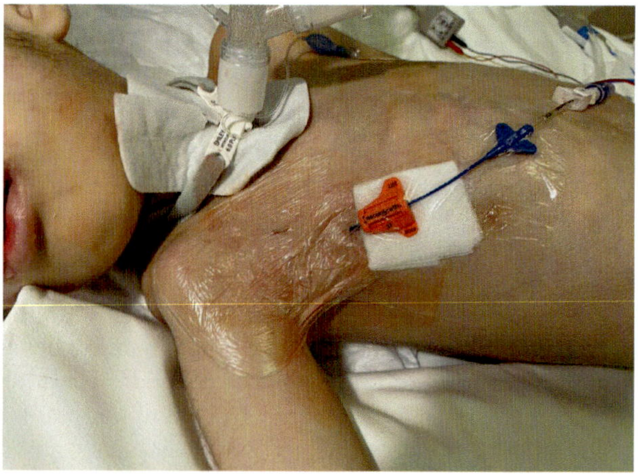

Fig. 21.3 CICC tunneled to the chest after infraclavicular venipuncture (access to the axillary vein) in child with tracheostomy

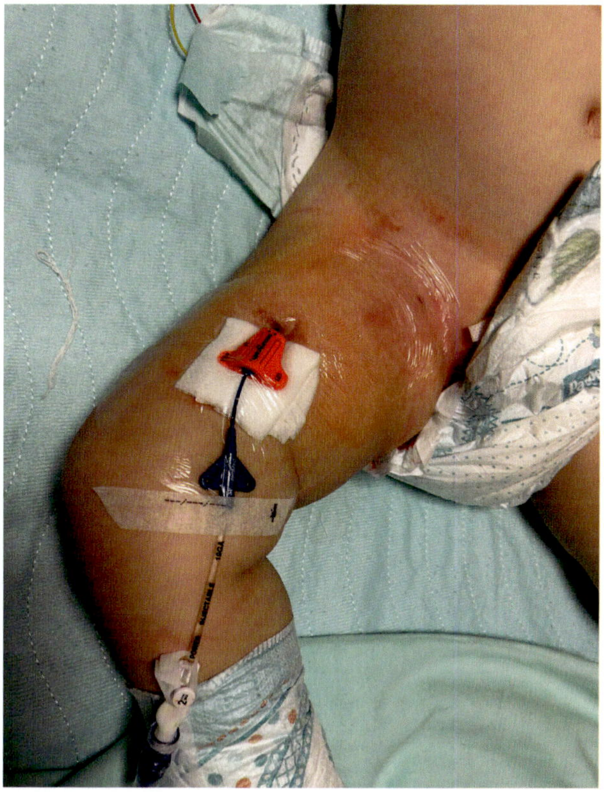

Fig. 21.4 FICC tunneled to mid-thigh after puncture of the common femoral vein

bly—at mid-thigh: this is possible either by direct puncture of the superficial femoral vein at mid-thigh or by puncture of the common femoral vein at the groin and subsequent tunnelling to mid-thigh (Fig. 21.4).

- Hand hygiene. Any maneuver of insertion (of any type of VAD) and any manipulation of any VAD (from dressing change to handling of the infusion line to blood sampling) should be preceded by proper hand hygiene, preferably by alcohol-based rub, but also with antiseptic soap and water, in selected cases (visible dirt; risk of contamination by spores).
- Skin antisepsis. Before the insertion of any type of peripheral or central VAD (including ECC and UVC in neonates), or during dressing change of any type of VAD, or before accessing a totally implantable device with a Huber needle, the skin must be appropriately disinfected with 2% chlorhexidine in 70% isopropyl alcohol (Fig. 21.5). The only exception is the known/proven allergy of the child to chlorhexidine: in this case, skin antisepsis with iodine povidone in 70% isopropyl alcohol is indicated. Though, iodine povidone is contraindicated in pre-term neonates, due to potential disturbance of growth because of interaction with thyroid function. Considering that no neonate is possibly allergic to chlorhexidine, 2% chlorhexidine in 70% isopropyl-alcohol is the antiseptic of

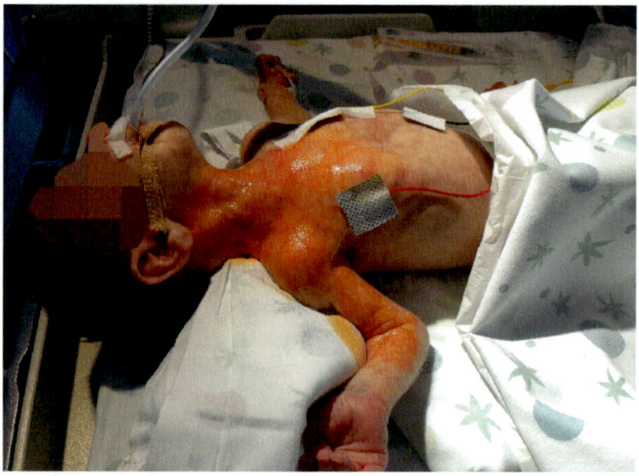

Fig. 21.5 Skin antisepsis with 2% chlorhexidine before CICC insertion

choice also in neonates, but it must be used with caution: (a) the amount of antiseptic must be proportioned to the skin area to be disinfected (which implies that an applicator with a known volume of solution is mandatory); (b) the antiseptic must be applied for 30 s, letting it dry for additional 30 s; (c) then, the excess of antiseptic still in place must be removed by rinsing with sterile saline or by wiping with sterile gauzes. Excessive amounts of chlorhexidine, with 'pooling' of the antiseptic, may be associated with severe chemical damage to the skin of the neonate (Fig. 21.6).

- Maximal barrier precautions. All central VADs, with no exception (i.e., including also ECC and UVC), must be inserted with maximal barrier precautions (i.e.: cap, mask, sterile gloves, sterile gown, sterile field, wide sterile drapes over the child, long sterile cover for the ultrasound probe) (Figs. 21.7 and 21.8). Such recommendation extends also to peripheral VADs that are meant to stay in place for more than a week, such as long peripheral catheters ('mini-midlines') and midline catheters. On the other hand, the insertion of a short peripheral cannula does not require maximal barrier precautions, though it requires proper hand hygiene and skin antisepsis with 2% chlorhexidine; sterile gloves are preferred, even if—using a proper no-touch technique—non-sterile, clean gloves are also acceptable; when non-sterile gloves are used, maximal attention should be paid in avoiding touching the puncture site during and after disinfection. If a central VAD has been inserted without maximal barrier precautions (for example, in emergency/urgency), it should be considered contaminated and removed within 24–48 h. The use of insertion packs surely facilitates the systematic adoption of the maximal barrier precautions (Fig. 21.9).
- Cyanoacrylate glue. Cyanoacrylate glue (either butyl-cyanoacrylate or octyl-butyl-cyanoacrylate) is recommended for sealing the exit site and for closing all skin incision required during VAD insertion. As a sealing tool, glue has the triple advantage of securing the catheter, stopping any bleeding/oozing from the skin breech, and avoiding bacterial contamination of the breech. As a skin-closing

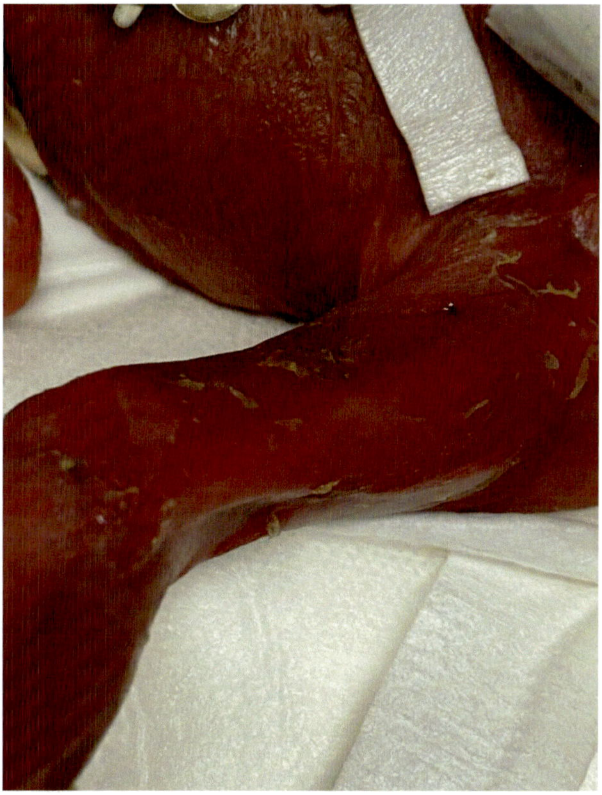

Fig. 21.6 Skin damage due to chlorhexidine (Courtesy of Matthew Ostroff)

tool (for instance, for closing the pocket of a totally implantable venous access device, or the skin incisions necessary for tunneling the VAD), it protects the subcutaneous tissues from bacterial invasion, while transcutaneous skin sutures create communications between the skin surface and the underlying tissues. Cyanoacrylate glue is completely safe, and it should be used on the exit site on any central VAD (including ECC in preterm neonates), except for UVC (though some recent evidence suggests that glue may improve securement of UVC). We recommend the use of glue also on peripheral venous access devices, where its role as securement is especially evident. The only contraindication to glue is the use of silicon catheters, that are very fragile and could be damage by cyanoacrylate. Though, as explained in several chapters of this handbook, silicon catheters should be abandoned in the clinical practice, for many reasons.

- Securement using sutureless devices. According to all current guidelines, venous access devices must not be secured using stitches. Transcutaneous skin sutures—when used for securing the wings of the catheter—are a clear and demonstrated cause of catheter-related infection: the sutures create a communication between the skin surface and the subcutaneous tissue, allowing bacterial invasion of the tissues; all stitches inevitably cause a chronic infective granuloma (one granuloma

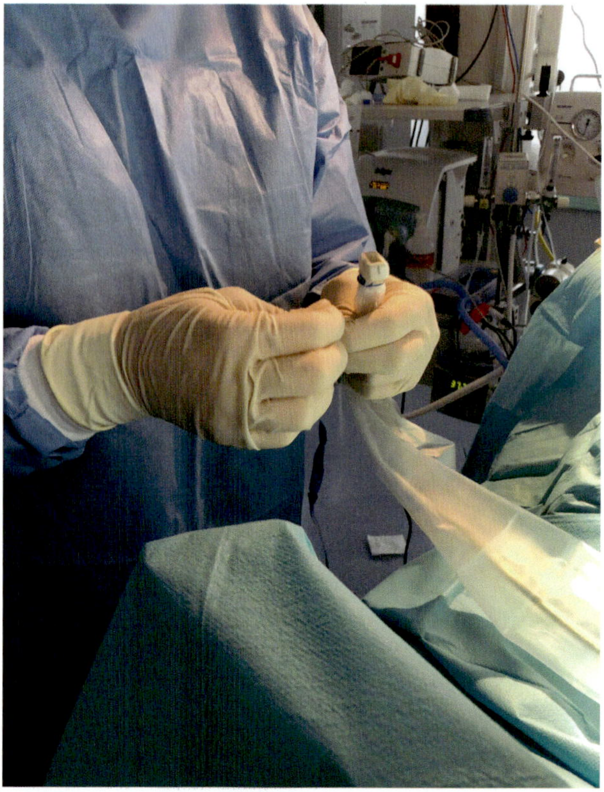

Fig. 21.7 Sterile cover for the probe

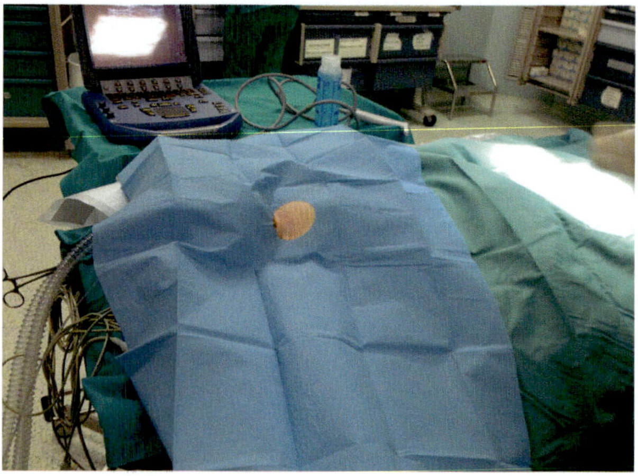

Fig. 21.8 Sterile field

for each skin passage of each stitch), which contaminates for days or weeks the exit site located in its proximity (Fig. 21.10). Furthermore, stitches are cause of pain during placement and maintenance, as well as cause of accidental needle

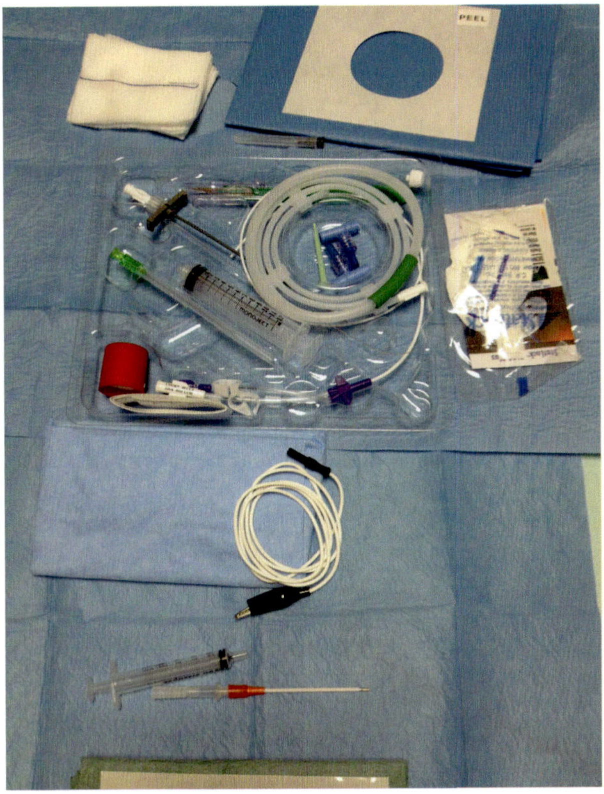

Fig. 21.9 Insertion pack

injury for the operator. Considering the variety of sutureless devices currently available on the market, both skin-adhesive and subcutaneously anchored, the use of stitches is not acceptable anymore.

- Transparent semipermeable membranes. The exit site of any VAD—either peripheral o central—should be covered and protected with a transparent semipermeable membrane, and not with gauze-and-tape dressing. The membrane is the only real barrier against contamination of the exit site from environmental bacteria (Fig. 21.11). The gauzes offer no protection; even if initially sterile, they rapidly become colonized and favor the overgrowth of bacteria over the exit site. When choosing a membrane, it is important to select membraned with high permeability (moisture vapor transfer rate, MVTR > 1500), so to avoid accumulation of fluid and skin maceration below the dressing.
- Chlorhexidine-releasing sponge dressings. Many randomized control studies have demonstrated the efficacy of chlorhexidine sponge dressings in reducing the risk of exit site contamination—and subsequent catheter-related blood stream infection—in non-tunneled central VADs (except for ECC and UVC). Their use for peripheral venous access devices or for tunneled central VADs is questionable. Considering that they are not effective in stopping the bleeding for the exit

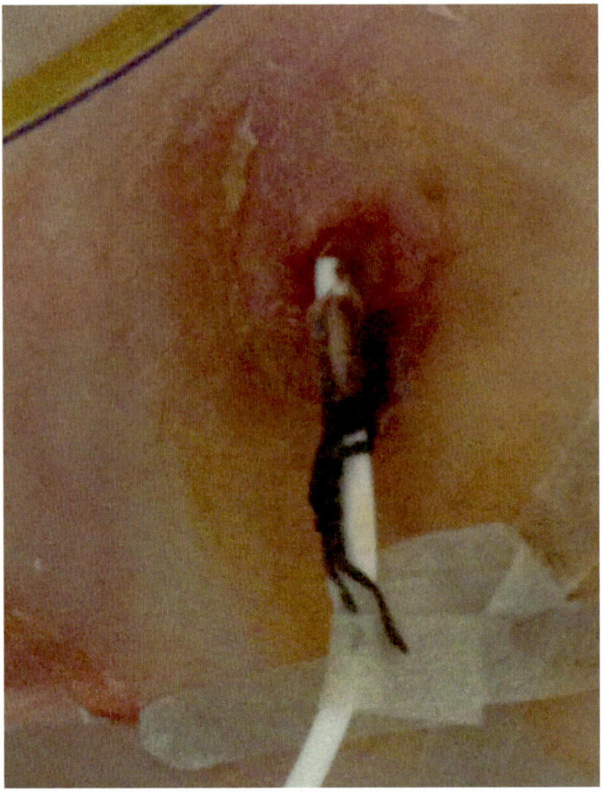

Fig. 21.10 Exit site infection caused by securement with stitches

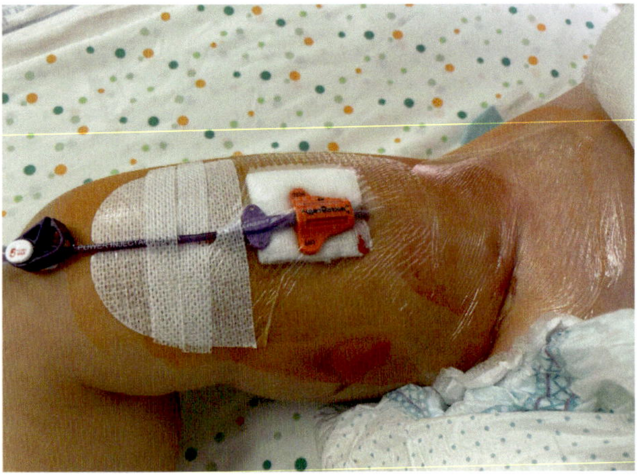

Fig. 21.11 Transparent membrane with high MVTR over the exit site

site, at the time of the insertion we recommend to place glue on the exit site (which is both a protection against bacterial contamination and against bleeding). When the dressing is changed, a week later, the operator may choose between replacing the glue with the sponge dressing or sealing again the exit site with glue. However, chlorhexidine releasing sponge dressing should not be used in preterm neonates (due to possible skin damage from the prolonged exposure to chlorhexidine) and used with caution in neonates at term. We recommend avoiding the use of transparent dressing with chlorhexidine-releasing gel pads: their use is not indicated in the pediatric patient.

- Proper policy of dressing change. Last, the exit site is protected by contamination when a proper policy of dressing change is adopted. In children, the transparent membranes (and other devices that must be replaced weekly) should be changed every 7–10 days or even earlier, if the dressing is soiled or damaged; in neonates and infants, the same dressing can stay in place also for longer times if there are no signs or symptoms of infection or of skin irritation.

21.1.2 Tunnel Infection

Both cuffed and non-cuffed tunneled catheters may be complicated by a tunnel infection, which may be the result of an uncontrolled infection of the exit site or start directly from the cuff. Infection is more likely to occur if the cuff has been placed inappropriately close to the exit site (less than 2.5 cm): this error of implantation is often associated with tunnel infection and/or expulsion of the cuff, both of which are inevitably associated with loss of the device. The diagnosis of tunnel infection is made by inspection: tenderness, reddening and swelling of the tunnel are the main finding. Tunnel infection may also be associated with purulent secretions: in this case, a swab culture of the secretions is recommended. Bacteremia is not always present.

The treatment of tunnel infection is removal of the device plus systemic antibiotic therapy, either directed on the germs isolated by the culture or against staphylococcus, the germ most frequently responsible of this complication.

The prevention is based on the same strategies described above for prevention of exit site infection. Furthermore, if the tunneled catheter is cuffed, it is important to place the cuff at appropriate distance from the exit site: such precaution is known to be effective in preventing cuff infection and subsequent tunnel infection.

21.1.3 Pocket Infection

This infective complication occurs exclusively with totally implantable venous access devices (ports). The usual cause is inappropriate antisepsis of the skin before accessing the reservoir with the Huber needle. The diagnosis is established by inspection: the pocket where the reservoir is placed appears swollen, reddened, and tender. The infection rapidly becomes purulent, and a fluid area around the reservoir can be palpated or detected by ultrasound.

The treatment is inevitably the removal of the system: if pus is present, the pocket should be left open after removal of the device and allowed to heal secondarily.

The prevention is the adoption of an appropriate policy of access to the port: hand hygiene, sterile gloves, skin antisepsis with 2% chlorhexidine in 70% isopropyl-alcohol, sterile infusion sets, removal of the Huber needle after the infusion, leaving it place no more than 7 days.

21.1.4 Catheter-Related Blood Stream Infection

Catheter-related bloodstream infection (CRBSI) is the one of the most severe complications of VADs, being associated with high morbidity, loss of the device, and increased healthcare costs. It is typically associated with central VADs, but it may occur also with peripheral VADs (short cannulas, long peripheral catheters, midline catheters). CRBSI should not be confused with CLABSI (central-line associated blood stream infection); CLABSI describes the occurrence of a bloodstream infection in a patient who has a central VAD, while CRBSI is a bloodstream infection directly caused by the germs that colonize the central VAD. While CLABSI is useful in epidemiological retrospective studies, the proper care of the patient with a central VAD requires a precise and reliable diagnosis of CRBSI. The only method that allows an accurate diagnosis of CRBSI without removing the device is the simultaneous culture of the blood drawn from the catheter and of the blood drawn from a peripheral vein. The two cultures are compared either considering the quantity of colony-forming units or the time to positivity. The latter method (Differential Time to Positivity = DTP) is easier and less expensive; it can be applied to all central VADs, if blood withdrawal is feasible (therefore, it is not usually applicable to ECCs). If the culture of catheter blood becomes positive at least 2 h before the culture of peripheral blood (with the same micro-organism), the diagnosis of CRBSI is established; if only the culture of catheter blood is positive and the peripheral blood culture is negative, there is no evidence of infection, but the catheter is colonized; if both blood cultures become positive simultaneously or if peripheral blood becomes positive before catheter blood, the bacteremia is not caused by the VAD. To interpretate the DTP appropriately, the technique of blood culture is of paramount importance: a frequent occurrence is a positive culture of peripheral blood with negative catheter culture, a situation that can only be interpretated as a false positive due to inappropriate blood sampling (for example, inadequate skin antisepsis before venipuncture).

In most cases, treatment of CRBSI include the removal of the device. When a bloodstream infection is detected in a neonate with an ECC, as DTP is not possible, the ECC must be removed based on the presumption of CRBSI. Also, in children with severe septic shock (hemodynamical instability), central VADs should be removed without hesitation, in the suspicion of a catheter-related sepsis. Apart these two exceptions, in absence of exit site infection, it is strongly recommended to remove a central VAD only after a proper diagnosis of CRBSI is established by

DTP. If the DTP suggests a bloodstream infection not related to the central VAD, the VAD should be left in place and used for the antibiotic therapy. If the DTP suggests a CRBSI, the VAD should be removed and antibiotic treatment delivered inserting a new peripheral or central VAD, depending on the prescribed antibiotic (i.e., if the antibiotic is compatible with the peripheral route or not). In some very selected situations, it is acceptable to try to treat the CRBSI without removing the device: this strategy should be adopted only (a) if the venous patrimony of the child is critically reduced and/or if a new VAD insertion is regarded as difficult or dangerous, and (b) if there is no evidence of metastatic seeding of the germs (for example, on the cardiac valves). This 'conservative' treatment—not recommended for yeast infection or for infection by Staph. Aureus or Gram-negative germ—consists in systemic antibiotic treatment (specifically directed against the germ cultured in the blood), delivered through the VAD plus a 'therapeutic lock' of the catheter for some hours each day. The traditional therapeutic lock is a lock of the catheter with a solution containing antibiotics active against the germ cultured in the blood; recently, a therapeutic lock with a solution with 2% taurolidine has also been tested. Taurolidine lock has many advantages over antibiotic lock: taurolidine is active against all micro-organisms and demolish the biofilm; it is inexpensive, completely safe even if accidentally infused in the blood; it does not induce bacterial resistance and it is not associated with any risk of allergic reactions. The therapeutic lock with taurolidine should stay inside the catheter for 8–10 h, daily. Taurolidine lock may also be used for treating a colonized central VAD, as an alternative option to VAD removal.

Prevention of CRBSI is based on the prevention of bacterial contamination by the extraluminal and intraluminal routes. The strategies for preventing extraluminal contamination are the same above described (proper choice of the exit site; hand hygiene; skin antisepsis; maximal barrier precautions; cyanoacrylate glue; sutureless securement; chlorhexidine-releasing sponge dressing; transparent semipermeable membranes; proper policy of dressing change). The evidence-based strategies directed to minimize intraluminal contamination are the following:

Hand hygiene. Proper hand hygiene and use of clean non-sterile gloves are recommended before any manipulation of the infusion lines (including bolus injections, change of the primary or secondary lines, blood sampling, etc.).

Use of needle-free connectors and port protectors. All hubs not used continuously should be closed with a needle-free connector. Hubs and stopcocks represent the most frequent cause of bacterial contamination of the infusion line. While the presence of needle free connectors does not automatically exclude the possible entrance of germs, their design and structure allow the possibility of appropriate disinfection before any connection with infusion lines or syringes. Disinfection may be 'active' (i.e., performed by the operator: this means 5–15 s scrub of the connector with an antiseptic) or 'passive' (i.e., covering the needle free connector—when not connected—with 'disinfecting caps', also known as 'port protectors'). The latter strategy has been proven to be easier, less expensive, and more effective than the former, having the great advantage of eliminating the variability in the modality of disinfection.

Proper policy of change of the infusion line. As recommended by current guidelines, infusion lines should be changed within few hours if used for blood or blood derivatives and every 24 h if used for lipid-based parenteral nutrition. Infusion lines used only for 'clear' fluids may stay in place 96 h or more.

Prophylactic lock with taurolidine. In children at high risk for CRBSI, especially if their venous patrimony is scarce and if the intravenous treatment is expected to last for prolonged time, periodic lock with 2% taurolidine (at least 3 times per week, for at least 1 h) is proven to be safe and effective. As taurolidine has a powerful antibacterial activity, but no anticoagulant effect, in the case of a catheter used for dialysis or apheresis, a solution with taurolidine and citrate should be used as prophylactic lock.

21.2 Venous Thrombosis

Catheter-related venous thrombosis may occur with both peripheral and central VADs, though its clinical consequences may be relevant especially when the thrombosis affects the great veins close to the heart. The pathogenesis of venous thrombosis is related to any kind of endothelial damage of the vein wall, either traumatic or chemical. As all VADs (except for UVCs) are inserted by penetrating the vein wall, venous thrombosis is inevitable at the site where the catheter enters the vein. Though, in most cases such thrombosis (which should be regarded as a highly specialized tissue that attempts to repair the damage of the vein wall) is so limited that it cannot be detected with ultrasound. In some other cases, the thrombosis may be evident at ultrasound scan but not associated with clinical signs or symptoms (asymptomatic thrombosis). In a small percentage of cases, the thrombosis might become clinically evident (symptomatic thrombosis) and in an even smaller number of cases, if not treated, it may be associated with pulmonary embolism. Another cause of catheter-related thrombosis (CRT) is chemical damage to the endothelium. For example, many thrombotic events associated with peripheral VADs are caused by direct chemical irritation of the endothelium when solutions that are not compatible with the peripheral route are inappropriately administered via a short cannula or a midline. In such cases, the thrombosis occurs at the tip of the catheter. The same phenomenon may occur when the tip of a central VAD is not placed correctly (primary or secondary malposition). Apart from these two mechanisms, other factors may facilitate the formation of the thrombus: (a) the instability of the catheter, associated with micro-movements that cause a friction on the endothelium; (b) the presence of a catheter occupying too much space inside the vein lumen (more than 33–45%), so to induce venous stasis; (c) the existence of a thrombophilia related to the disease or to possible congenital disorders of the child.

21.2.1 CRT and Peripheral VADs

In short peripheral cannulas, it is difficult to differentiate between venous thrombosis (growth of a repair tissue inside the vein) and phlebitis (inflammation of the vein wall), so that it is possible to name the phenomenon, regardless of its pathogenesis, as 'thrombophlebitis'. Also, it is difficult to differentiate bacterial vs. chemical vs. mechanical thrombophlebitis, all of which may have the same clinical presentation (pain, swelling, redness, loss of function of the device). The diagnosis of thrombophlebitis is based on the clinical findings. Treatment is simply the removal of the device.

On the other hand, CRT associated with long peripheral catheters and midline catheters is usually secondary to inappropriate use of the device for infusion of solutions not compatible with the peripheral route, and they occur at the tip of the catheter. As midline catheters have their tip located in the axillary vein or in the subclavian vein, CRT occurs very close to the central veins and is especially dangerous in terms of risk of pulmonary embolism. Diagnosis of CRT associated with long peripheral catheters and midline catheters is suspected by clinical signs (swelling of the arm) and by malfunction of the VAD and is confirmed by ultrasound scan. Treatment includes removal of the VAD and—in the case of CRT extended to the axillary vein or to the subclavian vein—anticoagulant treatment (low molecular weight heparin, 100 units/kg/12 h).

As regards CRT associated with peripheral VADs, the most important prevention strategy is to avoid the infusion of solutions not compatible with the peripheral route.

21.2.2 CRT and Central VADs

Thrombosis associated with ECC and UVC in the neonates has been discussed in Chaps. 9, 10, 11, and 12.

CRT associated with PICC, CICC and FICC is usually of two different types: (a) CRT at the site of VAD insertion; (b) CRT at the tip.

The first type of CRT is more common, and it has a multiple pathogenesis (excessive damage of the vein at the time of insertion; catheter exceedingly large if compared to the diameter of the vein; instability of the catheter at the exit site; thrombophilia of the patient). Many of such CRT are asymptomatic, and they may affect the deep veins of the arm or the axillary vein or the subclavian vein (in case of PICCs), or the veins of the supra/infraclavicular area or the brachiocephalic vein or the superior vena cava (in case of CICCs), or the femoral vein or the iliac veins or the inferior vena cava (in case of FICCs). This type of thrombosis is not associated with malfunction of the VAD. When CRT is symptomatic, the suspicion is based on the local clinical signs (swelling, pain) and is confirmed by ultrasound scan. CT scan is indicated only when the thrombosis extends to tracts of the vasculature that cannot be explored by ultrasound. In neonates and infants, CT scan is

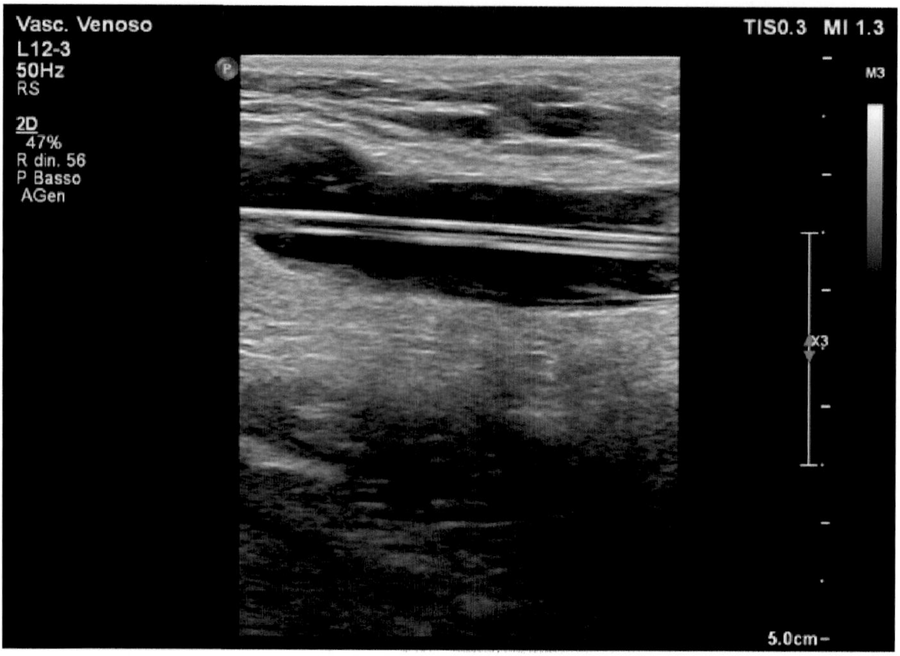

Fig. 21.12 CRT obstructing the lumen (view in long axis)

seldom indicated, as all veins can be easily scanned by ultrasound. When scanning the veins, it is of paramount importance to discriminate between CRT and fibroblastic sleeve (FS). CRT appears initially as an anechoic mass adherent to the vein wall, obstructing the flow partially or completely (Figs. 21.12 and 21.13). FS is a pathophysiological phenomenon that occurs consistently after insertion of any VAD. FS is a connective tissue that is produced by macrophages as a reaction of the tissue (the blood) to the foreign body (the catheter); its production is stimulated by fibronectin, a circulating protein. Interestingly, though FS has been erroneously named 'fibrin sleeve', it has no connection with CRT: it is a cellular tissue containing fibroblasts and smooth muscle cells, plus a matrix of collagen; it is harmless, except for a few cases where it may interfere with the catheter function (if the FS engulfs the tip) and is never associated with any risk of pulmonary embolism. At ultrasound examination, FS can be seen as a hyperechoic sheath all around the catheter (Fig. 21.14). Treatment of symptomatic CRT is proper anticoagulant therapy (low molecular weight heparin, 100 units/kg/12 h); the central VAD can be left in place and used for the scheduled purpose. In fact, removal of the central VAD does not accelerate the reabsorption of the thrombus, and early removal of a recent thrombus may be associated with risk of pulmonary embolism. The only reasons for removing the central VAD are the simultaneous diagnosis of CRBSI, or the malfunction of the VAD, or the end of use. If removal is indicated, it can be performed safely only after few days of anticoagulant treatment.

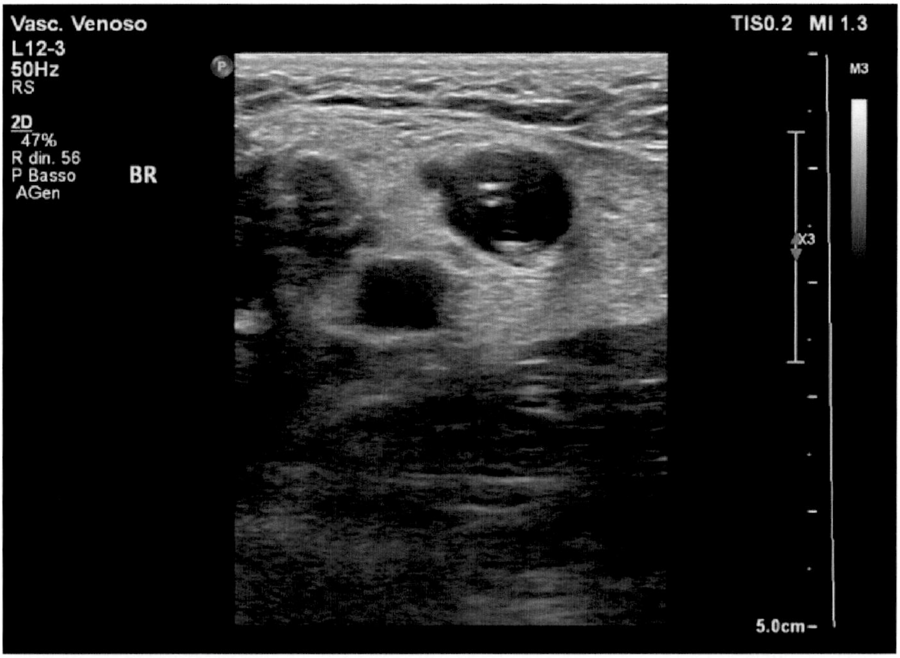

Fig. 21.13 CRT obstructing the lumen (view in short axis)

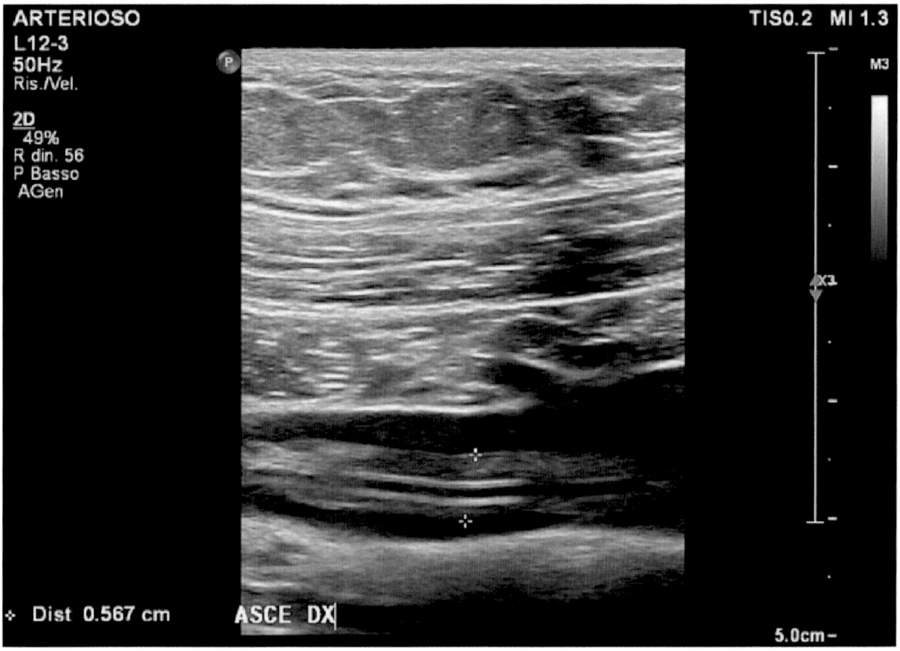

Fig. 21.14 FS as a hyperechoic sleeve around the catheter

The second type of CRT (thrombosis at the tip) is invariably associated with an incorrect position of the tip. The pathogenesis is related to the traumatic injury of the tip of the catheter over the vein wall, but also to the chemical injury of the infusate against the endothelium. Diagnosis requires ultrasound scan of the central veins and sometimes echocardiography. With this type of CRT, the catheter is usually not functioning, and it must be removed after a few days of anticoagulant treatment.

As regards central VADs, prevention of CRT is based on the following strategies:

1. Choose appropriately the catheter, matching the caliber of the catheter with the inner diameter of the vein, so that the catheter may not occupy more than 33%–45% of the vein lumen (Figs. 21.15, 21.16, 21.17 and 21.18).
2. Minimize the trauma to the vein, using ultrasound-guided venipuncture (Fig. 21.19) and micro-introducer kits for venipuncture.
3. Assess the correct position of the tip of the catheter during the procedure, preferably using intracavitary ECG and ultrasound-based tip location, both accurate, safe, and easily feasible in most infants and children.
4. Stabilize the catheter as much as possible, choosing an appropriate exit site and securing with sutureless devices, glue, and transparent membranes.

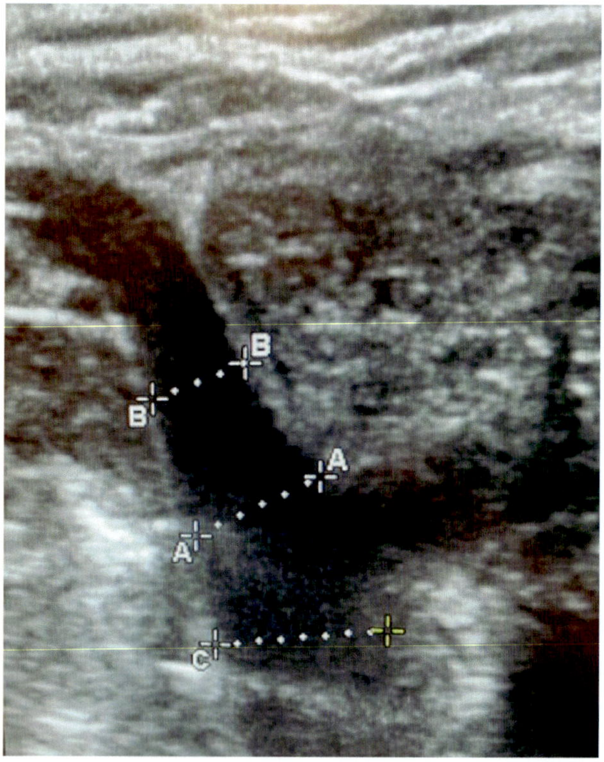

Fig. 21.15 Measurement of right brachio-cephalic vein and superior vena cava

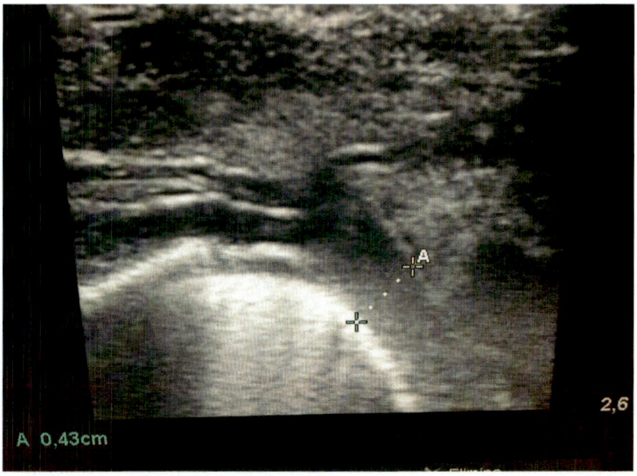

Fig. 21.16 Measurement of right brachio-cephalic vein

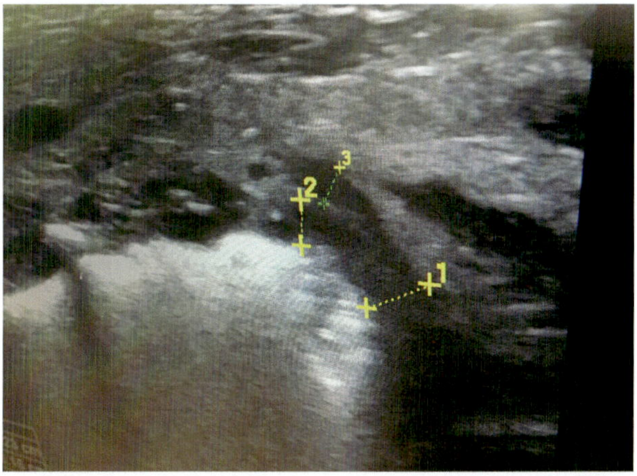

Fig. 21.17 Measurement of external jugular vein, subclavian vein, and brachio-cephalic vein

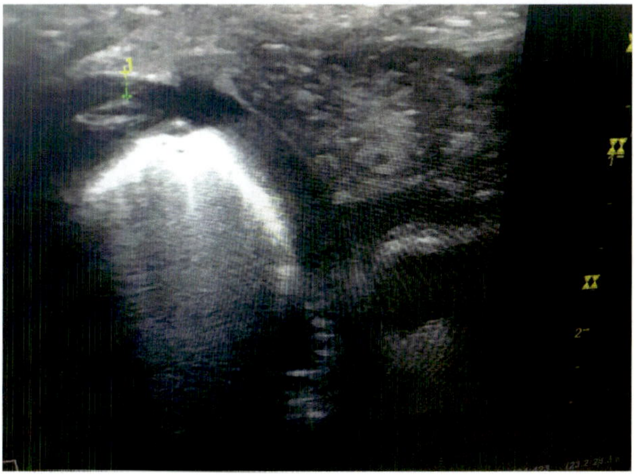

Fig. 21.18 Measurement of external jugular vein

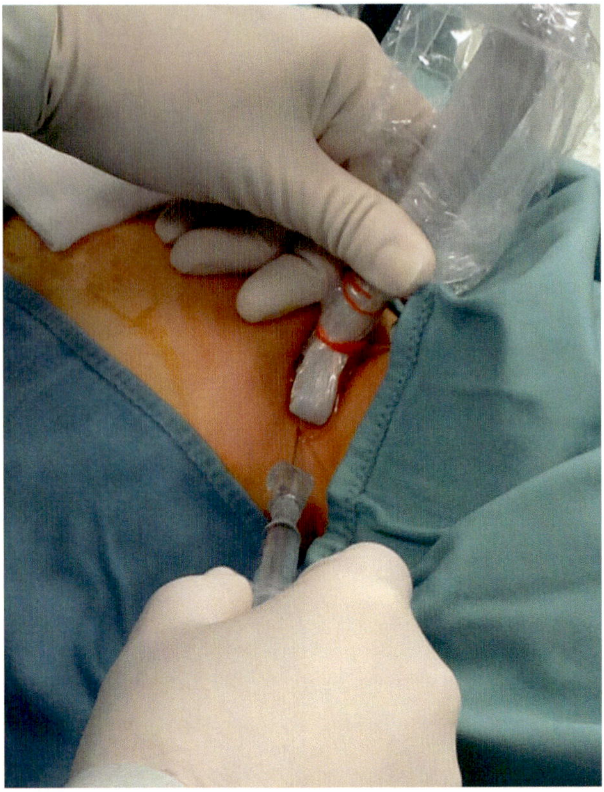

Fig. 21.19 Ultrasound guided venipuncture

Applying all these strategies, the risk of CRT cannot be completely nullified (as the risk factors related to the patient cannot be abolished), but certainly minimized. Pharmacological prevention with prophylactic dosage of anticoagulants (low molecular weight heparin, 100 units/kg/24 h) is indicated only in children with previous history of CRT or of deep venous thrombosis related to neoplastic disease.

21.3 Dislodgment

Peripheral VADs. Dislodgment of peripheral VADs is usually associated with loss of the device. Causes of dislodgment include poor securement, inappropriate choice of the exit site, non-collaborative, restless or agitated children. As already explained, short cannulas inserted on the back of the hand or in the antecubital fossa are prone to accidental dislodgment. Prevention of dislodgment of peripheral VADs include the following strategies: proper choice of the exit site, sealing of the exit site with cyanoacrylate glue, securement with sutureless devices and coverage with transparent semipermeable membranes.

Central VADs. Dislodgment may be partial or complete. Complete dislodgment means loss of the device. After a minor dislodgment (1–2 cm) a central VAD may still have the tip in a central position in a child; though, in a neonate or small infant even a minimal dislodgment may move the tip of the catheter away from the cavo-atrial junction. Major dislodgments (>2 cm) require a new assessment of the position of the tip (using ultrasound or X-ray). Assessment by ultrasound is performed using the 'bubble test' (as described in Chap. 6). Assessment by X-ray is performed by an anterior-posterior chest X-ray: if the tip appears to be above the level of the tracheal carina, the catheter has become too short and should be replaced (Fig. 21.20).

When partial dislodgment occurs and the tip is not centrally located anymore, the best treatment is replacement of the catheter over guidewire. Though, there are some contraindications to guidewire replacement (suspected CRBSI or presence of CRT or of FS around the catheter); furthermore, guidewire replacement of a tunneled catheter—especially if cuffed—may be technically difficult, so that removal and placement of a new central VAD may be preferred.

Prevention of dislodgment of central VADs include the following strategies: proper choice of the exit site, sealing of the exit site with cyanoacrylate glue, securement with sutureless devices and coverage with transparent semipermeable membranes. The best sutureless securement is the subcutaneous anchorage: we recommend adopting it in all PICCs, CICCs and FICCs inserted in neonates, infants,

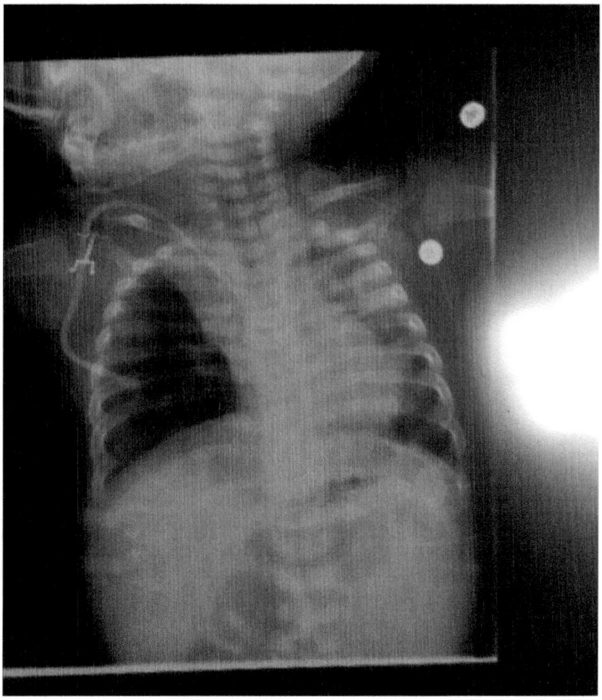

Fig. 21.20 Short central catheter (tip above the level of the tracheal carina)

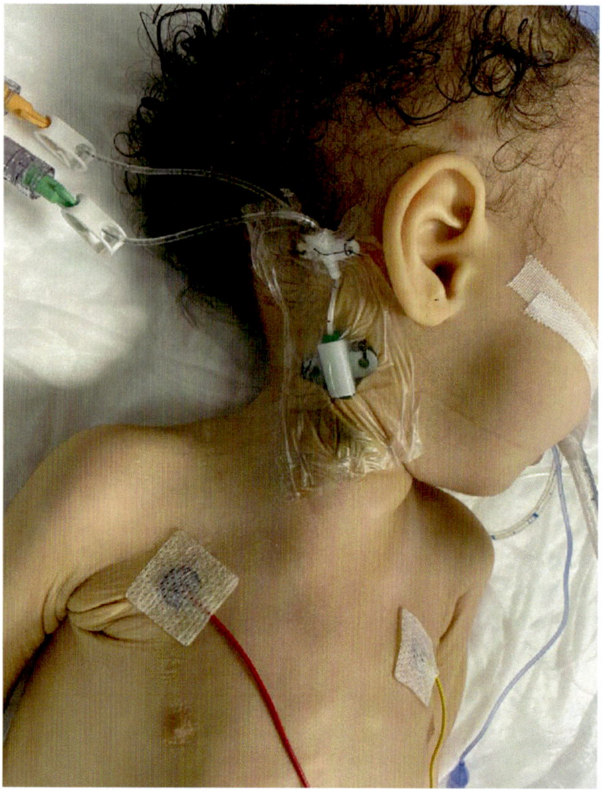

Fig. 21.21 CICC inserted in an inappropriate area (the neck) and inappropriately secured with stitches

and children, as long as the caliber of the catheter ranges between 3Fr and 12Fr, with the only possible exception of central lines inserted in emergency (and thus scheduled to be removed within 48 h). Securement with stitches must always be avoided in any pediatric patient, for any central lines (the only possible exception being the UVC). Stitches are far less effective than subcutaneous anchorage, they increase the risk of infection, and they are associated with local pain, skin damage and risk of accidental needle injury (Fig. 21.21).

21.4 Lumen Occlusion

Malfunction of the catheter may be secondary to extraluminal or intraluminal causes.

Extraluminal causes are (a) CRT at the tip of the catheter, (b) FS around the tip, (c) primary or secondary malposition with the tip pressing against the vein wall or blocked in a small vein, (d) use of a catheter with a distal valve, or (e) 'blind' insertion of a CICC by infraclavicular approach to the subclavian vein (which is a frequent cause of 'pinch-off' syndrome, invariably associated with compression of the catheter, sometimes leading to permanent catheter damage: see below). All these extraluminal causes are typically associated with the malfunction known as 'persistent withdrawal occlusion' (PWO) (i.e., infusion is feasible, but blood sampling is impossible).

Proper diagnosis of the cause of the PWO requires the following steps:

1. Check the type of catheter (valved vs. non-valved, silicon vs. polyurethane); valved catheters (especially with distal valve) are associated with malfunction and should be replaced. Silicon catheters are more prone to be damaged by the 'pinch-off' syndrome.
2. Verify whether the catheter has been inserted according to the obsolete technique of 'blind' subclavian puncture by the infraclavicular approach. If a pinch-off is suspected, the device must be removed.
3. Assessment of the position of the tip, either by ultrasound and 'bubble test' (see Chap. 6) or by X-ray. If a malposition is detected, the catheter must be removed or replaced over guidewire (see below).
4. If the position of the tip is apparently appropriate, the next step is to perform an echocardiography, which may detect the presence of FS or of CRT around the tip of the catheter. CRT at the tip is treated by anticoagulant treatment and subsequent removal of the catheter (few days later); the immediate removal of the device is not recommended, as it may be associated with pulmonary embolism; in very selected cases, if the thrombus is very recent, local thrombolysis can be tried, infusing slowly rTPA (half of the full dose) directly inside the catheter.
5. Last, radiologic study by infusing contrast medium through the catheter (so-called 'line-o-gram') may discriminate between pinch-off syndrome, FS, and CRT around the tip. The presence of a FS causing PWO is usually an indication to VAD removal, as FS is a connective tissue and—as such—is not affected by heparin of by thrombolytic drugs.

Most of the extraluminal causes of malfunction are preventable by adopting the current recommendations of good clinical practice in selecting and inserting the central VAD: use of non-valved catheters; adoption of ultrasound-guided venipuncture; intraprocedural assessment of the position of the tip by intracavitary ECG or ultrasound.

On the contrary, occlusion of the lumen is secondary to inappropriate policies of catheter maintenance, such as inadequate flushing/locking of the catheter. Occlusion may be incomplete (resistance to infusion) or complete. Most lumen occlusions are due to blood clots, or lipid aggregates, or drug precipitates, or contrast media. The diagnosis of lumen occlusion is based on the collection of anamnestic data. The recent history of blood sampling or of infusion of blood products usually indicates an occlusion by clots. Lipid emulsions are typically associated with an occlusion that develops slowly and progressively. The history of multiple drugs infused together mixed in the same bottle, or infused simultaneously through the same lumen, is highly suspicious for an occlusion due to drug precipitates. If the blockade of the VAD has occurred soon after its use for infusion of contrast medium for a CT scan or a MRI, the cause of the occlusion is obvious.

Treatment of lumen occlusion includes at first attempts to overcome the block by forcing the infusion with syringes filled with saline. In this situation, the infusion of heparin is useless; heparin has no effect on blood clots, and—being an acid drug—may further facilitate the local precipitation of lipids, contrast media, and drugs with high pH. If the device is power injectable, small caliber syringes (that exert bigger pressure) can be used safely (2–5 ml). If the catheter is not power injectable, it is recommended to use only 10 ml syringes, that exert lower pressure: though, the maneuver of unblocking will be less effective. If hydraulic unblocking fails, there is indication for pharmacological maneuvers. Blood clots may be solved by thrombolytic drugs (rTPA or urokinase). If occlusion due to lipid aggregates is suspected, 45–55% ethanol is used. Occlusion by contrast media can be solved by 8.4% sodium bicarbonate; this solution is also sometimes effective in the case of drugs aggregates. Other unblocking solutions used in adults for solving drug precipitates (chlorohydric acid and sodium hydroxide) are not recommended in neonates and children. If the occlusion is complete, the unblocking solution can be sent passively inside the device by using the method of the two syringes: two syringes are connected to the catheter through a three-way stopcock (one with the unblocking solution and one empty); connecting the empty syringe with the catheter, a strong aspiration is performed, creating negative pressure inside the system; switching the stopcock from one syringe to another, the unblocking solution is passively aspirated inside the catheter. The maneuver is repeated every 15–20 min, until blood is withdrawn when aspirating with the empty syringe. This method has the double advantage (a) of not creating excessive pressure inside the device, and (b) of avoiding the infusion of the clots or drug precipitates into the bloodstream. As regard this last aspect, it is important to clarify that the accidental infusion of blood clots (or other inert material) inside the bloodstream is never associated with pulmonary embolism; still, it should be avoided because the material occluding the lumen is often a mixture of blood cells, drugs, biofilms, bacteria, etc., so that its infusion into the blood stream may be associated with chills and fever, either due to transient bacteremia or to the pyrogenic effect of inert material.

If the hydraulic and pharmacological methods are ineffective, the device must be removed. As a rule, the sooner these maneuvers are performed after lumen blockade, the higher the chances of success; also, power injectable devices in polyurethane are easy to unblock than silicon catheters. Catheters of small caliber (3Fr PICCs and CICCs; ECCs) may be difficult or impossible to unblock.

As for many other complications, prevention is more cost-effective than treatment. The current evidence-based strategies for prevention of lumen occlusion are the following:

- *Implementation of a strict policy of saline flushing* of all venous access devices, before the use, after the use, and between different infusions; flush should be made with 10 ml syringe operated by hand (gravity infusion of saline is not effective for flushing); the volume of each flushing should be at least twice the priming volume (dead space) of the system, but this amount should be increased to 3–4 times the priming volume, in special cases (after blood sampling and after infusion of lipid-based emulsions, blood products or contrast media). Flushing should be performed preferably with the 'push-pause' technique, so to create turbulent flow and increase the effectiveness of flushing. Flushing with heparin should be discouraged: heparin is not more effective than saline and is dangerous in the pediatric patient, as inappropriate dilution or incorrect estimation of the priming volume may be associated with excessive infusion of heparin into the bloodstream; furthermore, heparin can facilitate the precipitation of lipids and of drugs with high pH.

- *Lock with saline all non-dialysis catheters and lock with anticoagulants only the devices used for apheresis and dialysis.* Evidence has shown that heparin lock has no advantage over saline lock; on the contrary, it may facilitate obstruction. Catheters used for dialysis or apheresis are an exception, since anticoagulant lock is needed, either as heparin lock or citrate lock. Lock with 4% citrate appears to be as effective as heparin lock, but safer and less expensive.
- *Use of neutral displacement needle-free connectors.* Needle-free connectors (NFCs) may be associated with relevant blood reflux during connection (positive displacement NFCs) or during disconnection (negative displacement NFCs); in the pediatric patient, considering the small caliber of the catheters, it is mandatory to use NFCs with neutral displacement (less than 8–10 ml), so to minimize blood reflux during the maneuvers of connection and disconnection with the infusion line. Valved NFCs are commercially available, with reflux close to zero, but their cost-effectiveness is still questionable.
- *Use of power injectable polyurethane devices.* Recent studies suggest that power injectable polyurethane devices are less prone to lumen occlusion than silicon devices. Also, in case of obstruction, hydraulic unblocking is more successful for power injectable devices, since small syringes (which exert high pressures) can be used.
- *Use of non-valved catheters.* Valved catheter, especially if the valve is placed at the tip (Groshong valve) should be abandoned, since characterized by high risk of malfunction. The typical malfunction of these devices is PWO.
- *Proper technique of removal of Huber needles.* When removing a Huber needle from a port, the silicon septum of the reservoir is drawn upward, creating a negative pressure inside the system and thus some blood reflux into the catheter. We recommend removing the Huber leaving a positive pressure inside the port; this can be achieved with two methods, (a) either withdrawing the needle while infusing saline into it (this maneuver may require two operators, (b) or adopting special Huber needles (commercially available since a few years) that create a positive pressure inside the system during removal.
- *Avoidance of multiple drug infusion, unless specifically authorized by the pharmacist.* Mixing different drugs in the same solution is never recommended unless the stability of the solution is certified by a pharmacist (such as, for instance, in the case of the parenteral nutrition). Many drugs are incompatible when mixed, and precipitation is not uncommon.
- *Administration of parenteral nutrition in a specific lumen.* Parenteral nutrition is an emulsion of several compounds (amino-acids, glucose, triglycerides, electro-

lytes), in very delicate equilibrium. Such equilibrium is easily unbalanced when some drugs is added to the bag of parenteral nutrition, or when parenteral nutrition is administered into the same lumen simultaneously with other solution. This leads very quickly to precipitation of lipid aggregates inside the catheter. For the prevention of this phenomenon, parenteral nutrition should be administered separately from the other infusion and preferably using an intravenous pump.

- *Surveillance of infusion lines.* The proper functionality and flow rate of each infusion line should be checked several times a day. Irregularity of flow and unexpected end of the infusion may be associated with blood reflux inside the catheter.

21.5 Mechanical Complications

The mechanical post procedural complications regard central VADs, and are tip migration (secondary malposition), pinch-off syndrome, fracture of the catheter.

Tip migration is defined as dislodgment of the tip and of the intravascular tract of the catheter. This can happen even if the position of the tip was correctly verified at the end of the procedure. Several factors which increase the intrathoracic pressure (cough, vomiting, strong exercise, etc.) may dislodge the tip from the cavo-atrial junction and propel it back into the brachio-cephalic vein (Fig. 21.22) or into the internal jugular vein (ipsilateral or contralateral) (Fig. 21.23), or create loops inside the superior vena cava. This complication occurs most easily with very soft catheters (typically, in silicon) or of small caliber (3–4 Fr or less); in some cases, an acceptable but sub-optimal position of the tip at the time of insertion (for example, in the middle third of the superior vena cava) is a co-factor facilitating this

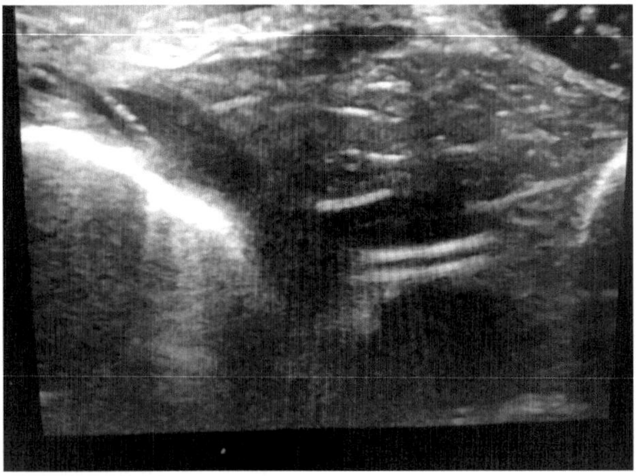

Fig. 21.22 Catheter misplaced to the contralateral brachio-cephalic vein

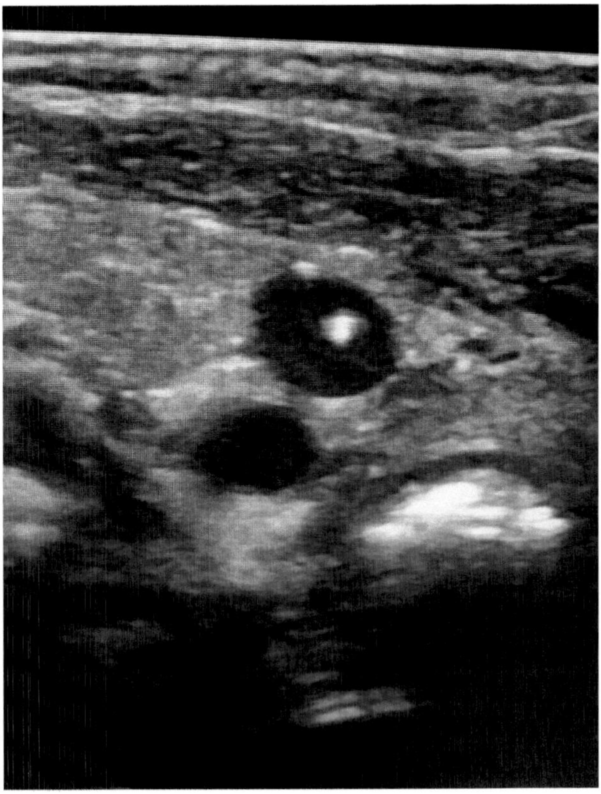

Fig. 21.23 Tip of the catheter migrated to the internal jugular vein

complication. Such secondary malpositions are often discovered because of malfunction of the system or the detection of venous thrombosis around the malpositioned tip.

If the tip migration is diagnosed early, before the occurrence of venous thrombosis, an attempt of non-invasive repositioning (by 'jet injection' through the catheter) is justified. If this vigorous and rapid injection of saline does not bring the tip back to its original position, guidewire replacement is indicated. Guidewire replacement should be performed only after ruling out venous thrombosis.

Prevention of tip migration is based on few principles: (a) systematic adoption of polyurethane catheters, abandoning the use of silicon catheters; (b) appropriate intraprocedural assessment of the position of the tip, using ultrasound and/or intracavitary ECG, so that the final location is the cavo-atrial junction; (c) periodic ultrasound control of neonates and children with catheters that are at high risk for tip migration (UVC, ECC, 3Fr central VADs): ultrasound scan of the supraclavicular area may detect abnormal position of the tip, while ultrasound-based tip location with bubble test (see Chap. 6) may confirm the correct position.

Pinch-off syndrome consists in the pinching of the CICC in its subcutaneous extravascular tract between the first rib and the clavicle; this causes catheter damage (especially if the catheter is made of silicon) with consequent risk of extravasation and of embolization of catheter fragment into the blood stream. This phenomenon is exclusively associated with the 'blind' puncture of the subclavian vein with an infraclavicular approach. As 'blind' venipuncture is unacceptable today, we hope that this complication may disappear soon from the clinical scene.

Partial or complete fracture of the catheter, due to damage of the catheter wall, may happen in the intravascular or in the extravascular tract; it may occur because of excessive pressure exerted during attempts of unblocking the lumen, or it may occur accidentally during the maneuvers of removal of the catheter (most typically, when removing a cuffed catheter or a totally implantable venous access device). In almost all cases, the fractured catheter is a silicon catheter. With the progressive reduction of the use of silicon catheters and the widespread use of power injectable polyurethane catheters, this type of complication will become infrequent.

Bibliography

1. Barone G, Pittiruti M, Biasucci DG, Elisei D, Iacobone E, La Greca A, Zito Marinosci G, D'Andrea V. Neo-ECHOTIP: a structured protocol for ultrasound-based tip navigation and tip location during placement of central venous access devices in neonates. J Vasc Access. 2021;5:11297298211007703. https://doi.org/10.1177/11297298211007703.
2. Biasucci DG, Pittiruti M, Taddei A, Picconi E, Pizza A, Celentano D, Piastra M, Scoppettuolo G, Conti G. Targeting zero catheter-related bloodstream infections in pediatric intensive care unit: a retrospective matched case-control study. J Vasc Access. 2018;19(2):119–24. https://doi.org/10.5301/jva.5000797.
3. Cellini M, Bergadano A, Crocoli A, Badino C, Carraro F, Sidro L, Botta D, Pancaldi A, Rossetti F, Pitta F, Cesaro S. Guidelines of the Italian Association of Pediatric Hematology and Oncology for the management of the central venous access devices in pediatric patients with onco-hematological disease. J Vasc Access. 2020;10:1129729820969309. https://doi.org/10.1177/1129729820969309.
4. Crocoli A, Martucci C, Sidro L, Delle Donne D, Menna G, Pittiruti M, De Pasquale MD, Strocchio L, Natali GL, Inserra A. Safety and effectiveness of subcutaneously anchored securement for tunneled central catheters in oncological pediatric patients: a retrospective study. J Vasc Access. 2021;4:11297298211009364. https://doi.org/10.1177/11297298211009364.
5. D'Andrea V, Barone G, Pezza L, Prontera G, Vento G, Pittiruti M. Securement of central venous catheters by subcutaneously anchored suturless devices in neonates. J Matern Fetal Neonatal Med. 2021;9:1–4. https://doi.org/10.1080/14767058.2021.1922377.
6. D'Andrea V, Pezza L, Barone G, Prontera G, Pittiruti M, Vento G. Use of cyanoacrylate glue for the sutureless securement of epicutaneo-caval catheters in neonates. J Vasc Access. 2021;8:11297298211008103. https://doi.org/10.1177/11297298211008103.
7. Dawson R. PICC zone insertion method™ (ZIM™): a systematic approach to determine the ideal insertion site for PICCs in the upper arm. Journal of the Association for Vascular Access. 2011;16(3):156–65.
8. Gilardi E, Piano A, Chellini P, Fiori B, Dolcetti L, Pittiruti M, Scoppettuolo G. Reduction of bacterial colonization at the exit site of peripherally inserted central catheters: a comparison between chlorhexidine-releasing sponge dressings and cyano-acrylate. J Vasc Access. 2021 Jul;22(4):597–601. https://doi.org/10.1177/1129729820954743.
9. Giustivi D, Gidaro A, Baroni M, Paglia S. Tunneling technique of PICCs and midline catheters. J Vasc Access. 2021;16:11297298211002579.

10. Gorski L, Hadaway L, Hagle M, et al. Infusion therapy standards of practice. J Infus Nurs. 2021;44(1S Suppl 1):S1–S224.
11. Ostroff MD, Moureau N, Pittiruti M. Rapid assessment of vascular exit site and Tunneling options (RAVESTO): a new decision tool in the management of the complex vascular access patients. J Vasc Access. 2021;21:11297298211034306. https://doi.org/10.1177/11297298211034306.
12. Ostroff MD, Pittiruti M, Ostroff MD, Pittiruti M. Alternative exit sites for central venous access: Back tunneling to the scapular region and distal tunneling to the patellar region. J Vasc Access. 2020;9:1129729820940178.
13. Passaro G, Pittiruti M, La Greca A. The fibroblastic sleeve, the neglected complication of venous access devices: a narrative review. J Vasc Access. 2021 Sep;22(5):801–13. https://doi.org/10.1177/1129729820951035.
14. Pinelli F, Balsorano P, Mura B, Pittiruti M. Reconsidering the GAVeCeLT consensus on catheter-related thrombosis, 13 years later. J Vasc Access. 2021 Jul;22(4):501–8. https://doi.org/10.1177/1129729820947594.
15. Pinelli F, Pittiruti M, Van Boxtel T, Barone G, Biffi R, Capozzoli G, Crocoli A, Elli S, Elisei D, Fabiani A, Garrino C, Graziano U, Montagnani L, Prato AP, Scoppettuolo G, Zadra N, Zanaboni C, Zerla P, Konstantinou E, Jones M, Rosay H, Simcock L, Stas M, Pepe G. GAVeCeLT-WoCoVA consensus on subcutaneously anchored securement devices for the securement of venous catheters: current evidence and recommendations for future research. J Vasc Access. 2020;2:1129729820924568. https://doi.org/10.1177/1129729820924568.
16. Pittiruti M, Scoppettuolo G, Dolcetti L, Celentano D, Emoli A, Marche B, Musarò A. Clinical experience of a subcutaneously anchored sutureless system for securing central venous catheters. Br J Nurs. 2019;28(2):S4–S14. https://doi.org/10.12968/bjon.2019.28.2.S4.
17. Pittiruti M, Van Boxtel T, Scoppettuolo G, Carr P, Konstantinou E, Ortiz Miluy G, Lamperti M, Goossens GA, Simcock L, Dupont C, Inwood S, Bertoglio S, Nicholson J, Pinelli F, Pepe G. European recommendations on the proper indication and use of peripheral venous access devices (the ERPIUP consensus): a WoCoVA project. J Vasc Access. 2021;4:11297298211023274. https://doi.org/10.1177/11297298211023274.
18. Zito Marinosci G, Biasucci DG, Barone G, D'Andrea V, Elisei D, Iacobone E, La Greca A, Pittiruti M. ECHOTIP-ped: a structured protocol for ultrasound-based tip navigation and tip location during placement of central venous access devices in pediatric patients. J Vasc Access. 2021;13:11297298211031391. https://doi.org/10.1177/11297298211031391.

Chapter 22
Compatibility of Drugs

Mauro Pittiruti and Giancarlo Scoppettuolo

22.1 Drugs Appropriate for Central vs. Peripheral Infusion

Venous access devices (VADs) are commonly used for the infusion of solutions with extremely variable characteristics in terms of pH, osmolarity, viscosity, and so on. Some of these solutions have the potentiality of bringing damage to the endothelium, by very different mechanisms; though, this damage is not likely to occur when the solution is rapidly diluted in the blood flow. This concept is at the basis of the differentiation between solutions 'compatible' with the peripheral route and solutions that—on the contrary—require to be administered via a central line. The blood flow in the superior vena cava (approximately 2 L/min) may be 200 times higher than the blood flow in a superficial vein of the forearm (approximately 10 mL/min), so that an irritant or vesicant solution infused in a central VAD that has the tip in the superior vena cava is immediately diluted and does not exert any damage on the endothelium of the vein wall; on the other hand, the same solution—if administered by a short cannula into a small superficial vein of the forearm—is likely to interact with the endothelium causing local inflammation and thrombosis (i.e., a thrombophlebitis). There is a long list of solutions that should be preferably infused via central VADs, i.e., VADs with their tip in the superior vena cava (SVC), or right atrium (RA), or inferior vena cava (IVC):

- Solutions with pH lower than 5 or higher than 9: a category that includes many antibiotics, anticonvulsants, vasopressors, and other drugs

M. Pittiruti (✉)
Department of Surgery, Catholic University Hospital, Rome, Italy

G. Scoppettuolo
Department of Infective Diseases, Fondazione Policlinico Universitario "A. Gemelli" IRCCS, Rome, Italy
e-mail: giancarlo.scoppettuolo@policlinicogemelli.it

D. G. Biasucci et al. (eds.), *Vascular Access in Neonates and Children*,
https://doi.org/10.1007/978-3-030-94709-5_22

- Very hyper-osmolar solutions (more than 850 mOsm/L), i.e., emulsions of parenteral nutrition
- Vesicant solutions, typically represented by antiblastic drugs
- Many other drugs that—by mechanisms that may be different from pH and osmolarity—have the potential of causing damage to the endothelium.

If these solutions are administered by a peripheral route for a prolonged period, local complications such as phlebitis and thrombosis are very likely to occur. Thrombosis secondary to chemical damage is a very frequent cause of catheter failure for any peripheral VAD, not only short cannulas but also long peripheral catheters and midline catheters. Repeated episodes of thrombophlebitis of the superficial veins lead to a progressive depletion of the venous patrimony, which is particularly feared in the pediatric patient. In any patient, but particularly in infants and children, whenever the prolonged intravenous infusion of an irritant/vesicant solution is planned, a central VAD should also be planned.

It is recommended that each clinical unit should have a list of drugs/solutions potentially associated with endothelial damage that require a central VAD. Many lists are available on the web, provided by GAVeCeLT (the Italian Group of Long-Term Venous Access Devices), by the Infusion Nursing Society, and by other associations. Ideally, such a list should also be included in the hospital policies for intravenous infusion. Also, each neonatal and pediatric unit should implement a proper policy of adoption of central venous access in the four situations that we have discussed in Chap. 1:

1. Prolonged infusion (>48 h) of solutions not compatible with the peripheral route
2. Repeated daily blood sampling
3. Hemodynamic monitoring
4. Hemodialysis

Any central venous access device—epicutaneo-cava catheter (ECC), umbilical venous catheter (UVC), centrally inserted central catheter (CICC), peripherally inserted central catheter (PICC) and femorally inserted central catheter (FICC)—is expected to be appropriate for (1).

Though, ECCs are not appropriate for (2) and (3). FICCs are appropriate for (3) only if the tip is not in the IVC but at the junction IVC/RA or inside the RA. The last indication to central access (4) requires a CICC or a FICC specifically designed for dialysis.

22.2 Incompatibility Between Drugs

Many drugs commonly infused intravenously may be incompatible, i.e., they may precipitate if infused together and/or they may inactivate each other. A typical example is the incompatibility between heparin (an acid compound) vs. lipid emulsion (which have high pH): heparinization of central VADs used for administration of parenteral nutrition used to be a frequent cause of lumen occlusion due to lipid aggregates (this is bound to disappear now that heparin lock is not recommended anymore).

Some drugs are potentially incompatible, but they can be infused together after a careful stepwise preparation of the final solution, respecting certain ratios of concentration: typical example is the emulsion of parenteral nutrition, where lipids, glucose, amino acids, and electrolytes are in a temporary balance among each other, though this balance can be upset by inappropriate storage (exposure to light, high temperature, etc.) or by inappropriate addition of other drugs.

It is important to remember some key points:

(a) The issue of incompatibility between drugs exists only when the drugs are infused in the same bottle, and/or in the same lumen. Two incompatible drugs can be infused simultaneously in separate lumens of the same device.
(b) When two incompatible drugs are infused one after the other in the same lumen of the venous access device, appropriate flushing with saline is recommended between the two infusions. This must be an 'active' flushing (with a syringe, and not by gravity infusion), with a volume at least twice the priming volume of the device.
(c) The practice of preparing and administering 'cocktails' of different drugs should be discouraged. An infusion containing multiple drugs and meant to be administered intravenously is acceptable only if prepared under the supervision of a qualified pharmacist.

22.3 Interaction Between Drugs and Catheters

The most frequently materials used for VADs, polyurethane and silicon, can be affected or damaged by some drugs and compounds. This can happen either if the compound is inoculated inside the lumen, or if the compound is applied on the external surface of the device.

Alcohol may damage both silicon and old-generation polyurethanes; the magnitude of the damage depends on the type of alcohol (ethyl alcohol is more aggressive than isopropyl alcohol), on its concentration (50–70% is less dangerous than 90%) and on the time of exposure. Standard antisepsis with 2% chlorhexidine in 70% isopropyl alcohol is regarded as safe for all catheters in silicon or polyurethane, also considering that the time of exposure is limited to 1 min or less. On the other hand, antisepsis with solutions including ethyl alcohol should be discouraged.

Ethyl alcohol (usually, 45–55%) has also been used as antibacterial lock for prophylaxis of catheter-related infections; though, it is potentially associated with catheter damage—since the lock stays inside the catheter for hours—and also with other complications (lumen occlusion due to protein precipitation and neurological undesired side effects); therefore, ethanol lock it is currently discouraged in pediatric patients, where taurolidine lock has a wider margin of safety and the same efficacy.

High concentration of ethanol (55%) is also used for unblocking lumens with lipid precipitates; the safety of the maneuver is acceptable in children, considering the short time of exposure, as long as the ethanol is not accidentally inoculated into the bloodstream, but it is not recommended in neonates and infants.

Some antiblastic drugs are also administered in alcohol-based solutions, but no adverse effect has ever been reported, either in silicon or in polyurethane catheters.

Interestingly, new-generation polyurethanes (Carbothane, Chronoflex, etc.), with urethanes mixed with carbonates, structured with aliphatic links rather than with aromatic links, are proven to be resistant to the action of alcohols.

Other drugs that may damage the material of the device are iodine (which may be incorporated inside the catheter wall) and ether (which is particularly aggressive against most thermoplastic materials). Though, iodine is not used as frequently as before, since iodine povidone has been replaced by chlorhexidine in alcohol; ether has been abandoned in the clinical practice.

Last, cyanoacrylate glue has been reported to damage silicon, but not polyurethanes. Considering that silicon catheters are being progressively abandoned in favor of polyurethane catheters, this is not a relevant issue.

In conclusion:

(a) the best strategy is to adopt systematically power injectable venous access devices, which are mostly made with new generation polyurethane. For venous access devices that are not available in new generation polyurethanes (such as ECC and UVC), standard polyurethane should always be preferred to silicon
(b) 2% chlorhexidine in 70% isopropyl alcohol is proven to be safe for all devices
(c) Intraluminal use of ethanol should be limited or discouraged in the pediatric patient, not much for the potential catheter damage, but because of the possible neurological adverse effect when it enters accidentally the blood stream
(d) The use of ether for 'cleaning' the skin or the device must be abandoned
(e) Cyanoacrylate glue is proven to be safe on all polyurethane catheters.

Bibliography

1. Cellini M, Bergadano A, Crocoli A, Badino C, Carraro F, Sidro L, Botta D, Pancaldi A, Rossetti F, Pitta F, Cesaro S. Guidelines of the Italian Association of Pediatric Hematology and Oncology for the management of the central venous access devices in pediatric patients with onco-hematological disease. J Vasc Access. 2020;10:1129729820969309. https://doi.org/10.1177/1129729820969309.
2. Crocoli A, Tornesello A, Pittiruti M, Barone A, Muggeo P, Inserra A, Molinari AC, Grillenzoni V, Durante V, Cicalese MP, Zanazzo GA, Cesaro S. Central venous access devices in pediatric malignancies: a position paper of Italian Association of Pediatric Hematology and Oncology. J Vasc Access. 2015;16(2):130–6. https://doi.org/10.5301/jva.5000314.
3. Di Puccio F, Gallone G, Baù A, Calabrò EM, Mainardi S, Poli P, Scocca A. Experimental investigation on the mechanical behavior of polyurethane PICCs after long-term conservation in in vivo-like conditions. J Vasc Access. 2017;18(6):522–9. https://doi.org/10.5301/jva.5000772.

4. Di Puccio F, Giacomarro D, Mattei L, Pittiruti M, Scoppettuolo G. Experimental study on the chemico-physical interaction between a two-component cyanoacrylate glue and the material of PICCs. J Vasc Access. 2018 Jan;19(1):58–62. https://doi.org/10.5301/jva.5000816.
5. Gorski L, Hadaway L, Hagle M, et al. Infusion therapy standards of practice. J Infus Nurs. 2021;44(1S Suppl 1):S1–S224.
6. Pittiruti M, Scoppettuolo G. The GAVeCeLT manual of PICC and midlines. Milan: Published by EDRA; 2016.
7. Pittiruti M, Van Boxtel T, Scoppettuolo G, Carr P, Konstantinou E, Ortiz Miluy G, Lamperti M, Goossens GA, Simcock L, Dupont C, Inwood S, Bertoglio S, Nicholson J, Pinelli F, Pepe G. European recommendations on the proper indication and use of peripheral venous access devices (the ERPIUP consensus): a WoCoVA project. J Vasc Access. 2021;4:11297298211023274. https://doi.org/10.1177/11297298211023274.
8. Poli P, Scocca A, Di Puccio F, Gallone G, Angelini L, Calabrò EM. A comparative study on the mechanical behavior of polyurethane PICCs. J Vasc Access. 2016;17(2):175–81. https://doi.org/10.5301/jva.5000452.

Chapter 23
Organization of a Hospital-Based Vascular Access Team

Massimo Lamperti and Mauro Pittiruti

Pediatric vascular access teams are a dedicated multidisciplinary group of physicians, nurses and allied-health specialists involved in the proactive vascular, planning, insertion and management of any intravenous access that is required in children. The team should be composed of expert members with specific training managing pediatric patients and dedicated equipment for children such as specific ultrasound probes, a near-infrared visualizers, and intracavitary ECG systems should be present to allow the optimal insertion and check of the catheter before its use. The team should also be responsible for the maintenance of catheters and management of complications. As many of the children who need intravenous vascular access require sedation, it is important to perform these procedures in a safe environment with emergency equipment and medications. In cases where there is a need for deep sedation, it should be managed by a dedicated pediatric anesthesiologist.

Organization is the key to success in any company and institution, even in the healthcare setting. The concept of creating a dedicated multidisciplinary team for vascular accesses was introduced in 2004 by the World Health Organization in a broader concept of reduction of hospital acquired infections (HAI) in which, vascular catheter related infections was one of the main reasons for increased mortality and morbidity during the hospital journey. From this concept of prevention of HAI, many institutions started creating specific units inside their hospitals dealing with any indication, implantation, and care-problems related with vascular accesses.

M. Lamperti
Anesthesiology Institute, Cleveland Clinic, Abu Dhabi, UAE
e-mail: lamperm@clevelandclinicabudhabi.ae

M. Pittiruti (✉)
Department of Surgery, Catholic University Hospital, Rome, Italy

D. G. Biasucci et al. (eds.), *Vascular Access in Neonates and Children*,
https://doi.org/10.1007/978-3-030-94709-5_23

23.1 Definition of Vascular Access Specialist Team (VAST)

The term Vascular Access Specialist Team (VAST) is quite new and was provided by Carr et al. as: "any grouping of caregivers involved in vascular access devices (VAD), with synonymous names (such as: infusion teams, intravenous teams, or intravenous therapy teams) as well as individual vascular access specialists (nurse, doctor, therapist, technician, and physician assistant) who have advanced skills and who frequently insert or manage (or both) VADs". Examples of VASTs are reported in critical care areas where nurses and advanced-nurse practitioners are successfully inserting these devices with an increased first-attempt insertion success rate and reduced catheter-related complications. This new model has completely changed the approach to VAD management that was traditionally handled by physicians and nurses from different departments without a central coordination and care to the indication and management of complications related to the VADs.

The VAST is not only composed of nurses, advanced practitioners, and physicians, but also by hospitalists, infectious disease control, and pharmacy. Each member brings to the team their specific expertise in dealing with prevention and care of vascular catheters and their related problems. Everyone in the team has a clear role in the management of the VADs from the indication for insertion, to the management of long-term complications such as catheter-related thrombosis and catheter-related infections.

The pediatric IV team has a specific role that is mainly to follow the patients from the beginning of their medical journey in the hospital when the indication for intravenous therapy is placed. The main goal of the pediatric IV team is to not only to minimize the child's psychological trauma by avoiding the multiple punctures that come from multiple catheter insertions and attempts, but also to optimize the needs of the patient, providing the appropriate form of vascular access according to the length and type of therapy that is required. If successful, hopefully such interventions can prevent patients from becoming needle-phobic in the future.

In some pediatric hospitals, there is a further division of the VAST into different roles: the peripheral intravenous (PIV) team, the peripherally inserted central venous catheters (PICC) team, and the central venous catheters (CVC) team.

23.2 Evidence from the Literature

The literature reports different examples of VASTs applied in different areas (e.g., emergency department, operating theatres, oncology) where a VAD is required; though, there are few papers published on a dedicated pediatric VAST.

A study from Da Silva et al. showed that the introduction of an IV team in a mid-sized hospital made possible performing control measures of punctures through a follow-up record where every venipuncture was noted. The benefits achieved by the IV team were successful in decreasing the number of venipuncture attempts, decreasing the rate of phlebitis (from 0.47 to 0.35%), optimizing the team's time, and a 29.47% reduction in the use of PIV catheters.

In another paper from Santolim and colleagues, the authors presented an algorithm to guide nurses in choosing the best intravenous device by considering the main variables of drug therapy. The adoption of this guideline lead to a decrease in the incidence of phlebitis from 0.77 to 0.17% in a one-year period, with a tendency to reduce overall complications. The team appeared more satisfied regarding the choice of the catheters; there was also a reduction in the distress related to multiple punctures and failure placing the venous catheters.

A specific pediatric vascular access program has been studied by Pitts, in which the author analyzed the effect of the introduction of a nurse-led PICC team in a group of 669 patients. The authors found a success rate of 94% in the insertion of PICC lines in pediatric patients by using an ultrasound guided and modified Seldinger technique. The main result found was a reduction in catheter-related infection from 9.12 per 1000 catheter line days to 2.0 per 1000 catheter line days during the first 18 months of the program. The requirement for sedation and even general anesthesia was significantly reduced, with 49% of patients receiving an oral anxiolytic dose of midazolam and the integration of certified child life specialists helping the nurse during insertion of the PICC. These data are encouraging the introduction of a structured dedicated team model in children but there is still a lack of evidence on which requirements are needed to define competences in pediatric vascular placement and maintenance.

23.3 Organization and Structure

The milestone of a business, even in healthcare, is its organization. There are some general characteristics related to the organization of a pediatric IV team that are similar to adults but there are specific needs that a pediatric team will require.

The organization is based on two foundations: human resources and environment.

An IV team, as mentioned before, requires a collaborative group of people able to secure vascular access for the proper indication, with the correct equipment, at the right time. There are different points to consider when intravenous therapy is indicated in a pediatric patient. One of the main points is the need to minimize the maintenance of the catheter allowing the patient to do about their daily life in a normal fashion. Most pediatric patients requiring long-term intravenous vascular access are oncological patients so the team should involve the referring oncologist to discuss the length of therapy to determine which kind of vascular access would be best suited for the proposed treatment plan.

From a practical point of view, to create a 24/7 IV team needs a minimum of 6 team members to account for the placement of an average of 10 catheters per day, care, and maintenance of the catheters, as well as dealing with any complications.

The IV team should also include an infectious disease control specialist, an epidemiologist, and the availability of a vascular surgeon or an interventional radiologist to consult for special cases. Albeit there is no evidence for having specific training in pediatric vascular access, it is common sense that the pediatric IV team should be composed by members with experience in pediatric patients and with advanced skills in placement of different types of catheters (from peripheral IV lines to tunneled catheters). It is also important to involve a pediatric anesthesiologist as many of the children require moderate to deep sedation to allow the placement of a catheter.

It is mandatory that all the pediatric IV teams should be trained in pediatric advanced life support (PALS) as during sedation or catheter placement there may be the need to treat the patient for life-threatening emergencies such as airway obstruction, pneumothorax, or cardiac dysrhythmias.

It's important that all the IV team personnel should keep their skills to allow always having someone able to solve the possible complications related to vascular accesses.

The second important part in organizing a pediatric IV team is the environment. This includes not only the space where vascular access will be performed but also the materials and equipment needed to provide this kind of service. Most of the times, the IV team will place vascular access in a dedicated area. It is not mandatory that this area be the operating room as this will dramatically increase the costs per procedure. Some hospitals have a dedicated area on the pediatric ward or in the infusion center where it is possible to perform sterile procedures such as PICCs or tunneled intravenous catheters. It is mandatory that those areas be properly equipped with all the pediatric catheters required and with a dedicated pediatric resuscitation cart. If a pediatric anesthesiologist is not involved in the sedation process, there should be immediate availability of an anesthesiologist in case of an emergency. Office-based sedation and insertion should not be performed. There should be a dedicated storage room to stock all possible catheters; the minimum needed to be available include peripheral intravenous catheters from 24 to 20G, single and double-lumen PICC lines from 3Fr to 4Fr, including polyurethane power-injectable types, tunneled catheters (4–5Fr), short-term central venous lines (4.5–5–6Fr), port catheters (4–5Fr), and nitinol guidewires. Smaller catheters (1–2.9Fr) are usually inserted by a neonatal specialist and are not part of the typical responsibilities of the pediatric IV team.

Special equipment that a pediatric IV team should have include a dedicated ultrasound machine with a hockey-stick linear probe or a linear high-frequency (8–15 MHz) probe with Doppler and color Doppler function and a near-infrared (NIR) visualizer.

An ECG monitor and equipment to allow detection of the catheter tip position in PICC or central venous line placement is highly recommended. Intracavitary ECG has been shown to be a reliable tool for central venous line tip detection. A phase-array probe to perform a trans-thoracic echocardiogram should also be available as it allows to detect the central venous catheter tip.

It is important to underline that most of the vascular access devices in pediatric patients are peripheral IV catheters and the usual environment where they are required is on the pediatric ward. For this reason, the core part of the pediatric IV team should be comprised of pediatric nurses. A mobile insertion kit or cart should be prepared should there be need for vascular access outside the pediatric department.

From a financial perspective, a dedicated IV team has been proven to be cost saving with a net reduction of hospital acquired infection costs such as hospital-length of stay and the increased cost for antibiotic therapy. The initial costs for setting up the equipment and the environment for a pediatric IV team will have positive returns once the system is working and a reduction of postoperative complications can be measured. Another important point to be considered is the patients' and parents' perspective as the pediatric IV team creates trust, enhances the quality of healthcare delivered, and improves patient satisfaction.

The IV team should create specific care-paths to enhance patients' involvement and education on how to handle catheters if they are discharged home or if catheter-related problems arise. Simple and clear information is the key to success.

23.4 Tips and Tricks

Do not treat a pediatric patient as a small adult. Children are a different and specific category of patients and sometimes they are treated as small adults. It is important that the pediatric IV team should handle the specific needs of these patients as to play and be distracted from the procedure they must undergo and to have a parent or relative always with the child reassuring him/her.

Children are needle-phobic or can become. A needle stick represents a trauma for pediatric patients, and we should do any effort to minimize this trauma reducing the number of attempts required to get the IV cannulation done. Some of these patients require a prolonged intravenous therapy with the need for multiple blood samplings for weeks or months. It is important to do a proper proactive vascular planning to plan for a catheter that should minimize the patient to receive needle punctures but also, we should consider the requirement for having a normal lifestyle. In this case, the debate should be for choosing a PICC line more than a port in case of a prolonged chemotherapy.

Children are an 'everything or null' world. When considering an IV-line placement, we should consider the potential risks and benefits for it. Peripheral IV lines can be considered a low-risk procedure and placement of mid-to-long term catheters is typically associated with the need for procedural sedation. It has been demonstrated that procedural sedation done outside the operating room with propofol in children has quite a high incidence of operative complications. Children can start having intraoperative problems suddenly. For this reason, it is safer to have a separate person performing sedation with adequate skills to resuscitate a pediatric patient. A pediatric anesthesiologist must handle the sedation when deep sedation is required.

Create your own protocols. Every IV team should adhere to international standards, but it is important to adapt the standards and guidelines to the local needs and different cultural differences. Protocols are important as the presence of checklists allow the team to ensure all the correct steps are followed to avoid complications.

Analyze your data. A critical appraisal of every IV team's patient population is necessary to understand if the introduction of the IV team has improved the quality of care. The IV team should revisit and revise data at least four times a year. It is also important to have an objective look into individual cases when complications occur to provide a root-cause analysis that will help the team to change and improve care in the future.

23.5 Conclusions

IV teams are part of the quality improvement process to reduce hospital acquired complications and enhance patients' experiences. The pediatric IV teams should represent a subgroup of the IV team able to handle children and it should be based in the pediatric departments. Specific equipment and a separate environment are necessary to create a safe setting. Given the requirement for sedation in most of these patients, a pediatric anesthesiologist should be part of the team or readily available when sedation is performed.

Bibliography

1. Alexandrou E, Spencer TR, Frost SA, et al. Central venous catheter placement by advanced practice nurses demonstrates low procedural complication and infection rates - a report from 13 years of service. Crit Care Med. 2014;42:536–43.
2. Carr PJ, Glynn RW, Dineen B, et al. A pilot intravenous cannulation team: an Irish perspective. Brit J of Nursing. 2010;19:s19–27.
3. Carr PJ, Higgins NS, Cooke ML, et al. Vascular access specialist teams for device insertion and prevention of failure. Cochrane Database Syst Rev. 2014;12:CD011429.
4. Cravero J, Beach M, Blike G, et al. The incidence and nature of adverse events during Pediatric sedation/Anesthesia with propofol for procedures outside the operating room: a report from the Pediatric sedation research consortium. Anesth Analg. 2009;108:795–804.
5. Da Silva G, Priebe S, Dias F. Benefits of establishing an intravenous team and the standardization of peripheral intravenous catheters. J Infus Nurs. 2010;33:156–60.
6. Dennis MM, Ours JL, Competent i.v. management, Part 2. Nurs Manag. 2001;32:21–3.
7. Dhar S, Cook E, Oden M, et al. Building a successful infection prevention program: key components, processes, and economics. Infect Dis Clin N Am. 2016;30:567–89.
8. Gopal K, Fitzsimmons L, Lawrance JA. Nurse-led central venous catheter service: Christie experience. Brit J Radiol. 2006;79:762–5.
9. Graves N. Economics and preventing hospital-acquired infection. Emerg Infect Dis. 2004;10:561–6.
10. Kokotis K. Cost containment and infusion services. J Inf Nurs. 2005;28:S22–32.
11. Pitts S. Retrospective analysis of a Pediatric vascular access program and clinical outcomes. JAVA. 2013;18:114–20.

12. Rossetti F, Pittiruti M, Lamperti M, et al. The intracavitary ECG method for positioning the tip of central venous access devices in pediatric patients: results of an Italian multicenter study. J Vasc Access. 2015;16:137–43.
13. Santolim TQ, Santos LA, Giovani AM, et al. The strategic role of the nurse in the selection of IV devices. Br J Nurs. 2012;21:S28–30-2.
14. Tomford JW, Hershey CO, McLaren CE, et al. Intravenous therapy team and peripheral venous catheter-associated complications. A prospective controlled study. Arch Int Med. 1984;144:1191–4.
15. Vezzani A, Manca T, Vercelli A, et al. Ultrasonography as a guide during vascular access procedures and in the diagnosis of complications. J Ultrasound. 2013;16:161–70.
16. World Health Organization. Practical Guidelines for Infection Control in Health Care Facilities. 2004: ISBN 92 9022 238 7. http://www.wpro.who.int/publications/docs/practical_guidelines_infection_control.pdf. Accessed 1 Aug 2017.
17. Yacopetti N, Alexandrou E, Spencer TR, et al. Central venous catheter insertion by a clinical nurse consultant or anaesthetic medical staff: a single-Centre observational study. Crit Care and Resuscit. 2010;12:90–5.

Chapter 24
Special Problems of Venous Access in Intensive Care and Emergency

Daniele G. Biasucci

Establishing the right vascular access device (VAD), either central or peripheral, in the right patient in a specific clinical condition is crucial, especially in emergency and critical care, and it can be even more challenging in critically ill neonates and children. Emergency, urgency, and intensive care are different clinical settings in which different kind of VADs and different techniques of placement have their own specific role. First, a difficult venous access score (DIVA score) should be always applied, so to quickly recognize the neonate or the child in whom a difficult access is anticipated. Then, an evidence-based algorithm must be adopted, so to rapidly choose the appropriate venous access device using the appropriate strategy. Finally, each operator should be proficient in using cost-effective vascular imaging techniques, such as ultrasound and near-infrared technology, to facilitate VADs placement and avoiding failure and complications. All these above-mentioned tools must be appropriately used in an adequate and timely manner so to anticipate any problem and prevent any complication which is essential in critical conditions.

In this chapter an evidence-based algorithm for the choice of the most appropriate VAD in emergency and urgency conditions and in intensive care will be reviewed. Usefulness of DIVA scores in these settings will also be discussed. Then, the importance of imaging techniques like ultrasound and the near-infrared technology will be addressed. Finally, some specific settings like ECMO cannulas will be commented.

D. G. Biasucci (✉)
Intensive Care Unit, Department of Emergency, Anesthesiology and Intensive Care, Fondazione Policlinico Universitario "A. Gemelli" IRCCS, Rome, Italy
e-mail: danieleguerino.biasucci@policlinicogemelli.it

D. G. Biasucci et al. (eds.), *Vascular Access in Neonates and Children*,
https://doi.org/10.1007/978-3-030-94709-5_24

24.1 The Critically Ill Child in the Emergency Room, 'On the Scene' or in the Ward

VADs generally indicated in emergency and urgency conditions are: short peripheral cannulas; long peripheral cannulas (also defined "mini midline"); non-tunneled central VADs like CICC or FICC. PICCs and traditional Midlines have no role in this setting. It is of crucial importance to highlight that every VADs placed in emergency or urgency conditions, especially 'on the scene' or during resuscitation maneuvers, must be removed within 24–48 h. In fact, in most cases, in emergency conditions, procedures are not performed with an appropriate adherence to the international recommendations for infection prevention.

First, it is necessary to early identify those children with difficult peripheral venous access (superficial veins difficult to visualize or palpate). This category of patients has recently been described with the acronym 'DIVA' (Difficult Intra-Venous Access), normally referred to the difficulty of accessing the superficial veins of the upper limbs. It has been described that DIVA patients are up to 15% of children presenting to the emergency room. Yen, Rikers and coworkers have developed a difficult intravenous access (DIVA) score based on four variables: vein palpability, vein visibility, patient age, and history of prematurity. This score has been validated to be effective in predicting failure of peripheral VADs placement in children. A DIVA score major or equal to 4 has been defined as the cut-off value for predicting failure. Also, a simpler score based on three variables (vein palpability, vein visibility, patient age) has been proved to be predictive of peripheral VADs placement on first attempt as the four-variable rule.

DIVA score is a powerful tool, with high value in daily practice, allowing the clinician to accurately plan the strategy so to anticipate any problem and prevent any complication. In fact, when a patient has been identified as a DIVA, depending on clinical conditions, healthcare personnel must use all technologies available to obtain the appropriate venous access as rapidly as possible and avoiding complications. In presence of a DIVA patient, the personnel must utilize an appropriate bedside technology for vascular imaging, like near-infrared technology (NIR) or ultrasound guidance. Both these techniques are described elsewhere in this book. The Infusion Nursing Society (INS), in its latest guidelines released in the 2021, states that each operator expert in the field of vascular access should become proficient in the appropriate use of NIR and, obviously, ultrasound. NIR allows to visualize not visible/not palpable superficial veins at a maximum depth of 7–8 mm. Ultrasound allows to visualize and puncture veins deeper than 8 mm.

In emergency conditions, especially 'on the scene', intra-osseous (IO) access can be used. This kind of VAD is very useful during territorial life-threatening emergencies or mass casualties. The European Resuscitation Council guidelines on pediatric cardiac arrest recommend using a IO device when, during resuscitation of an infant or child, a venous access is not readily established within 1 minute. The ATLS (Advances Trauma Life Support) guidelines, released by the American College of Surgeons (ACS), suggest considering an IO device before placing a central venous access in trauma victims younger than 6 years of age. IO access is quite well tolerated; however, given the well described related complications, it must be promptly removed as soon as the patient's conditions will allow, but no later than 48 h after placement.

Finally, once the patient has been stabilized, an appropriate peripheral or central venous access must be established and any VAD which had been placed in emergency should be promptly removed within 24 or 48 h at maximum.

24.2 The Critically Ill Newborn in the Delivery Room

Many factors may influence the choice of the most appropriate VAD in the newborn: (a) the exact moment of the need of the VAD, if immediately after birth or more than 24 h after birth; (b) the clinical conditions of the patient, if stable or not; (c) the expected indwelling time of the VAD; (d) the type of solutions to be infused and drugs to be administered.

During those emergencies commonly occurring in the delivery room, there is indication for placement of an umbilical venous catheter (UVC), preferably double lumen, in most cases. The most common conditions include: (a) a neonate with hypoxic-ischemic encephalopathy due to perinatal asphyxia; (b) a premature newborn with a gestational age of less than 28 weeks; (c) newborns older than 29 weeks of gestational age or at term and suffering from respiratory failure needing CPAP with FiO2 > 40% or endotracheal intubation, and/or presenting hemodynamic instability, or in case of difficult peripheral venous access.

In the remaining conditions, a short peripheral cannula may be placed, with the aid of NIR technology if a difficulty in obtaining a peripheral access exists.

More than 48 h after birth, it may not be possible to insert an UVC and the choice of the right VAD mainly depends on the duration of the intravenous therapy and the type of drugs and solution to be infused.

24.3 The Child in the Pediatric Intensive Care Unit (PICU)

Infusion of drugs with pH > 9 or < 5 or hyperosmolar solutions (> 800 mOsm/L), hemodynamic monitoring, dialysis, need of repeated central venous blood samples, are all well-known and common indications to central venous catheters.

Central VADs commonly used in PICU are the following: (a) CICCs, centrally inserted central catheters, inserted through ultrasound guided direct puncture of a central vein; (b) PICCs, peripherally inserted central catheters, inserted through ultrasound guided puncture of a deep vein of the arm; (c) FICCs, femoral inserted central catheters, inserted through ultrasound guided puncture of a vein at the groin (deep femoral vein, superficial femoral vein or great saphenous vein).

Ultrasound evaluation of all possible venous options must be always performed to choose the safest and the most appropriate vein to be punctured. In the PICU setting, planning the exit site location is of outmost importance to minimize risks of infection and thrombotic complications. Disregarding the puncture site, the exit site must be in an area with the lowest bacterial colonization and where the dressing is optimal.

The exit site of a PICC must be at the third medium of the arm. If a deep vein of the arm cannot be directly punctured at the mid arm, a vein close to the axilla or into the axilla may also be punctured but it should be tunneled at the third medium of the arm.

The ideal exit site of a CICC should be in the infra-clavicular area on the chest wall (Fig. 24.1). An exit site in the supra-clavicular area may be acceptable even if not ideal. Exit site at the neck should be absolutely avoided (Figs. 24.2 and 24.3). If a direct puncture of a vein in the infraclavicular area (i.e., axillary vein or cephalic vein), is not possible because veins in this area are too small, a direct ultrasound guided puncture of the brachiocephalic vein or, as second option, of the subclavian vein in the supraclavicular area, is recommended. After a puncture of a vein in the supraclavicular area, if the exit site appears to be not acceptable in terms of infection and thrombosis prevention since dressing and nursing may not be optimal, the tunneling of the catheter is recommended so to move the exit site to the infra-clavicular area (Fig. 24.4) or even to the chest wall (Fig. 24.5). For this purpose, it is suggested to use, off-label, power injectable PICCs as multi-purpose CICCs. The PICC is ideal for tunneling because it is longer than the traditional CICC and can be trimmed; it can be easily inserted through a central vein, and then also easily tunneled. Furthermore, power injectability has the additional advantage of tolerating high-pressure injection (up to 300–350 psi) of contrast media during radiological procedures and allows delivery of high flows of fluids for resuscitation. Moreover, disregarding the puncture site, 5 Fr power injectable double lumen catheters may be safely used also for apheresis in critically ill infants. Using such

Fig. 24.1 Double lumen CICC in pediatric patient, inserted by ultrasound-guided puncture of the axillary vein

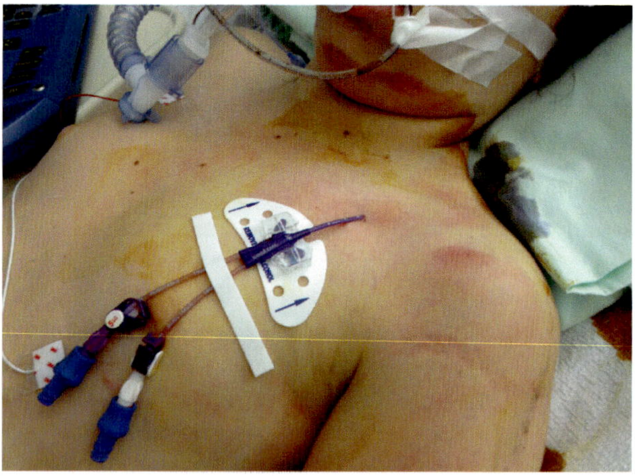

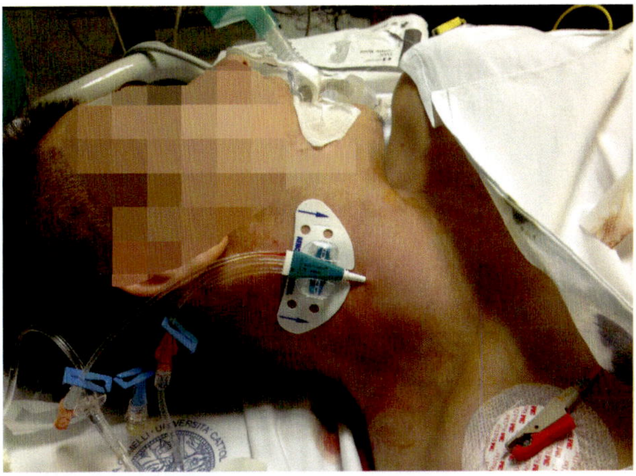

Fig. 24.2 Exit site of CICC at the neck in pediatric patient: unacceptable

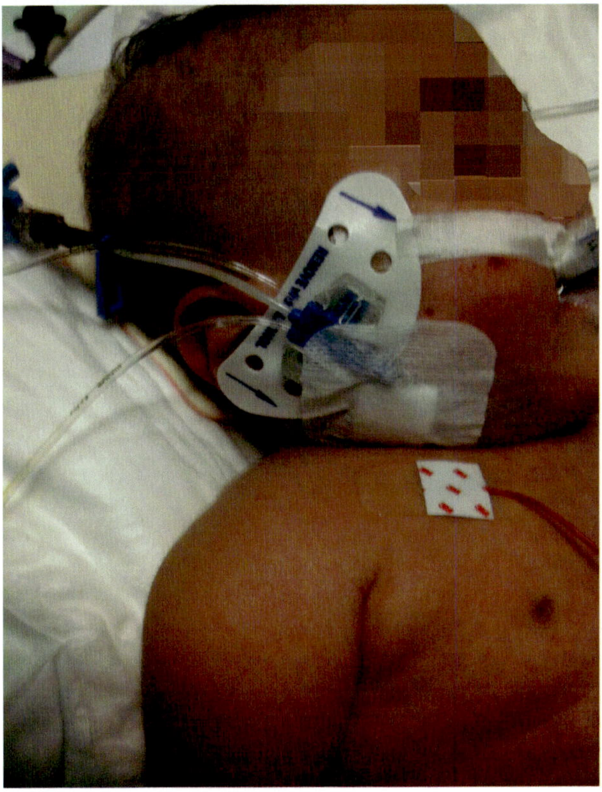

Fig. 24.3 Exit site of CICC at the neck in neonate: unacceptable

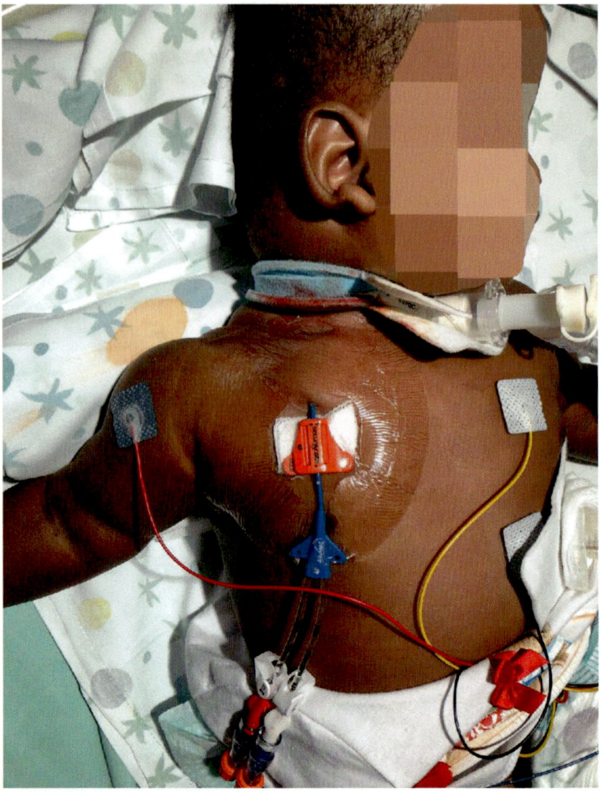
Fig. 24.4 CICC tunneled to the infraclavicular area, after ultrasound-guided puncture of the brachio-cephalic vein

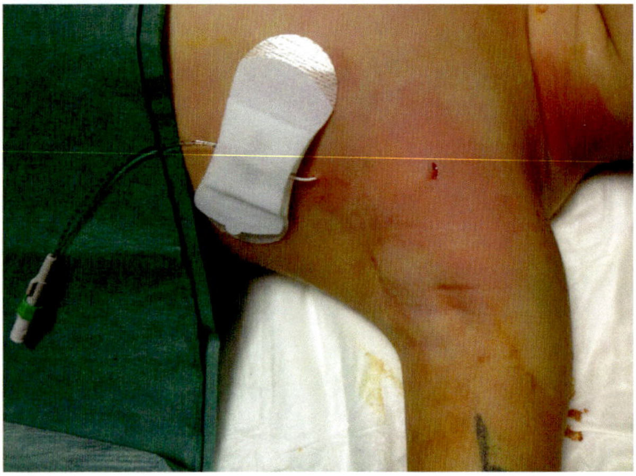
Fig. 24.5 CICC tunneled to the lateral side of the chest

VADs, up to 25–30 ml/min can be obtained, enough for extra-corporeal blood purification techniques.

When inserting central catheters with a modified Seldinger technique in hypovolemic and/or spontaneously breathing patients, the operator should pay particular attention to the risk of venous embolism during inspiration. To avoid this complication in critically il neonates and children, spontaneous breathing, if present, must be abolished using apneic sedation or pharmacologic paralysis (if not contraindicated), and hypovolemia must be corrected. Moreover, as soon as the wire and the dilator are removed, the operator must close the introducer with a thumb and then insert the catheter very quickly.

A long trimmable catheter should be also used as a FICC (Fig. 24.6). In fact, to be considered a central catheter and to be used also for hemodynamic monitoring, the tip of a FICC should reach the junction between the inferior vena cava and the right atrium. For dialysis or apheresis, it may be adequate a FICC whose tip lies in the inferior vena cava after the confluence of the two common iliac veins.

The ideal exit site of a FICC should be at the mid-thigh. To obtain an exit site in this area, the catheter must be tunneled after a groin puncture so to move the exit site to the mid-thigh (Figs. 24.7, 24.8, 24.9 and 24.10). Alternatively, a direct ultrasound guided puncture of the superficial femoral vein at the mid-thigh may be performed if this vein does not appear too small nor too superficial.

If a central venous catheter is not indicated and a peripheral venous access is adequate, the type of peripheral VAD to be placed depends on the expected duration

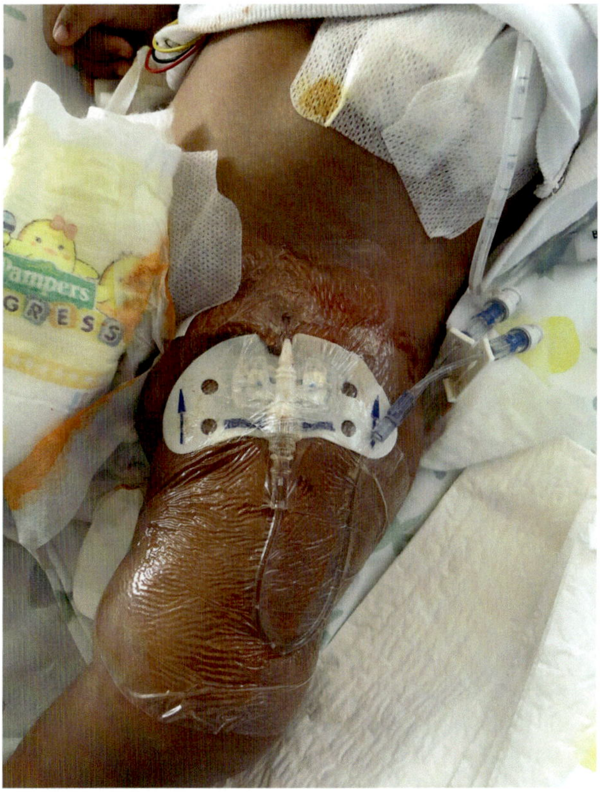

Fig. 24.6 Non-tunneled FICC inserted in the common femoral vein (exit site at the groin)

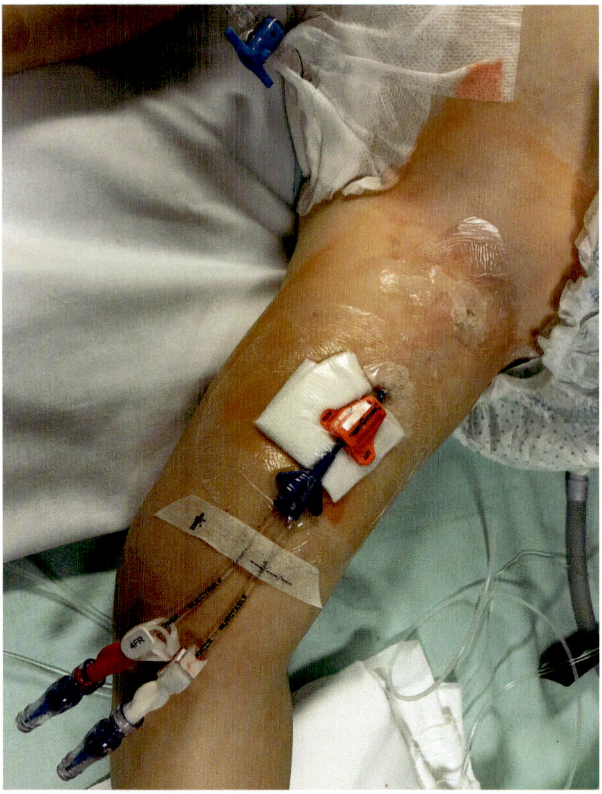

Fig. 24.7 Double lumen FICC tunneled to mid-thigh

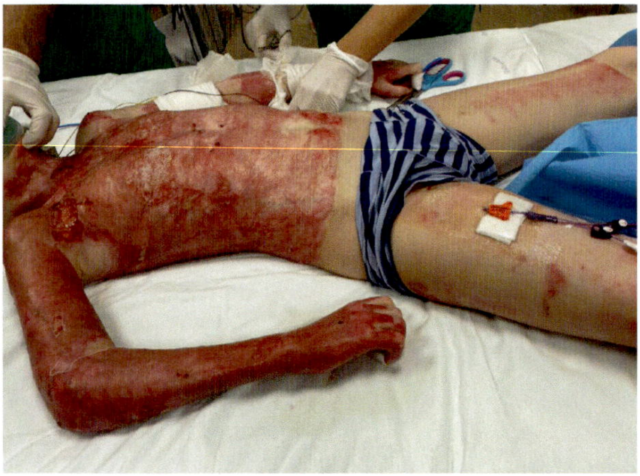

Fig. 24.8 Double lumen FICC tunneled to mid-thigh in burned child

of a given intravenous therapy and on the expected indwelling time of the VAD itself. If the duration of the intravenous therapy is expected to be longer than 1 week, ultrasound guided placement of a long peripheral cannula, also called '*mini-midline*', is recommended. If duration of intravenous therapy is shorter than 7 days,

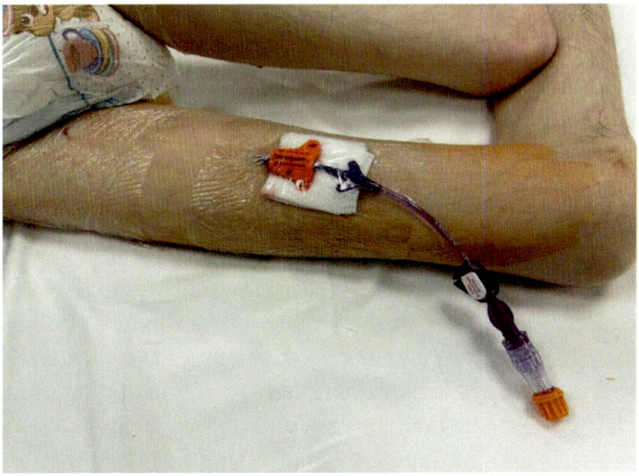

Fig. 24.9 Single lumen FICC tunneled to mid-thigh

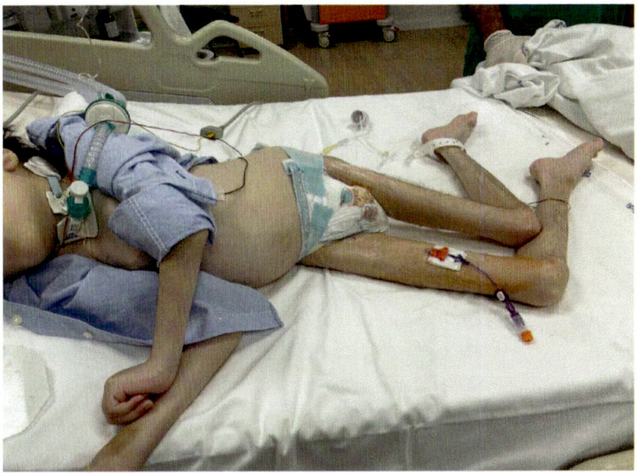

Fig. 24.10 Single lumen FICC tunneled to mid-thigh in child with complex chronic syndrome

a short peripheral cannula is indicated. In case of a DIVA score > 4 suggesting a difficult peripheral venous access, NIR technology should be used to aid superficial vein cannulation. In case of failure in obtaining a peripheral venous access using NIR, ultrasound guidance should be used, and the placement of a mini midline should be considered.

24.4 The Newborn in the Neonatal Intensive Care Unit (NICU)

Critically ill newborns need central venous catheters for many clinical purposes which include: (a) infusion of fluids with different kind of osmolarity; (b) bolus of fluids for volume replacement and/or continuous infusion of inotropes or vasopressors when hemodynamically unstable; (c) blood products transfusions; (d) hemodynamic monitoring including pre-load assessment and determination of oxygen saturation in mixed venous blood; (e) frequent blood samples for lab tests. For all these purposes, in absence of an UVC or when it must be removed or it cannot be placed, single-lumen 3 Fr or dual-lumen 4 Fr, polyurethane power injectable central venous catheters, placed by ultrasound guided puncture of the brachiocephalic vein (CICC—Centrally Inserted Central Catheter) or of the femoral vein (FICC—Femoral Inserted Central Catheter) are highly indicated.

CICCs and FICCs are also indicated in the stable premature newborn with the need of intravenous treatments for more than 14 days. In the same category of patients with a duration of intravenous therapy lasting less than 14 days but more than 1 week, epicutaneo-caval catheters are indicated. Finally, if VAD is needed for less than 7 days, a short peripheral cannula can be used.

In case of difficult peripheral venous access, NIR technology must be used in neonates and premature newborns so to choose the most suitable vein for peripheral cannulation.

24.5 'Targeting Zero' Complications in PICU and NICU: A Bundle of Recommendations

VADs related complications, especially infections and thrombosis still represent a relevant cause of morbidity and mortality both in the PICU and the NICU. It has been shown that most VAD related complications are multifactorial but preventable. An evidence-based insertion and care bundle aimed at reducing all risk factors is associated with a significant decrease in the rate of catheter-related bloodstream infections (CRBSI) and catheter-related thrombosis (CRT) (Fig. 24.11). Costello and coworkers, in a retrospective interventional study, showed a reduction in CR-BSI rate from 7.8/1000 catheter-days to 2.3/1000 catheter-days after a systematic intervention. In adult patients, Pronovost et al. demonstrated that an evidence-based intervention resulted in an effective and sustained reduction of the CR-BSI rate.

A bundle of recommendations for preventing VADs-related early and late complications must be systematically adopted by each PICU and NICU staffs. It must include the following evidence-based recommendations: (1) Hand washing and maximal barrier precautions; (2) Skin antisepsis with 2% chlorhexidine; (3) Ultrasound pre-puncture evaluation; (4) Ultrasound-guided venipuncture; (5) Tunneling of the catheter so to obtain an exit site in the infraclavicular area; (6) Tip location technique using intracavitary ECG and/or echocardiography; (7) Sealing of the exit site with glue; (8) Securement with sutureless device (adhesive ones or subcutaneously anchored); (9) Coverage with transparent semipermeable dressing (10) Chlorhexidine-impregnated sponges on the exit site after the first week; (11) Use of neutral NFC and port protectors; (12) Timely removal of central lines no

Insertion and maintenance bundle
1. Hand washing and maximal barrier precautions
2. Skin antisepsis with 2% chlorhexidine in 70% alcohol
3. Ultrasound pre-puncture evaluation through RaCeVA and RaPeVA
4. Ultrasound guided venipuncture
5. Tunneling of the catheter so to obtain exit site in infraclavicular area
6. Tip location technique using intracavitary ECG and/or echocardiography
7. Sealing of the exit site with cyanoacrylate glue for the first week
8. Securement with sutureless device
9. Coverage with transparent semipermeable dressing
10. Use of chlorhexidine sponge dressing from the 7th day on
11. Use of neutral NFC and Port Protectors
12. Timely removal of central lines no longer necessary
13. Simulation-based standardized training program
14. Planned clinical audit with all physicians and nurses

Fig. 24.11 Bundle for insertion and maintenance of central venous access in children

longer necessary; (13) Simulation-based standardized training program; (14) Planned clinical audit with all physicians and nurses.

Several guidelines recommend the use of ultrasound to reduce both early mechanical complications and late infective and thrombotic complications. In fact, it has been proved that facilitating CICC placement by reducing the number of attempts and, subsequently, both the risk of possible break-down of aseptic technique and the risk of hematoma formation, ultrasound guidance may indirectly reduce the incidence of CRBSI and CRT.

As already discussed above in the previous paragraphs, current guidelines and some studies place emphasis on exit site selection. CRBSIs are related to the contamination risk at the exit site. It should be considered that different areas of the skin have different degrees of bacterial colonization. Furthermore, moisture, warmer areas of body, hair distribution, failure of dressing to adhere, are among relevant risk factors. On the other hand, various studies have demonstrated that when a long indwelling time is expected, tunneled catheters are preferred because of the lower risk of infection. Disregarding the puncture site, tunneling the catheter allows to move the exit site to the chest, a dry, stable area with low bacterial colonization, where dressing is optimal, and the risk of infection is low. Moreover, by stopping bacteria spread along the catheter, the tunnel avoids their entrance into the vein.

Also, sealing the exit site of catheters with cyanoacrylate glue reduces the risk of extraluminal contamination, presumably by reducing bacterial entrance through the skin breech. Furthermore, the glue reduces bleeding at the exit site and at the puncture site, and by stabilizing the catheter, the glue may decrease local damage to the endothelium and the risk of thrombosis. Sutures are no longer recommended and should be avoided since they cause disruption of the skin around the catheter exit site, causing inflammation and bacterial colonization. Published evidence and guidelines recommend sutureless devices to stabilize the catheter.

Finally, each bundle should be implemented using a simulation-based training program aimed at education and assessment of procedural competence of the staff, which has been shown to have important implications for the quality of care. All medical and nursing staffs must be trained according to evidence-based recommendations of the World Congress on Vascular Access (WoCoVA) consensus conference.

24.6 Special Feature: ECMO Cannulas

The use of extracorporeal membrane oxygenation (ECMO) has increased over recent years providing respiratory and cardiac support. Particularly, ECMO can be veno-arterial (VA-ECMO) for both cardiocirculatory and respiratory support and veno-venous (VV-ECMO) for respiratory support. Optimal cannula placement is essential for a successful procedure and for reducing complications. Multiple cannulation strategies may be employed depending on age and weight and on underlying conditions.

VV-ECMO should be considered the preferred modality for respiratory support in pediatrics because of the significant reduction in the morbidity compared to veno-arterial access. Today, veno-venous double-lumen cannula for respiratory failure is much more frequently utilized, accounting for 18.9% of all neonatal cases and 17.0% of all pediatric ones. The last generation of cannulas is best suitable for percutaneous placement. This kind of cannulas allows to minimize recirculation, which is a well-known problem with femoral-jugular cannulation, since aspiration ports are in the superior and inferior vena cava (SVC, IVC), while the infusion port is directed toward the tricuspid valve (TV).

In fact, globally ultrasound guided, percutaneous, bi-caval double-lumen cannulation in neonates and infants has been recently proved to be safe and effective, even performed at bedside and in emergency conditions. After ultrasound guided puncture of a central vein (Internal Jugular Vein or Brachiocephalic Vein), the guidewire first and then the cannula is advanced under echocardiographic guidance to the IVC using a subcostal bi-caval view (Fig. 24.7). The wire must be guided into the IVC, excluding and avoiding guidewire loops into the right atrium and tip wedge into the hepatic veins. Ultrasound guidance is of paramount importance for the entire procedure, to ensure correct positioning of the bicaval double-lumen cannula for a successful treatment without complications. In fact, the cannula infusion port must face the tricuspid valve with its distal end into the IVC to avoid recirculation. Distal aspiration port into the IVC should lie beyond the merge of the hepatic veins, to avoid the inadvertent displacement of the cannula into them which might cause ECMO flow limitation or obstruction of the venous drainage from the liver with a subsequent acute Budd-Chiari syndrome. These above-mentioned complications do not occur if the cannula is advanced under echocardiographic guidance through a subcostal view, both the four-chambers one and the bi-caval view, so to have the infusion port facing the tricuspid valve and the distal end of the cannula into the IVC beyond hepatic veins. After the cannula is placed, ECMO support is started, and the correct position of the cannula must be confirmed again by echocardiography demonstrating that the flow is effectively directed from the infusion port toward the tricuspid valve. Then, the cannula is secured to the skin. The correct position of the cannula must be checked by echocardiography every 8 h or in the case of ECMO flow decrease in constant revolutions per minute or increase in the negative aspiration pressure.

In case of indication of VA-ECMO, a cannula is placed through the right internal jugular vein into the right atrium, the blood is drained to a venous reservoir and then actively pumped through the oxygenator where gas exchange occurs. Then, the blood is warmed to body temperature by the heat exchanger before returning to the patient through a cannula placed through the right carotid artery into aortic arch or into descending aorta through a femoral artery. In peripheral VA-ECMO, the venous cannula can be placed by the intensivist through a percutaneous ultrasound guided puncture of the right internal jugular vein or a femoral vein, whilst the arterial cannula is usually inserted by a surgeon with an open surgical technique.

24.7 Conclusions: Algorithm for VADs Choice in the Critically Ill Children and Neonates

Figure 24.12 shows the algorithm for choosing the appropriate VAD in the critically ill children both in emergency conditions and ICU stay. It should be a guide for clinicians and all healthcare operators. The algorithm has been already commented and described above in the previous paragraphs.

Figure 24.13 shows the algorithm for choosing of the appropriate VAD in the critically ill neonate both in emergency conditions in the delivery room and during NICU stay.

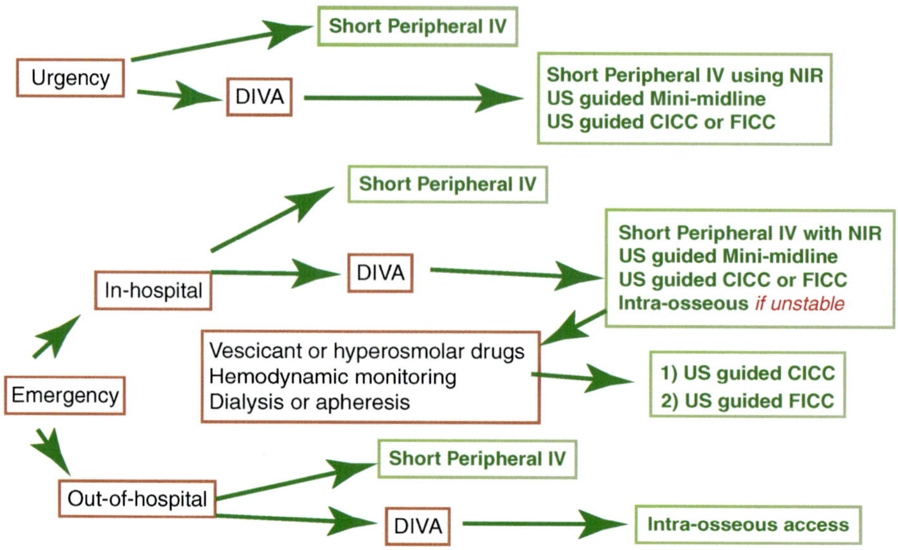

Fig. 24.12 Algorithm for choosing the venous access in children

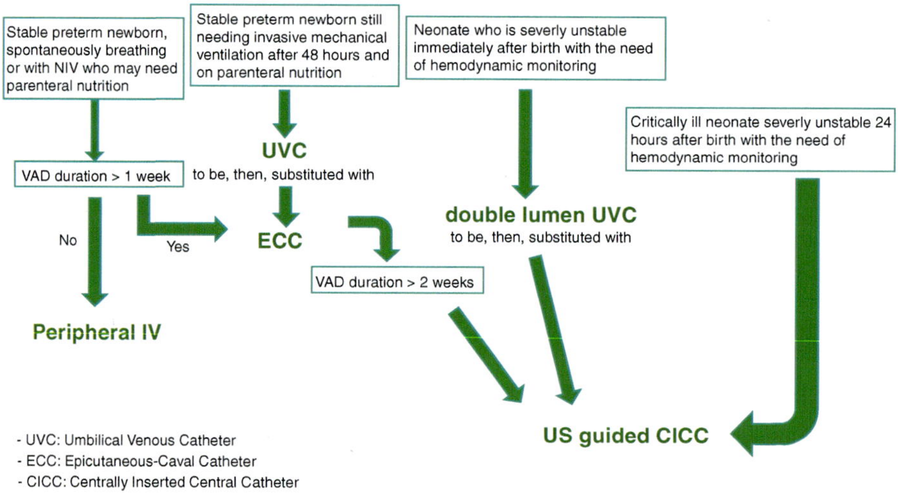

Fig. 24.13 Algorithm for choosing the venous access in neonates

Bibliography

1. ATLS Subcommittee; American College of Surgeons' Committee on Trauma; International ATLS Working Group. Advanced trauma life support (ATLS®): the ninth edition. J Trauma Acute Care Surg. 2013 May;74(5):1363–6. https://doi.org/10.1097/TA.0b013e31828b82f5.
2. Benkhadra M, Collignon M, Fournel I, Oeuvrard C, Rollin P, Perrin M, Volot F, Girard C. Ultrasound guidance allows faster peripheral IV cannulation in children under 3 years

of age with difficult venous access: a prospective randomized study. Paediatr Anaesth. 2012 May;22(5):449–54. https://doi.org/10.1111/j.1460-9592.2012.03830.x.
3. Biasucci DG, Pittiruti M, Taddei A, Picconi E, Pizza A, Celentano D, Piastra M, Scoppettuolo G, Conti G. Targeting zero catheter-related bloodstream infections in pediatric intensive care unit: a retrospective matched case-control study. J Vasc Access. 2018 Mar;19(2):119–24. https://doi.org/10.5301/jva.5000797.
4. Costello JM, Morrow DF, Graham DA, Potter-Bynoe G, Sandora TJ, Laussen PC. Systematic intervention to reduce central line-associated bloodstream infection rates in a pediatric cardiac intensive care unit. Pediatrics. 2008;121(5):915–23.
5. Elward AM, Hollenbeak CS, Warren DK, Fraser VJ. Attributable cost of nosocomial primary bloodstream infection in pediatric intensive care unit patients. Pediatrics. 2005;115(4):868–72.
6. Fallon SC, Shekerdemian LS, Olutoye OO, et al. Initial experience with single-vessel cannulation for venovenous extracorporeal membrane oxygenation in pediatric respiratory failure. Pediatr Crit Care Med. 2013;14(4):366–73.
7. Gorski LA. The 2016 infusion therapy standards of practice. Home Healthc Now. 2017;35(1):10–8. Review
8. Hallas P, Brabrand M, Folkestad L. Complication with intraosseous access: scandinavian users' experience. West J Emerg Med. 2013 Sep;14(5):440–3. https://doi.org/10.5811/westjem.2013.1.12000.
9. Henneberg SW, Jungersen D, Hole P. Durability of central venous catheters. A randomized trial in children with malignant diseases. Paediatr Anaesth. 1996;6(6):449–51.
10. Javidfar J, Brodie D, Wang D, et al. Use of bicaval dual-lumen catheter for adult venovenous extracorporeal membrane oxygenation. Ann Thorac Surg. 2011;91(6):1763–9.
11. Karakitsos D, Labropoulos N, De Groot E, et al. Real-time ultrasound-guided catheterisation of the internal jugular vein: a prospective comparison with the landmark technique in critical care patients. Crit Care. 2006;10(6):R162.
12. Lamperti M, Bodenham AR, Pittiruti M, et al. International evidence-based recommendations on ultrasound-guided vascular access. Intensive Care Med. 2012;38(7):1105–17.
13. Lamperti M, Moureau N, Kelly LJ, et al. Competence in paediatric central venous lines placement. Br J Anaesth. 2014;112(2):383.
14. Lamperti M, Pittiruti M. II. Difficult peripheral veins: turn on the lights. Br J Anaesth. 2013 Jun;110(6):888–91. https://doi.org/10.1093/bja/aet078.
15. Lazar DA, Cass DL, Olutoye OO, et al. Venovenous cannulation for extracorporeal membrane oxygenation using a bicaval dual-lumen catheter in neonates. J Pediatr Surg. 2012;47(2):430–4.
16. Loveday HP, Wilson JA, Pra RJ, et al. UK Department of Health. epic3: national evidence-based guidelines for preventing healthcare-associated infections in NHS hospitals in England. J Hosp Infect. 2014;86(Suppl 1):S1–S70.
17. Maconochie IK, de Caen AR, Aickin R, Atkins DL, Biarent D, Guerguerian AM, Kleinman ME, Kloeck DA, Meaney PA, Nadkarni VM, Ng KC, Nuthall G, Reis AG, Shimizu N, Tibballs J, Pintos RV, Pediatric Basic Life Support and Pediatric Advanced Life Support Chapter Collaborators. Part 6: Pediatric basic life support and pediatric advanced life support: 2015 International Consensus on Cardiopulmonary Resuscitation and Emergency Cardiovascular Care Science with Treatment Recommendations. Resuscitation. 2015 Oct;95:e147–68. https://doi.org/10.1016/j.resuscitation.2015.07.044.
18. Marschall J, Mermel LA, Fakih M, et al. Strategies to prevent central line-associated bloodstream infections in acute care hospitals: 2014 update. Infect Control Hosp Epidemiol. 2014;35(Suppl 2):S89–S107.
19. Moscatelli A, Buratti S, Gregoretti C, Lampugnani E, Salvati P, Marasini M, et al. Emergency percutaneous, bicaval double-lumen, ECMO cannulation in neonates and infants: insights from three consecutive cases. Int J Artif Organs. 2015 Sep;38(9):517–21. https://doi.org/10.5301/ijao.5000432.
20. Moureau N, Lamperti M, Kelly LJ, et al. Evidence-based consensus on the insertion of central venous access devices: definition of minimal requirements for training. Br J Anaesth. 2013;110(3):347–56.

21. Nahum E, Levy I, Katz J, et al. Efficacy of subcutaneous tunneling for prevention of bacterial colonization of femoral central venous catheters in critically ill children. Pediatr Infect Dis J. 2002;21(11):1000–4.
22. OGrady NP, Alexander M, Burns LA, et al. Healthcare Infection Control Practices Advisory Committee. Guidelines for the prevention of intravascular catheter-related infections. Am J Infect Control. 2011;39(Suppl 1):S1–S34.
23. OGrady NP, Alexander M, Burns LA, et al. Healthcare Infection Control Practices Advisory Committee (HICPAC). Guidelines for the prevention of intravascular catheter-related infections. Clin Infect Dis. 2011;52(9):e162–93.
24. Olaussen A, Williams B. Intraosseous access in the prehospital setting: literature review. Prehosp Disaster Med. 2012 Oct;27(5):468–72. https://doi.org/10.1017/S1049023X12001124.
25. Pittiruti M. Ultrasound guided central vascular access in neonates, infants and children. Curr Drug Targets. 2012;13(7):961–9.
26. Pronovost P, Needham D, Berenholtz S, et al. An intervention to decrease catheter-related bloodstream infections in the ICU. N Engl J Med. 2006;355(26):2725–32.
27. Riker MW, Kennedy C, Winfrey BS, Yen K, Dowd MD. Validation and refinement of the difficult intravenous access score: a clinical prediction rule for identifying children with difficult intravenous access. Acad Emerg Med. 2011 Nov;18(11):1129–34. https://doi.org/10.1111/j.1553-2712.2011.01205.x.
28. Rollins MD, Hubbard A, Zabrocki L, Barnhart DC, Bratton SL. Extracorporeal membrane oxygenation cannula on trends for pediatric respiratory failure and central nervous system injury. J Pediatr Surg. 2012;47(1):68–75.
29. Rycus P. ECLS Registry Report. 2014 Jan 1; January 2014:1–26.
30. Schwab SJ, Buller GL, McCann RL, Bollinger RR, S ckel DL. Prospective evaluation of a Dacron cuffed hemodialysis catheter for prolonged use. Am J Kidney Dis. 1988;11(2):166–9.
31. Scoppettuolo G, Dolcetti L, Emoli A, La Greca A, Biasucci DG, Pittiruti M. Further benefits of cyanoacrylate glue for central venous catheterisation. Anaesthesia. 2015;70(6):758.
32. Shekelle PG, Pronovost PJ, Wachter RM, et al. The top patient safety strategies that can be encouraged for adoption now. Ann Intern Med. 2013;158(5 Pt 2):365–8.
33. Skinner SC, Hirschl RB, Bartlett RH. Extracorporeal life support. Semin Pediatr Surg. 2006;15(4):242–50.
34. Slonim AD, Kurtines HC, Sprague BM, Singh N. The costs associated with nosocomial bloodstream infections in the pediatric intensive care unit. Pediatr Crit Care Med. 2001;2(2):170–4.
35. Stolz LA, Stolz U, Howe C, Farrell IJ, Adhikari S. Ultrasound-guided peripheral venous access: a meta-analysis and systematic review. J Vasc Access. 2015 Jul–Aug;16(4):321–6. https://doi.org/10.5301/jva.5000346.
36. Victor K, Barre N, Glover G, Kapetanakis S, Langrish C. Acute Budd-Chiari syndrome during veno-venous extracorporeal membrane oxygenation diagnosed using transthoracic echocardiography. Br J Anaesth. 2012;108(6):1043–4.
37. Voigt J, Waltzman M, Lottenberg L. Intraosseous vascular access for in-hospital emergency use: a systematic clinical review of the literature and analysis. Pediatr Emerg Care. 2012 Feb;28(2):185–99. https://doi.org/10.1097/PEC.0b013e3182449edc.
38. Wilkinson JN, Chikhani M, Mortimer K, Gill SJ. The antimicrobial effect of Histoacryl skin adhesive. Anaesthesia. 2008;63(12):1382–4.
39. Yen K, Riegert A, Gorelick M. Derivation of the DIVA score: a clinical prediction rule for the identification of children with difficult intravenous access. Pediatr Emerg Care. 2008;24:143–7.

Chapter 25
Special Problems of Venous Access in Oncology and Hematology

Alessandro Crocoli and Mauro Pittiruti

Insertion and management of vascular access are critical concerns for children affected by malignancies. Prolonged course of disease, complexity, and variety of treatment protocols require long-lasting vascular access to provide an adequate route for administration of intravenous therapies as well as to allow routine blood sampling without repeated and painful venipunctures. For those reasons, central venous catheters are nowadays an important component in the care of this patient population, with a direct influence on outcome. In this respect, there are peculiar issues (techniques of insertion, management, complications etc.) which must be known to improve both quality of life over the course of the disease and outcome of children with cancer.

25.1 Introduction

Even though cancer is a rare condition in the pediatric population, it is the second most common cause of death in children older than 12 months. In 2017, the National Institute of Health—National Cancer Institute estimates that there will be 10,270 new diagnoses of cancer among children from 0 to 14 years of age, and 1190 patients are expected to die from the disease. Over the last 50 years, the overall survival for this population has dramatically increased, with the 5-year survival rate after diagnosis from 50% in late 70's to 85% in 2010. Interestingly, a more notable

A. Crocoli
Operative Unit of General and Thoracic Surgery, Bambino Gesù Children's Hospital IRCCS, Rome, Italy
e-mail: alessandro.crocoli@opbg.net

M. Pittiruti (✉)
Department of Surgery, Catholic University Hospital, Rome, Italy

D. G. Biasucci et al. (eds.), *Vascular Access in Neonates and Children*,
https://doi.org/10.1007/978-3-030-94709-5_25

improvement has been observed for some tumors like acute lymphoblastic leukemia (5% in early 50's to 90% in 2010), lymphomas (30% in 60's to around 80% in 2010) and Wilms tumor (20–90%). All those successes have been achieved since the concept of multidisciplinary treatment was introduced in the field of pediatric onco-hematology. Therefore, more intensive chemotherapy and radiation regimens, stem cell and bone marrow transplantation options, as well as different surgical procedures and techniques have been developed over the last decades, with specific roles in different treatment protocols, thus having a direct influence on the outcome. However, non-negligible side effects of therapies (severe pancytopenia, mucositis induced by radiotherapy and chemotherapy, different aspects of graft-versus-host disease etc.) led to development of more intense and challenging intravenous supportive treatments (blood component transfusions, apheresis, prolonged parenteral nutrition etc.). Moreover, the necessity to have a reliable way to obtain routine blood samples in children who have difficult vascular access as they are needle-phobic, or have reduced pain tolerance, or have coagulation disorders, or are at risk of progressive peripheral vein depletion, but are more likely to require repeated and painful venipuncture, was another crucial factor influencing the progressive popularity gained by central venous catheters in the modern treatment of children with cancer.

In 1973 Broviac et al. developed the first long-term silicon central venous catheter to deliver home parenteral nutrition in patients, while the first use for onco-hematological therapy was reported in 1979 by Hickman et al. Gyves et al. then proposed the use of a totally implanted device for patients with cancer in 1982, and in the following years many advances have been described in terms of materials, techniques, and care. However, despite the referenced literature with many protocols and guidelines that have been published over the last decades, there is far less evidence for children than for adults, especially considering cancer patients. Indications, techniques for placement and removal, choice of device, catheter care, and rate of complications require closer study to gain insight into their use in the oncological and hematological population.

25.2 General Principles

The patient's needs are the first and most important issue to consider for the choice of vascular access device (VAD), also considering duration, type, and previous history of onco-hematological treatment. There is a large and established consensus that every chemotherapy medication should be delivered through adequate central venous access, since the risk of infusion-related injuries of vesicant and irritant substances via a peripheral vein is no longer acceptable. This statement must be considered also for supportive care issues, as well as for management of advanced cancer stages with palliative measures.

One of the main concerns for practitioners who treat children with cancer is the high volume and number of medications, either drugs or blood components, administrated via the catheter. Therefore, the mistake of thinking that bigger lumens mean better performance and that more lumens mean easier management has lead to demand for large bore and multiple lumen catheters for all patients.

Regarding the caliber of the catheter, it is now well known that the bigger the catheter, the higher the risk of venous thrombosis. Also, larger catheters require a larger hole in the vein during placement. Therefore, the size of the device should be decided after measuring with ultrasound the diameter of the target vein. This consideration is more important for cancer patients, who are prone to coagulation disorders (both bleeding and hypercoagulation) depending on the phase of disease and the treatment they undergo. Preferably, the outer diameter of the catheter should not be larger than one-third of the diameter of the target vein chosen for placement: for example, a 3 Fr (1 mm) catheter is appropriate for a vein whose diameter is 9 Fr (3 mm) or larger.

On the other hand, multiple lumen catheters are indicated in patients undergoing intensive treatments or stem cell transplantation, because of the complexity of therapy; these patients require administration of multiple intravenous drugs and solutions which is accompanied with non-negligible risk of undesirable reactions between drugs and inappropriate diluent IV solutions and drug-drug incompatibility. For those reasons, dual lumen VADs are often preferred, and their placement is strongly encouraged by physicians. However, handling and caring of multiple lumen catheters is associated with higher risk of infection compared to single lumen devices due to more maneuvers and actions required, thus, their use as first-choice catheter is still debated (Table 25.1).

25.3 Indications

Short term catheters must be used in emergency settings—resuscitation, lifesaving apheresis procedures for hyper-leukocytic leukemia, acute graft versus host disease treatment, acute renal failure, acute hemolytic anemia—and only for intrahospital use. Most children require long-lasting and stable venous access for discontinuous outpatient use; toddlers and younger children prone to repeated and painful punctures, as well as patients undergoing intensive and prolonged chemotherapy regimens will benefit from a tunneled VAD (TVAD), which is easier to handle and allows repeated infusion and blood sampling without pain. Disadvantages include

Table 25.1 General Principles of Central Venous Catheterization in Pediatric Malignancies

1. Central venous catheters are mainstay in treatment and management of children with cancer
2. Therapies for malignancies increases risk of complications such as bleeding, thrombosis, and infections; strategies to reduce these events include correct choice of vein, size and lumens of catheter: The outer diameter of the catheter should be decided on the basis of the inner diameter of the target vein chosen for placement, to minimize risk of thrombosis
3. Multiple lumen catheters are not always the appropriate device (higher risk of infection, more complex management etc.)

disturbed body image, need for adequate care of the exit site with regular dressing changes, as well as limitations on physical activities such as bathing and swimming. On the other hand, adolescents, young adults, or children who undergo discontinuous therapies (3–6 weeks interval) are eligible for totally implanted devices (TID) such as port catheters. Main advantages of a TID are that because it is completely subcutaneous, there is no need to maintain care of any external catheter, no limitations on physical activities, as well as the preservation of body image. However, limits of TIDs are that access to the reservoir can be painful or difficult (for example, in obese patients) and that removal requires a surgical procedure. Consequently, TIDs are recommended only in patients who require intermittent and prolonged use while TVADs are recommended for prolonged but continuous/frequent vascular access.

It is worthwhile to note that peripherally inserted central catheters (PICC) nowadays represent a versatile, durable, and easy to use long-term vascular access which is gaining notable popularity in the pediatric population due to improvements in materials (new generation power injectable polyurethane), quick placement procedure (bedside under local anesthesia), and good patient compliance. In children with cancer, PICCs represent a good solution for children who require adequate vascular access and cannot undergo general anesthesia (large mediastinal mass with airway compression for example) as well as for patients who cannot tolerate the limitations of a TVAD. PICCs have also been validated for patients undergoing bone marrow transplantation. For those reasons, PICCs can essentially be considered as long-term VADs. Furthermore, the World Congress Vascular Access (WoCoVA) in 2013 proposed new VAD nomenclature and classification that is no longer based on device "time" but on the vein cannulated during insertion: Centrally Inserted Central Catheters (CICCs) are devices inserted through a vein in the upper part the body, in the supraclavicular or infraclavicular region. PICCs are those devices inserted through a deep vein of brachial region (basilic or cephalic vein), while Femorally Inserted Central Catheters (FICC) are placed with femoral vein puncture (Table 25.2).

Table 25.2 Indications

1. Short-term VADs must be used only in acute/emergency condition and in hospitalized patients
2. TVAD and TID, also known as long-term VAD, are indicated for all diagnostic and therapeutic issues of cancer patients over the course of the disease
3. TVAD are preferred for continuous/frequent use (high dose chemotherapy, hydration, blood components transfusion, nutrition etc.);
4. TID are preferred for discontinuous use or in patients who do not tolerate external devices (adolescents, patients with mental disorders etc.);
5. The new WoCoVA classification is based on vein cannulated by the catheter and includes
Centrally inserted central catheters—CICC
Peripherally -inserted central catheters—PICC
Femorally-inserted central catheters—FICC

25.4 Technique

Recent guidelines recommend abandoning open venous cut-down (OVCD) as the primary technique for VADs placement, especially in pediatric patients dealing with cancer. The OVCD procedure can be considered a historical legacy of pediatric surgeons of the last century. There are some authors who recommend OVCD even in children with platelet disorders, however, surgical preparation and cannulation of the vein and for vascular access nowadays is to be regarded as obsolete and contra-indicated especially for cancer patients. In fact, OVCD is associated with a high risk of hemorrhage (wide dissection of tissue to prepare the vein, incision of vein wall with subsequent suture), as well as early dislodgment and infection. Moreover, OVCD requires skills and knowledge of microsurgery and vascular surgery and in the case of catheter failure (both for end of treatment and for complications) there is a permanent loss of the venous patrimony.

Over the last decades, the concept of minimally invasive venous access has been rapidly adopted in adult patients, thus becoming the gold standard. Though the evidence in pediatric patients is still limited, most studies suggest that ultrasound guidance should become the standard of care for venipuncture in children and neonates, as it is already in adults. The most important advantage of ultrasound is to allow choosing the most appropriate vein after a scan of all possible options. By using ultrasound guidance, both puncture and cannulation of the vein are quicker and easier, with less risk of complications. The reduced invasiveness of the procedure consistently reduces the risk of infection at the insertion site, of peri-procedural bleeding, and of catheter-related thrombosis. It is also important to bear in mind that infective and hemorrhagic complications are more frequent in this population because of the cytopenia induced by chemo and radiotherapy (Table 25.3).

25.5 Prevention and Management of Complications

Considering the prolonged course of the disease and the dramatic improvement in survival rate for children affected by cancer, strategies to prevent both early and long-term complications, as well as to preserve vascular assets for any further use,

Table 25.3 Technique

1. OVCD is no longer recommended for VAD placement
2. OVCD requires high-level surgical skills and carries non-negligible risk of short- and long-term complications, especially in children with cancer
3. OVCD is contraindicated due to the higher risk hemorrhagic events related with procedure, which is significantly increased in patient with cancer
4. Minimally invasive ultrasound guided procedure is the gold standard procedure for VADs placement for different reasons: It allows real-time evaluation of the target vein; it is easier, less invasive, less painful; it has a lower complication rate

have direct influence on outcome and quality of life after the disease. It is then imperative to be aware of any possible complication, to adopt strategies for prevention, and to correct complications through prompt recognition and appropriate management.

As previously mentioned, minimally invasive ultrasound-guided procedures for VAD placement completely changed the approach to vascular access, especially in children. With adequate training and knowledge of materials (needles, wires, introducers, catheters, and probes) and technique, ultrasound is beneficial because of the high percentage of first-time success and the possibility of diagnosis of preexisting vascular anomalies (malformations, anatomic variants, or thrombosis/stenosis), thus reducing the incidence of early and peri-procedural complications (accidental arterial puncture, hematoma, extravasation, dissection of the vessel, or stenosis). Avoiding multiple punctures, the risk of post-operative bleeding is reduced, especially in cancer patients, who often have hemorrhagic diathesis as consequence of therapies (thrombocytopenia, liver failure in veno-occlusive disease). Use of ultrasound has also been validated for early diagnosis of pneumothorax, which was quite a common complication after subclavian vein cannulation using a blind technique.

Catheter dislodgment or tip migration may lead to malfunction, difficulty to infuse fluids or draw blood, and in worst cases, difficulty to remove the device. Children undergoing chemotherapy or high dose steroids are more prone to these complications for different reasons (reduced healing ability and coagulation, increased infection, skin and subcutaneous tissue disease such as graft-versus-host disease). Strategies to reduce such complications include the use of non-cuffed new generation polyurethane catheters (which are also less predisposed to rupture compared to silicon catheters) secured with either sutureless devices or subcutaneously anchored securement systems (SASS) (Fig. 25.1); the use of cyanoacrylate glue on the exit site has been also demonstrated to be valid option to reduce failure of VADs in a pediatric population (better securement, reduced infection rate for quick skin closure and healing, good hemostatic action) (Table 25.4).

25.6 Removal Procedure

Catheter removal is often incorrectly regarded as a simple procedure that can be performed by improperly trained staff members in different ways (bedside under local anesthesia, in a procedure room with mild sedation) according to personal or institutional experience, without adopting evidence-based protocols. However, in patients with long-term cuffed catheters, removal is a surgical procedure with a significant risk of complications (hemorrhage, catheter fracture with embolization). For children affected by cancer, catheter removal must be also considered as one of many painful procedures they undergo over the course of disease, with an additional stress for both the patient and the family. Because of these reasons, elective long-term cuffed catheter removal (e.g., for end of treatment), should be performed in a dedicated procedure room equipped with adequate facilities, under sedation, with trained medical and nursing staff, and according to institutional

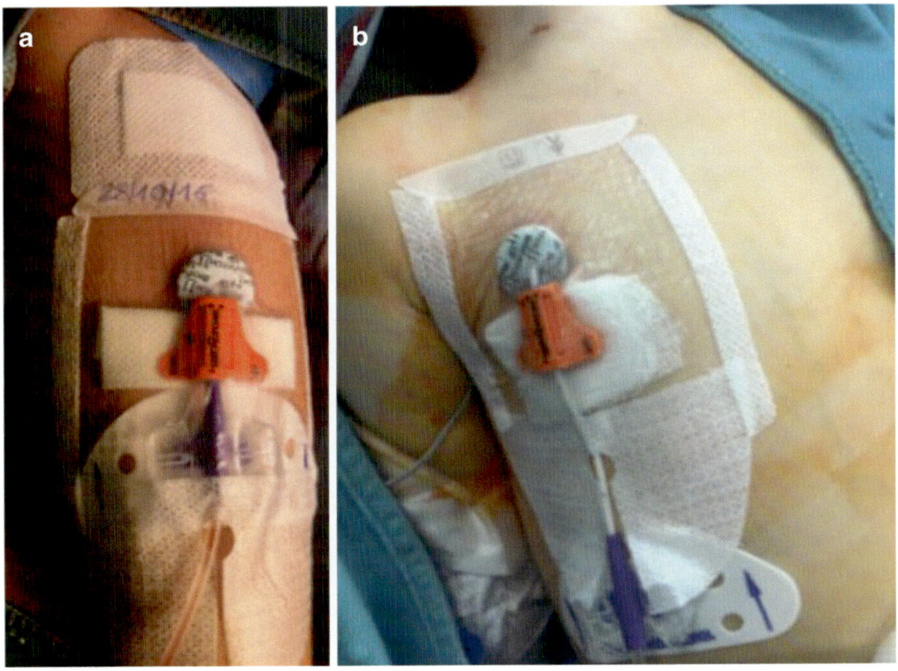

Fig. 25.1 (**a**) 14-year-old male affected by non-Hodgkin lymphoma with a PICC on the right arm and (**b**) 3-year-old male affected by Wilms tumor with a CICC (**b**); both VADs are secured with subcutaneous anchorage and with a skin-adhesive sutureless device; the exit sites are protected with a chlorhexidine-releasing sponge dressing and with transparent semi-permeable membranes

Table 25.4 Prevention and management of complications

1. Ultrasound-guided procedure reduces the risk of failure, multiple venipunctures, arterial puncture, perioperative/post-operative bleeding (often increased for thrombocytopenia or liver failure associated with treatment), and pneumothorax
2. Chemotherapy/steroids or skin issues (radiotherapy burns, cutaneous GVHD) may affect skin healing process.
3. Appropriate strategies to reduce risk of catheter dislodgment/removal include: Sutureless devices (including subcutaneous anchorage) and use of cyanoacrylate glue on exit-site

guidelines. Surgical technique must include blunt dissection and removal of the Dacron cuff together with the device. A retained cuff may remain as an innocuous foreign body, but it may have potential harmful consequences; as a nidus for infection or chronic inflammation (Fig. 25.2), create false images (calcification deposits or metastases) during diagnostic imaging, and last but not least it may be cosmetically unacceptable (Fig. 25.3). As a matter of fact, introduction of new devices with different securement systems (sutureless devices, cyanoacrylate glue, and SASS) allows for both easier fixation and removal of the catheter, if necessary, thus eliminating the use of cuffed catheters, especially in pediatric patients with cancer (Table 25.5).

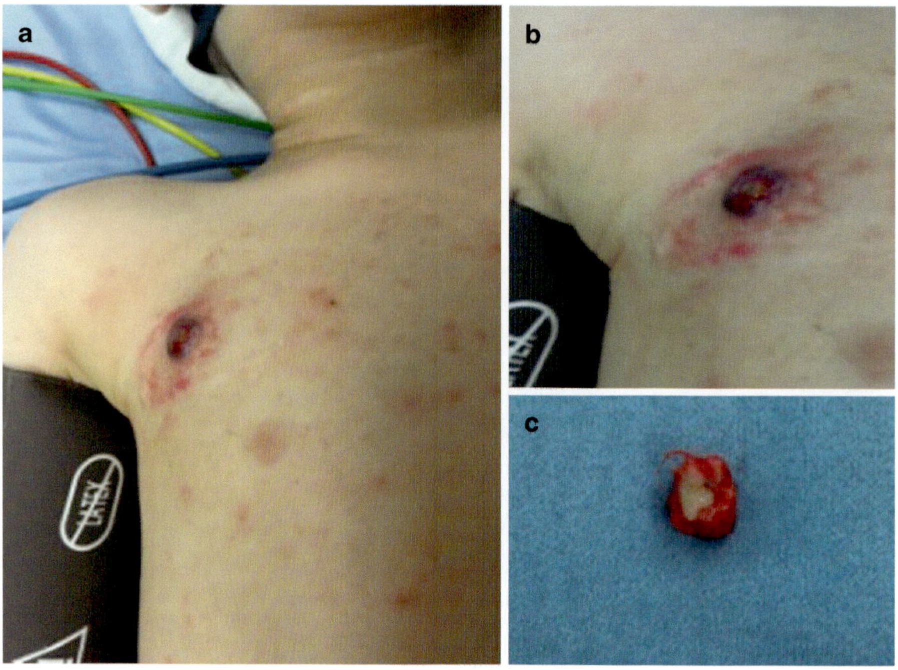

Fig. 25.2 Retained cuff. Chronic inflammatory reaction caused by foreign body infection is evident on the former exit site (**a**, **b**), and also on the cuff (**c**), its after removal

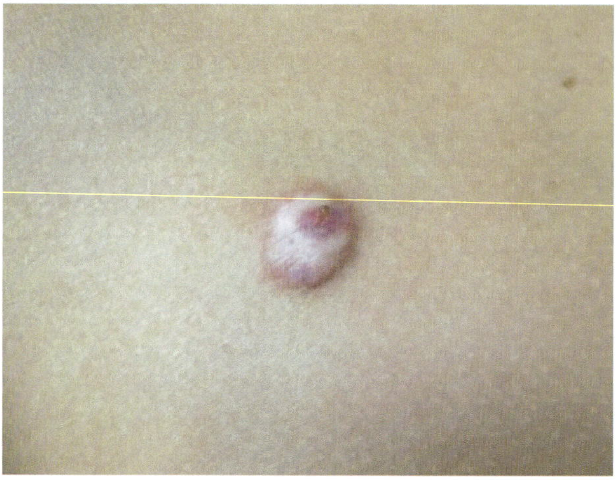

Fig. 25.3 retained cuff causing a chronic skin granuloma

Table 25.5 Removal

1.	Removal procedure must be performed in an adequate setting, under general anesthesia/deep sedation, by experienced medical/nurse staff
2.	In case of cuffed catheters, the cuff must be removed together with the device

Bibliography

1. Avanzini S, Guida E, Conte M, Faranda F, Buffa P, Granata C, Castagnola E, Fratino G, Mameli L, Michelazzi A, Pini-prato A, Mattioli G, Molinari AC, Lanino E, Jasonni V. Shifting from open surgical cut down to ultrasound-guided percutaneous central venous catheterization in children: learning curve and related complications. Pediatr Surg Int. 2010;26:819–24.
2. Bellesi S, Chiusolo P, de Pascale G, Pittiruti M, Scoppettuolo G, Metafuni E, Giammarco S, Sorà F, Laurenti L, Leone G, Sica S. Peripherally inserted central catheters (PICCs) in the management of oncohematological patients submitted to autologous stem cell transplantation. Support Care Cancer. 2013;21:531–5.
3. Borretta L, Macdonald T, Digout C, Smith N, Fernandez CV, Kulkarni K. Peripherally inserted central catheters in Pediatric oncology patients: a 15-year population-based review from Maritimes, Canada. J Pediatr Hematol Oncol. 2017.
4. Broviac JW, Cole JJ, Scribner BH. A silicone rubber atrial catheter for prolonged parenteral alimentation. Surg Gynecol Obstet. 1973;136:602–6.
5. Bugden S, Shean K, Scott M, Mihala G, Clark S, Johnstone C, Fraser JF, Rickard CM. Skin glue reduces the failure rate of emergency department-inserted peripheral intravenous catheters: a randomized controlled trial. Ann Emerg Med. 2016;68:196–201.
6. Cameron GS. Central venous catheters for children with malignant disease: surgical issues. J Pediatr Surg. 1987;22:702–4.
7. Cesaro S, Corrò R, Pelosin A, Gamba P, Zadra N, Fusaro F, Pillon M, Cusinato R, Zampieri C, Magagna L, Cavaliere M, Tridello G, Zanon G, Zanesco L. A prospective survey on incidence and outcome of Broviac/Hickman catheter-related complications in pediatric patients affected by hematological and oncological diseases. Ann Hematol. 2004;83:183–8.
8. Cornillon J, Martignoles JA, Tavernier-tardy E, Gire M, Martinez P, Tranchan C, Vallard A, Augeul-meunier K, Hacquard B, Guyotat D. Prospective evaluation of systematic use of peripherally inserted central catheters (PICC lines) for the home care after allogeneic hematopoietic stem cells transplantation. Support Care Cancer. 2017.
9. Crocoli A, Martucci C, Leopardi E, Padua M, Serra A, Cacchione A, Coletti V, Palumbo G, Ciofi degli atti ML, Ravà L, Inserra A. A dedicated protocol and environment for central venous catheter removal in pediatric patients affected by onco-hematological diseases. J Vasc Access. 2014;15:486–91.
10. Crocoli A, Narciso A, Pardi V, Accinni A, Madafferi S, Bertocchini A, Inserra A. Removal of tunneled-cuffed catheters in children: is it safe to leave the cuff? J Vasc Access. 2017;18:e22–3.
11. Crocoli A, Tornesello A, Pittiruti M, Barone A, Muggeo P, Inserra A, Molinari AC, Grillenzoni V, Durante V, Cicalese MP, Zanazzo GA, Cesaro S. Central venous access devices in pediatric malignancies: a position paper of Italian Association of Pediatric Hematology and Oncology. J Vasc Access. 2015;16:130–6.
12. Dezfulian C, Lavelle J, Nallamothu BK, Kaufman SR, Saint S. Rates of infection for single-lumen versus multilumen central venous catheters: a meta-analysis. Crit Care Med. 2003;31:2385–90.
13. Farber S. Chemotherapeutic studies of tumors, including leukemia, in children. Am J Dis Child. 1950;79:961–2.
14. Farber S. Chemotherapy in the treatment of leukemia and wilms' tumor. JAMA. 1966;198:826–36.
15. Fratino G, Molinari AC, Parodi S, Longo S, Saracco P, Castagnola E, Haupt R. Central venous catheter-related complications in children with oncological/hematological diseases: an observational study of 418 devices. Ann Oncol. 2005;16:648–54.
16. Gallieni M, Pittiruti M, Biffi R. Vascular access in oncology patients. CA Cancer J Clin. 2008;58:323–46.
17. Gyves JW, Ensminger WD, Niederhuber JE, Dent T, Walker S, Gilbertson S, Cozzi E, Saran P. A totally implanted injection port system for blood sampling and chemotherapy administration. JAMA. 1984;251:2538–41.

18. Harter C, Ostendorf T, Bach A, Egerer G, Goldschmidt H, Ho AD. Peripherally inserted central venous catheters for autologous blood progenitor cell transplantation in patients with haematological malignancies. Support Care Cancer. 2003;11:790–4.
19. Hickman RO, Buckner CD, Clift RA, Sanders JE, Stewart P, Thomas ED. A modified right atrial catheter for access to the venous system in marrow transplant recipients. Surg Gynecol Obstet. 1979;148:871–5.
20. Hooper WC, Holman RC, Strine TW, Chorba TL. Hodgkin disease mortality in the United States: 1979–1988. Cancer. 1992;70:1166–71.
21. Hord JD, Lawlor J, Werner E, Billett AL, Bundy DG, Winkle C, Gaur AH, Network, C. S. H. A. C. C. A. B. D. Central line associated blood stream infections in pediatric hematology/oncology patients with different types of central lines. Pediatr Blood Cancer. 2016;63:1603–7.
22. Karalexi MA, Georgakis MK, Dessypris N, Ryzhov A, Zborovskaya A, Dimitrova N, Zivkovic S, Eser S, Antunes L, Sekerija M, Zagar T, Bastos J, Demetriou A, Agius D, Florea M, Coza D, Bouka E, Dana H, Hatzipantelis E, Kourti M, Moschovi M, Polychronopoulou S, Stiakaki E, Pourtsidis A, Petridou ET. Mortality and survival patterns of childhood lymphomas: geographic and age-specific patterns in southern-eastern european and seer/us registration data. Hematol Oncol. 2016.
23. Kosloske AM, Klein MD. Techniques of central venous access for long term parenteral nutrition in infants. Surg Gynecol Obstet. 1982;154:394–9.
24. Kowalczyk JR, Samardakiewicz M, Pritchard-jones K, Ladenstein R, Essiaf S, Fitzgerald E, Petrarulo G, Vassal G. European survey on standards of care in paediatric oncology centres. Eur J Cancer. 2016;61:11–9.
25. Lamperti M, Bodenham AR, Pittiruti M, Blaivas M, Augoustides JG, Elbarbary M, Pirotte T, Karakitsos D, Ledonne J, Doniger S, Scoppettuolo G, Feller-kopman D, Schummer W, Biffi R, Desruennes E, Melniker LA, Verghese ST. International evidence-based recommendations on ultrasound-guided vascular access. Intensive Care Med. 2012;38:1105–17.
26. Lawrence H, Hacking M. Histoacryl((r)) for securing central venous catheters: not so sticky! Anaesthesia. 2014;69:1407–8.
27. Lee AC. Elective removal of cuffed central venous catheters in children. Support Care Cancer. 2007;15:897–901.
28. Marcy PY. Central venous access: techniques and indications in oncology. Eur Radiol. 2008;18:2333–44.
29. Matsuzaki A, Suminoe A, Koga Y, Hatano M, Hattori S, Hara T. Long-term use of peripherally inserted central venous catheters for cancer chemotherapy in children. Support Care Cancer. 2006;14:153–60.
30. Moureau N, Lamperti M, Kelly LJ, Dawson R, Elbarbary M, van Boxtel AJ, Pittiruti M. Evidence-based consensus on the insertion of central venous access devices: definition of minimal requirements for training. Br J Anaesth. 2013;110:347–56.
31. Nardi N, Wodey E, Laviolle B, de la Briere F, Delahaye S, Engrand C, Gauvrit C, Dessard S, Defontaine A, Ecoffey C. Effectiveness and complications of ultrasound-guided subclavian vein cannulation in children and neonates. *Anaesth crit care*. Pain Med. 2016.
32. Newton DW. Drug incompatibility chemistry. Am J Health Syst Pharm. 2009;66:348–57.
33. Niederhuber JE, Ensminger W, Gyves JW, Liepman M, Doan K, Cozzi E. Totally implanted venous and arterial access system to replace external catheters in cancer treatment. Surgery. 1982;92:706–12.
34. Nifong TP, Mcdevitt TJ. The effect of catheter to vein ratio on blood flow rates in a simulated model of peripherally inserted central venous catheters. Chest. 2011;140:48–53.
35. Noone AM, Cronin KA, Altekruse SF, Howlader N, Lewis DR, Petkov VI, Penberthy L. Cancer incidence and survival trends by subtype using data from the surveillance epidemiology and end results program, 1992–2013. Cancer Epidemiol Biomark Prev. 2017;26:632–41.

36. O'grady NP, Alexander M, Burns LA, Dellinger EP, Garland J, Heard SO, Lipsett PA, Masur H, Mermel LA, Pearson ML, Raad II, Randolph AG, Rupp ME, Saint S. Guidelines for the prevention of intravascular catheter-related infections. Clin Infect Dis. 2011;52:e162–93.
37. Olivieri C, Crocoli A, de Pasquale MD, Inserra A. Central venous catheter placement in children with thrombocytopenia. Minerva Pediatr. 2016;68:398–403.
38. Perdikaris P, Petsios K, Yasilatou-kosmidis H, Matziou V. Complications of Hickman-broviac catheters in children with malignancies. Pediatr Hematol Oncol. 2008;25:375–84.
39. Pinon M, Bezzio S, Tovo PA, Fagioli F, Farinasso L, Calabrese R, Marengo M, Giacchino M. A prospective 7-year survey on central venous catheter-related complications at a single pediatric hospital. Eur J Pediatr. 2009;168:1505–12.
40. Pittiruti M. Ultrasound guided central vascular access in neonates, infants and children. Curr Drug Targets. 2012;13:961–9.
41. Pritchard-jones K, Moroz V, Vujanic G, Powis M, Walker J, Messahel B, Hobson R, Levitt G, Kelsey A, Mitchell C, Group, C. S. C. A. L. G. C. R. T. Treatment and outcome of wilms' tumour patients: an analysis of all cases registered in the ukw3 trial. Ann Oncol. 2012;23:2457–63.
42. Raman D, Sharma M, Moghekar A, Wang X, Hatipoglu U. Utilization of thoracic ultrasound for confirmation of central venous catheter placement and exclusion of pneumothorax: a novel technique in real-time application. J Intensive Care Med. 2017;885066617705839.
43. Riella MC, Scribner BH. Five years' experience with a right atrial catheter for prolonged parenteral nutrition at home. Surg Gynecol Obstet. 1976;143:205–8.
44. Schiffer CA, Mangu PB, Wade JC, Camp-sorrell D, Cope DG, El-rayes BF, Gorman M, Ligibel J, Mansfield P, Levine M. Central venous catheter care for the patient with cancer: american society of clinical oncology clinical practice guideline. J Clin Oncol. 2013;31:1357–70.
45. Schrøder H, Malchau E, Larsen LN, Bugge K, Olsen H, Kamperis K. Tunnelled central venous catheters in children with cancer. Removal and duration. Ugeskr Laeger. 2008;170:343–7.
46. Scoppettuolo G, Dolcetti L, Emoli A, La Greca A, Biasucci DD, Pittiruti M. Further benefits of cyanoacrylate glue for central venous catheterisation. Anaesthesia. 2015;70:758.
47. Shulman RJ, Smith EO, Rahman S, Gardner P, Reed T, Mahoney D. Single- vs double-lumen central venous catheters in pediatric oncology patients. Am J Dis Child. 1988;142:893–5.
48. Skinner R, Koller K, Mcintosh N, Mccarthy A, Pizer B, (UKCCSG), U. K. C. S. C. S. G. & Group, P. O. N. F. P. S. C. Prevention and management of central venous catheter occlusion and thrombosis in children with cancer. Pediatr Blood Cancer. 2008;50:826–30.
49. Smith MA, Seibel NL, Altekruse SF, Ries LA, Melbert DL, O'leary M, Smith FO, Reaman GH. Outcomes for children and adolescents with cancer: challenges for the twenty-first century. J Clin Oncol. 2010;28:2625–34.
50. Ward E, Desantis C, Robbins A, Kohler B, Jemal A. Childhood and adolescent cancer statistics, 2014. CA Cancer J Clin. 2014;64:83–103.
51. Zerla PA, Canelli A, Cerne L, Caravella G, Gilardini A, de Luca G, Aricisteanu AM, Yenezia R. Evaluating safety, efficacy, and cost-effectiveness of picc securement by subcutaneously anchored stabilization device. J Vasc Access. 2017;18:238–42.

Chapter 26
Special Problems of Venous Access in Parenteral Nutrition

Mauro Pittiruti and Giancarlo Scoppettuolo

26.1 Introduction

Parenteral nutrition is sometimes required in neonates and children, every time there is the impossibility of meeting the nutritional requirements by the oral or enteral route. Typical situations are:

- Preterm, low weight neonates in neonatal intensive care unit
- Infants and children in pediatric intensive care unit, whereas tube feeding is contraindicated
- Nutritional support during the perioperative course of children undergoing major surgery
- Temporary home parenteral nutrition in children with inflammatory bowel disease
- Long term home parenteral nutrition in infants and children with acquired or congenital disorders associated with severe and irreversible intestinal malabsorption.

In most cases, parenteral nutrition is delivered via a central line. In some very selected cases, parenteral nutrition may be administered via a long peripheral catheter or a midline catheter, for a short period of time (one-two weeks), exclusively in hospitalized children, and consistently using lipid-based emulsions with osmolarity between 700 and 850 mOsm/L.

M. Pittiruti (✉)
Department of Surgery, Catholic University Hospital, Rome, Italy

G. Scoppettuolo
Department of Infective Diseases, Fondazione Policlinico Universitario "A. Gemelli" IRCCS, Rome, Italy
e-mail: giancarlo.scoppettuolo@policlinicogemelli.it

D. G. Biasucci et al. (eds.), *Vascular Access in Neonates and Children*,
https://doi.org/10.1007/978-3-030-94709-5_26

As in adults, also in children the risk of catheter-related bloodstream infection (CRBSI) is increased when the vascular access device is used for parenteral nutrition, since the components of the emulsion (in particular, the triglycerides and the amino acids) represent an ideal nourishment for bacteria and yeasts. Parenteral nutrition without lipids is associated with the risk of yeast colonization; when lipids are added to the emulsion, bacterial growth may also occur. In short, minimal colonization of the infusion line and of the catheter may easily become the occasion for overgrowth of micro-organisms inside the device, with high risk of CRBSI.

Also, the parenteral nutrition emulsion is characterized by high viscosity and by a relatively unstable balance among its components. Thus, minimal changes in the composition (e.g., after addition of some other drugs, or because of a concomitant infusion of another solution in the same line) may be associated with lipid precipitation and lumen occlusion. This complication is especially frequent with the low caliber catheter used in the pediatric patient, and particularly difficult to treat.

Furthermore, children on long term home parenteral nutrition must keep the venous access device for very long time and sometimes indefinitely, so that special strategies for avoiding accidental dislodgment/removal of the device must be adopted.

26.2 Strategies for Reducing the Risk of Infection during Parenteral Nutrition

All the infection prevention strategies listed in Chap. 21 should be implemented and adopted systematically, in particular:

1. Parenteral nutrition emulsions should be prepared by a certified hospital pharmacy or—preferably—acquired as industrially prepared, commercially available emulsions.
2. Ideally, no drug or nutrient should be added to the bag of parenteral nutrition. Though the addition of multi-vitamin products is a common practice, there is some evidence that vitamins may favor bacterial growth: vitamins should be provided daily, if possible, by a different route.
3. Parenteral nutrition should be delivered via a dedicated device (or a dedicated lumen of a multiple lumen device). The less the manipulation of the line, the less the risk of contamination. The line dedicated to parenteral nutrition should not be used for bolus injection of drugs or for piggy-back infusion of other solutions.
4. The bag of parenteral nutrition must be replaced every 24 hrs. The practice of delivering the same bag for 48 hrs, at low speed, should be discouraged because associated with higher risk of contamination. This is valid also for parenteral nutrition without lipids, which may favor the growth of yeasts.
5. The infusion lines used for delivering parenteral nutrition containing lipids must be changed every 24 hrs.

6. Long term parenteral nutrition requires special strategies for reducing bacterial contamination. The simplest and most effective strategy for reducing contamination by the extra-luminal route—as already discussed in Chap. 8—is to use tunneled catheters. Interestingly, both cuffed tunneled catheters and non-cuffed tunneled subcutaneously anchored catheters are equally effective in this regard. As concerns bacterial contamination by the intra-luminal route, a recent and effective strategy is the prophylactic lock with 2% taurolidine. As already explained in Chap. 21, taurolidine is non-antibiotic antibacterial agent very active against the colonization of venous access devices. In the case of parenteral nutrition, a lock solution containing taurolidine alone should be preferred to taurolidine-citrate or taurolidine-heparin combination. For prophylaxis, taurolidine lock should be applied daily or at least three times per week, and each lock should stay inside the catheter for a minimum of 1 hr. The volume of the lock should be equal to the priming volume, plus a 20%; though, even if taurolidine is accidentally infused into the bloodstream, this is not associated with any adverse event, as this compound is harmless and rapidly metabolized to taurine.

26.3 Strategies for Reducing the Risk of Lumen Occlusion during Parenteral Nutrition

Venous access devices utilized for parenteral solution are at high risk of lumen occlusion, as above explained. For proper prevention of this complication, several aspects should be kept in mind:

1. Silicon catheters are more prone to lumen occlusion (as the internal diameter is lower than polyurethane catheters of the same external caliber) and they are more difficult to unblock since they are not power injectable. Though, also polyurethane catheters of very small inner caliber (less than 20G) are at risk of lumen occlusion: this is true for ECCs (which have a caliber of 22G or less) and for each lumen of a double lumen 4Fr catheter; single lumen 3Fr catheters in polyurethane (inner diameter 20G) have a higher risk of occlusion than single lumen 4Fr catheters (inner diameter 18G). Valved catheters also increase the risk of catheter malfunction and lumen occlusion. Totally implanted venous access devices are not appropriate for parenteral nutrition; if used for this purpose, they are associated with a high risk of lumen occlusion; also, a port with lumen occlusion is difficult or impossible to unblock. In infants and children, parenteral nutrition should be preferably delivered through single lumen 4Fr or single/double lumen 5Fr power injectable polyurethane non-valved external catheters. The choice between PICC, CICC and FICC depends on the age of the patient and on his/her venous patrimony, previously evaluated by ultrasound.
2. Parenteral nutrition must be delivered via an intravenous pump. Gravity infusion is inevitably associated with unpredictable variations of flow, which increase the risk of precipitation of lipid aggregates.

3. At the time of daily replacement of the bag of parenteral nutrition, the venous access device should be vigorously flushed with a volume of saline equal to three-four times the priming volume.
4. The interaction of the parenteral nutrition emulsions with other drugs or solution, as much as it increases the risk of infection (see above), it also increased the risk of lipid precipitation and lumen occlusion. Therefore, parenteral nutrition should be delivered via a dedicated device (or a dedicated lumen of a multiple lumen device).
5. For venous access devices used intermittently for parenteral nutrition (for example: home parenteral nutrition delivered in the night hours), heparin lock should never be used: not only because it is not effective in preventing lumen occlusion, but also because heparin favors the precipitation of triglycerides inside the lumen.

26.4 Strategies for Reducing the Risk of Catheter Dislodgment during Parenteral Nutrition

Long term parenteral nutrition should be preferably delivered by tunneled catheters, and not by totally implanted venous access devices (ports). While the tunnel is effective against bacterial contamination by the extraluminal route, it is not effective as securement. The only currently available options for catheter securement are (a) the use of cuffed catheters, (b) subcutaneous anchorage.

Recent evidence suggests that both strategies are equally effective: a cuffed-tunneled catheter with the cuff located in the proper position inside the tunnel (at least 2 cm far from the exit site) and a non-cuffed tunneled catheter secured by subcutaneous anchorage have the same risk of dislodgment. Though, subcutaneous anchorage has some practical advantages over the cuff:

- Subcutaneously anchored catheters are immediately secured soon after insertion, while the cuff secures the catheter only after a few weeks (the time required for the development of a sterile chronic inflammation around the cuff).
- Though complications either due to the cuff or to the subcutaneous anchorage may sometimes occur, cuff-related complications almost inevitably require the removal of the venous access device, while complications related to subcutaneous anchorage are usually associated with removal of the securement device, but not of the venous access device.
- Removal of a cuffed catheter requires a minor surgical procedure with local anesthesia and/or sedation, to be performed in a procedure room by qualified operators (see Chap. 25); on the contrary, a subcutaneously anchored tunneled catheter can be easily removed bedside without local anesthesia, and even sedation is not usually required.
- Last, a cuffed catheter is much more expensive than a non-cuffed catheter plus a subcutaneously anchored securement device.

Bibliography

1. Biasucci DG, Pittiruti M, Taddei A, Picconi E, Pizza A, Celentano D, Piastra M, Scoppettuolo G, Conti G. Targeting zero catheter-related bloodstream infections in pediatric intensive care unit: a retrospective matched case-control study. J Vasc Access 2018 Mar;19(2):119–124. https://doi.org/10.5301/jva.5000797. Epub 2018 Feb 19. PMID: 29148002.
2. Cellini M, Bergadano A, Crocoli A, Badino C, Carraro F, Sidro L, Botta D, Pancaldi A, Rossetti F, Pitta F, Cesaro S. Guidelines of the Italian Association of Pediatric Hematology and Oncology for the management of the central venous access devices in pediatric patients with onco-hematological disease. J Vasc Access 2020 Nov 10:1129729820969309. https://doi.org/10.1177/1129729820969309. Epub ahead of print. PMID: 33169648.
3. Crocoli A, Martucci C, Sidro L, Delle Donne D, Menna G, Pittiruti M, De Pasquale MD, Strocchio L, Natali GL, Inserra A. Safety and effectiveness of subcutaneously anchored securement for tunneled central catheters in oncological pediatric patients: a retrospective study. J Vasc Access 2021 Jun 4:11297298211009364. https://doi.org/10.1177/11297298211009364. Epub ahead of print. PMID: 34088245.
4. Crocoli A, Tornesello A, Pittiruti M, Barone A, Muggeo P, Inserra A, Molinari AC, Grillenzoni V, Durante V, Cicalese MP, Zanazzo GA, Cesaro S. Central venous access devices in pediatric malignancies: a position paper of Italian Association of Pediatric Hematology and Oncology. J Vasc Access 2015 Mar–Apr;16(2):130–136. https://doi.org/10.5301/jva.5000314. Epub 2014 Oct 14. PMID: 25362978.
5. Gorski L, Hadaway L, Hagle M, et al. Infusion therapy standards of practice. J Infus Nurs. 2021 Jan–Feb 01;44(1S Suppl 1):S1–S224.
6. Pinelli F, Pittiruti M, Van Boxtel T, Barone G, Biffi R, Capozzoli G, Crocoli A, Elli S, Elisei D, Fabiani A, Garrino C, Graziano U, Montagnani L, Prato AP, Scoppettuolo G, Zadra N, Zanaboni C, Zerla P, Konstantinou E, Jones M, Rosay H, Simcock L, Stas M, Pepe G. GAVeCeLT-WoCoVA consensus on subcutaneously anchored securement devices for the securement of venous catheters: current evidence and recommendations for future research. J Vasc Access. 2020 Jul 2:1129729820924568. https://doi.org/10.1177/1129729820924568. Epub ahead of print. PMID: 32613887.
7. Pittiruti M, Hamilton H, Biffi R, MacFie J, Pertkiewicz M; ESPEN. ESPEN guidelines on parenteral nutrition: central venous catheters (access, care, diagnosis and therapy of complications). Clin Nutr 2009 Aug;28(4):365–377. https://doi.org/10.1016/j.clnu.2009.03.015. Epub 2009 May 21. PMID: 19464090.

Chapter 27
Sedation and General Anesthesia for Vascular Access in Children

Elizabeth Prentice

27.1 Introduction

The ability to undertake peripheral or central venous access in children (awake or lightly sedated, with various types of topical or local anesthesia or general anesthesia) is multifactorial. The degree of sedation of anesthesia required will be dependent on the child, on the skills of the inserter, on the type of venous access, and on the local environment; specific resources should be available to help have the child happy, still, and cooperative during the procedure.

27.2 Choosing Sedation or General Anesthesia for Venous Access in Children

There are several components to consider in assessing the ability for a child to tolerate venous access non-sedated or lightly sedated. If all or the majority of these is not available, a safer and more acceptable alternative may be general anesthesia.

1. The infant or child must have suitable, easily accessible veins.
2. The infant does not need to be wrapped, comforted, and kept still.
3. Skilled help is not required to hold the child or the child's limb immobile.
4. Age and patient specific distraction therapy is available: a parent or nurse may suffice for peripheral access, but central access will usually require skilled health

E. Prentice (✉)
Department of Anesthesia, Royal Children's Hospital, Melbourne, VIC, Australia
e-mail: Liz.Prentice@rch.org.au

D. G. Biasucci et al. (eds.), *Vascular Access in Neonates and Children*,
https://doi.org/10.1007/978-3-030-94709-5_27

care personal (e.g., Play Therapists or Child Life Specialists) to apply age and patient specific distraction therapy. The child must be amenable to this distraction therapy.
5. The child should be able to lie flat and still for several minutes: 30 min if a PICC or CICC is required—slightly less for a midline.
6. Topical or local analgesia and sedation must be available.
7. The maneuver is performed by an experienced operator: experience to enter the vein using ultrasound at first pass is required. This degree of skill is usually only maintained by inserting at least 50–200 ultrasound guided venous catheters a year. If the inserter is still on the learning curve, and access may take longer, general anesthesia may be required.

Presence of several of the following may make general anesthesia a better or safer option in children:

1. Infants and younger children.
2. "Needle phobia" especially in children with chronic conditions requiring frequent venous access
3. Inability to lie still or flat for longer procedures because of pain, developmental delay, deformities
4. Skilled distraction therapy (to keep the child calm and still) is not available
5. The inserter is still on the learning curve, and access may take longer than usual
6. Type of access: insertion of CICCs, tunneled VADS or implanted ports will usually require general anesthesia in children. When inserting these devices, the child is required to be very still for 30 plus minutes, with the neck extended and 80–100% full body draping, with much of the face covered. Movement can make the use of wires and tunnellers more dangerous.

27.3 Considerations and Tips for Anesthesia for Venous Access

1. The sedation/anesthesia team should be different from the insertion team.
2. If peripheral venous access is required, needle phobic children may benefit from a premedication prior to anesthesia and induction by inhalation.
3. If central venous access is required due to depleted peripheral access, it may be necessary to perform the procedure with no other venous access. Ultrasound may help. In the case no peripheral access can be found, the most skilled operator should be chosen to undertake central venous access.
4. As regards the choice of airway for general anesthesia, it depends on different issues. Venous access devices such as CICCs, ports and tunneled CICCs often require neck extension, so that an endotracheal tube is recommended for infants and younger children. Also, intubation may be required if additional procedures

(e.g., broncho-alveolar lavage for respiratory patients) are also scheduled. If the child has pre-existing respiratory conditions, a laryngeal mask may be preferred.
5. As regards the position of the patient, insertion of CICCs often requires a rolled towel under the shoulders. In case of cervical trauma, intubation may be performed with proper inline stabilization of the neck, and alternative insertion techniques that do not require neck extension (for example, a low-lateral in-plane approach to the brachiocephalic vein) should be preferred.

27.4 Sedation

The mainstays of conscious sedation for venous access are benzodiazepines and nitrous oxide.

Midazolam is the most frequently used benzodiazepine in children. It can be used orally or intra-nasally; the onset is within 20–30 min and the offset within 60–90 min. It rarely causes airway problems in sedation doses. It is amnestic and anxiolytic, but it does not provide analgesia. As the taste is bitter, it can be combined with sucrose containing syrup. Occasionally, a paradoxical effect may occur, and the child may become hyperactive and restless.

Nitrous oxide delivery requires specifically trained personnel: training should include airway management, basic advanced life support, monitoring, suction, and knowledge of airway maintenance for breathing and oxygenation. Nitrous oxide can be effective for both sedation and analgesia. It requires a short period of fasting prior (usually 2 hours). It may not be tolerated due to nausea and mask phobia.

27.5 Topical Anesthetics

Topical anesthetics are used to numb the skin and reduce pain before the procedure. The choice of the topical anesthetic depends on availability, preferences, and allergies the child may have and the desired wait time from application until the procedure can be started. In a busy vascular access service, it may be impossible to wait 30–60 min after application until the procedure starts, so that topical anesthetics may be impractical.

Percutaneous local anesthetic creams are usually recommended only in children over 1 month of age. They must be applied to the skin before the procedure, and they are kept in place using an adhesive plastic dressing or polyurethane wrap and a bandage. They need to be covered to allow time for the anesthetic to be absorbed and effectively numb the skin. The cream should be applied to no more than three areas at the same time. There are several different types of local anesthetic cream that can be used.

Tetracaine gel must be applied 30 to 45 min beforehand and should not be left on for longer. The site remains numb for 4–6 hrs. It commonly causes vasodilation (it increases the size of the blood vessels) where it has been applied and can cause temporary redness.

Lidocaine + prilocaine cream is an eutectic mixture of two local anesthetics, lidocaine and prilocaine, combined with agents which allow the drugs to pass through the skin. (Carbomer 934P, polyoxymethylene hydrogenated castor oil and sodium hydroxide). It must be applied at least an hour before the procedure and the site remains numb for up 2 hrs. It causes vasoconstriction, with temporary whiteness of the skin. It is contraindicated in some cases (methemoglobinemia; glucose-6-phosphate dehydrogenase deficiency).

Amethocaine gel has an anesthetic action 30 min after application, with a median duration of 1.5 hrs (range 0.5–3.5 hours). If applied for 60 min, it has a longer duration of action (median duration 3 hrs with a range of 1–5 hours). It is thought to act more rapidly in children than in adults. It has a vasodilating action at the site of application, and this may be an advantage in making small veins on the dorsum of the hand more prominent. Several side effects have been described: mild transient erythema at the site of application (lasting 20 min after removal of the gel and sometimes for several hours), slight edema or pruritus, blistering of the skin. Several cases of sensitization have been described in adults, after repeated exposure to topical amethocaine. The para-aminobenzoic acid metabolite of this anesthetic is thought to be involved in the sensitization process. On the other hand, there have been no reports of methemoglobinemia directly associated with amethocaine.

For all these topical anesthetics, there is risk of allergic reaction (itching, swelling, or bruising where the cream or spray has been applied). Some change in skin color may occur, but this is normal. Some dressings may also cause irritation. In these cases, non-adhesive dressing can be used to keep the cream in place and covered with a bandage. Topical anesthetic creams/gels should not be used on the following areas: wounds, broken skin, dermatitis, and eczema; mucous membranes such as inside the mouth or nose; lips, ears, nose, or eyes; anus or genitals; area with molluscum contagiosum. They must not be used in premature babies and infants under one month of age.

27.6 Local Anesthetics

Injecting local anesthetic with a hypodermic needle prior to the procedure seems counterintuitive, however there are several advantages to this method, and using a 27G needles with distraction and the body part held firmly immobilized, the pain of the injection can be minimized. Lidocaine is frequently used but is associated with local burning pain because of its low pH; more recent products (e.g., ropivacaine) are safer, more powerful than lidocaine and associated with longer action and less local pain. Vasopressors such as epinephrine or adrenaline should never be added to the anesthetic; there is no evidence that they may decrease venous ooze from the exit site after the procedure. Also, sodium bicarbonate should never be added to the anesthetic, since it reduces the anesthetic action and is ultimately useless when using new generation anesthetics such as ropivacaine or mepivacaine or bupivacaine, which are not acidic as lidocaine.

Local anesthetics help to ensure that pain—and the resultant movement—is minimized during the often technically challenging part of ultrasound guided entry of the needle into the vein. The most effective anesthetics are ropivacaine, bupivacaine and levo-bupivacaine, which are active even at very low concentrations (0.2%). The rapidity of onset is depending on the concentration of the solution: when the effect must be rapid, 1% solutions are to be preferred. For example, ropivacaine 1% allows the procedure to commence immediately, instead of waiting up to 60 min, as it happens with topical anesthetics. This allows treatment to be commenced rapidly, and increased efficiency for a busy IV access team. Anesthesia is achieved for 30 min or even for many hours, depending on the anesthetic used (ropivacaine has a longer effect than mepivacaine).

27.7 Surface Anesthesia

Some technologies allow to obtain a superficial anesthesia without using creams and without subcutaneous needle punctures.

The J-tip device is a needle-free injection system that uses CO_2 gas to create a fine stream of liquid anesthesia that passes through the skin and into the subcutaneous tissue. Jet injection technology creates a spray like pattern of anesthetic once inside the subcutaneous tissue, which allows for broad dispersion and quick absorption. This method is completely needle free and virtually pain free. The drug takes 1–2 min to take effect and lasts for 15–20 min thereafter.

Instant topical anesthetic skin refrigerants or 'vapo-coolants' (for example, based on ethyl chloride) are also used. A thin film of liquid is sprayed topically onto the skin, which makes the skin cold and less sensitive as the liquid evaporates. Vapo-coolants work very quickly (in a few seconds) but the effect wears off quickly as the skin warms up again in a few minutes. Usually, they have no anesthetic properties. Though, vapo-coolants are useful to temporarily control the pain associated with needle procedures, minor surgical procedures, foreign body removal, suturing and suture removal, or insertion of short intravenous cannulas. They can be used prior to intra-dermal local anesthetic injections. Vapo-coolants can be applied to intact skin, minor open wounds, and intact oral mucous membranes. They may be useful when the child is allergic to topical anesthetic creams, or when the child gets very upset when the cream is applied, or when there is not time to apply topical cream. The vapo-coolant must be sprayed on a flat, horizontal surface, approximately 3 to 7 inches from the skin; it must be applied for 4 to 10 sec, or until the skin begins turning white (whichever comes first). It is recommended not to spray for longer than 10 sec. The venous access needle should be inserted within 30 sec. The operator should not repeatedly spray the same area as this may cause frostbite and pain.

The same method of reduced sensitivity secondary to refrigeration is used in a simple, hand-held patented device (*'CoolSense'*) that anesthetizes the site of injections by a 'cryo' system. When stored in a freezer compartment, the device is immediately ready for use. It numbs the site of injection within 3–5 sec. The applicator's head is temperature-controlled by an electronic component and prevents the skin from being harmed and burned during the injection. The unit includes a disinfection mechanism, containing an alcoholic gel. The gel is spread over the applicator's metal surface, serving as an additional protection against a skin cold burn. It can be used repeatedly as long as it is restored in a freezer. Also, it is suitable for all ages: neonates, infants, children, adults, and the elderly.

Another patented device (*'Buzzy'*) combines cold and vibration to reduce pain with temperature and movement. The premise is that when nerves receive non-painful signals such as vibration or cold, the brain closes the gate on pain signals. Also, intense cold activates a supra-spinal modulation raising the body's overall pain threshold. The device is not placed directly on the site at all due to the possibility of vasoconstriction: it is placed 2–3 cm proximal and left in place for the procedure.

27.8 Distraction Therapy

Distraction therapy is a way of helping a child cope with a painful or difficult procedure. It aims to take the child's mind off the procedure by concentrating on something else that is happening. Discomfort by crying or shouting is not only distressing for the child, but also for parents and caregivers, and the staff attempting treatment. There are various methods of distraction therapy—some very simple to do, and others that need more practice. Qualified hospital specialists or therapists usually know how to carry out distraction therapy, although any member of staff who has had specific training can do it.

In North America, this task is assigned to 'Certified Child Life Specialists' (CCLS), who are employed in the health care setting to provide evidence-based, appropriate interventions including therapeutic play, preparation and education that reduce fear, anxiety, and pain for infants, children, and youth. They encourage effective coping strategies for children and their families under stress. They are trained to recognize individuality in patients, and use a range of developmentally appropriate activities, including play, preparation for a medical procedure, education, self-expression, and family support to help cope with hospitalization, illness, or death and dying. Also, they are trained to consider the cognitive emotional, and physical development of each child in order to encourage optimum development of children facing a challenging experience, particularly one related to healthcare and hospitalization.

A recent systematic review of preparation effectiveness evidence concluded that children who were psychologically prepared for surgery experienced fewer negative symptoms than did children who did not receive formal preparation. In addition to reducing anxiety and providing a more positive experience for the patient and family, research demonstrates that preparation and coping facilitation interventions decrease the need for sedation in procedures such as MRIs, resulting in lower risks for the child and cost savings in personnel, anesthesia, and throughput-related expenses.

Preparation techniques, materials, and language must be adapted to the developmental level, personality, and unique experiences of the child and his or her family. Learning is enhanced with "hands-on" methods versus exclusively verbal explanations. Photographs, diagrams, tours of surgical or treatment areas, actual and pretend medical equipment, and various models (e.g., dolls, puppets) are used to reinforce learning and actively engage the child. Interpreter services are used as appropriate to ensure understanding in patients or families who do not speak English or for whom English is a second language. Most parents have a strong desire for comprehensive information about their child's care and should be included in the preparation process. In cases in which children demonstrate avoidant preferences or when preparation before the event is not possible, the CCLS's focus may change from that of imparting information to other supportive strategies, such as teaching behavioral coping skills and preparing parents to support their child during a medical procedure.

Before the procedure starts, the CCLS will spend time with parent and child, getting to know the child better. The procedure is explained. Dolls, DVDs or books may be used to explain further. The Therapist aims to find out if there is a particular aspect of the procedure worrying the child. Some children may be afraid of needles, whereas others are worried about anesthetics.

It is often helpful to bring an element of choice can be into the procedure. Choosing the site or side of venous access, the color of a dressing. Offering choice can allow a child an element of control over the situation. It can also be helpful to plan a reward. Rewards can be useful for providing a focus for after the procedure and thinking about it can be a distraction. A reward can be something small, such as a sticker or balloon, or larger, such as an outing.

There are many different methods of distraction therapy: some are more suitable for younger children while others work better for teenagers:

- Controlled breathing: this can be used for all ages and involves the child blowing an imaginary balloon or feather up in the area. Other things can also be used, like party blowers or blowpipes. Older children might want to just concentrate on their breathing.
- Books. There are lots of different books that can be used for distraction therapy—the type depends on your child's ages. For instance, a younger child may enjoy a pop-up book or a musical book, whereas an older child or teenager may prefer to listen to a CD.
- Games and puzzles. These are suitable for all ages, but the game or puzzle will need to be appropriate for the child's age. Younger children may prefer counting games, whereas older children or teenagers may be happier with an iPad, or hand-held computer game.
- Mobile Devices. There is emerging evidence that mobile devices can be effective in minimizing patient perceptions of pain and anxiety during distressing medical procedures.

- Music. Listening to or singing along with music can also be used successfully with all age groups. There are also ‘therapeutic’ music CDs available that use sounds from nature to give a calming effect.
- Touch and feel toys. These are suitable for all ages and can work very effectively for children with special needs. Playing with textured toys like squashy plastic balls or their own cuddly toys can be helpful. Toys that are attractive to look at, such as kaleidoscopes, mirrors or bubbles tubes can also work well.
- Make believe toys. These can work very well with younger children who can use them to act out a story during the procedure. For instance, hand or finger puppets, dolls, soft toys or toy cars can all be used.
- Coaching/talking. Older children and teenagers may prefer to talk through the procedure as it happens, or otherwise just talk about things that interest them. By concentrating on carrying out the conversation, their mind might be distracted from the procedure itself.
- “comfort kits”. CCLSs may also develop “comfort kits” for use in treatment areas to include age-appropriate distraction items such as bubbles, pop-up and sound books, light-up toys, and other visual or auditory tools.
- Welcoming environment in treatment and examination rooms. CCLSs can also advocate for a more welcoming environment in treatment and examination rooms on pediatric units as well as outpatient settings. Their background and training are helpful in designing settings that are appropriately stimulating, non-threatening, and interactive.
- Family Support. The presence and participation of family members is a fundamental component of patient- and family-centered care and has a significant positive effect on a child’s adjustment to the health care experience.
- Guided imagery. Another distraction technique used to give the child an element of choice and control.

The child is assessed prior to the procedure to tailor the distraction therapy to the child. During the procedure it is very important that the CCLS is the only person trying to distract the child. If multiple people are also trying to distract the child, it will take his or her concentration away. After the procedure, evaluate the type of distraction therapy used and whether it has worked or not. This will be useful for planning future procedures.

Distraction therapy does not work for every child. Some children cannot take their mind off the procedure, no matter what else is happening around them, in which case, a different approach needs to be used.

Some key points to remember:

- Physical comfort measures and distraction activities are more effective than verbal reasoning.
- Children do not have sufficient cognitive development to understand strangers trying to reassure them until age 5–7 years
- Interactive distraction (blowing bubbles, playing a game, or playing with an electronic device) is better passive distraction (story telling or showing a toy)

- Strategies such as swaddling, oral sucrose, vibratory stimulation, breathing techniques, distraction, and visual imagery have been shown to decrease behavioral distress and pain experience in children during invasive medical procedures.
- Research has demonstrated that children are less fearful and distressed when positioned for medical procedures in a sitting position, rather than supine.
- In addition to reducing the child's distress and gaining his or her cooperation, these techniques generally require fewer staff to be present in the room, facilitate safe and effective accomplishment of the medical procedure, decrease parent anxiety, and increase parent satisfaction.

Bibliography

1. Inal S., Kelleci M. The effect of external thermomechanical stimulation and distraction on reducing pain experienced by children during blood drawing. Pediatr Emerg Care 2017; Sep 5.
2. Lacey CM, Finkelstein M, Thygeson MV. The impact of positioning on fear during immunizations: supine versus sitting up. J Pediatr Nurs 2008;23(3):195–200. PMID:18492548.
3. Lamperti M, et al. International evidence-based recommendations on ultrasound-guided vascular access. Intensive Care Med. July 2012;38(7):1105–17.
4. Murray KK, Hollman GA. Non-pharmacologic interventions in children during medical and surgical procedures. In: Tobias JD, Cravero JP, editors. Procedural sedation for infants, children, and adolescents; section on anesthesiology and pain medicine. American Academy of Pediatrics; 2016.
5. Moureau N, Lamperti M, Kelly LJ, Dawson R, Elbarbary M, van Boxtel AJH, Pittiruti M. Evidence-based consensus on the insertion of central venous access devices: definition of minimal requirements for training. Br J Anaesth. 2013;110(3):347–56.
6. Potts D, Davis KF, Fein J. A vibrating cold device to reduce pain in the pediatric emergency department: a randomized clinical trial. Pediatr Emerg Care. 2017; Jan 24
7. Sahiner N, Inal S. The effect of combined stimulation of external cold and vibration during immunization on pain and anxiety levels in children. J Perianesth Nurs. 2015 Jun;30(3):228–35.